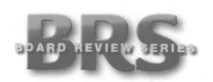

BOARD REVIEW SERIES

Biochemistry, Molecular Biology, and Genetics

FIFTH EDITION

Todd A. Swanson, M.D., Ph.D.
Resident in Radiation Oncology
William Beaumont Hospital
Royal Oak, Michigan

Sandra I. Kim, M.D., Ph.D.
Division of Nuclear Medicine and Molecular Imaging
Massachusetts General Hospital
Boston, Massachusetts

Marc J. Glucksman, Ph.D.
Professor, Department of Biochemistry and Molecular Biology
Director, Midwest Proteome Center
Rosalind Franklin University of Medicine and Science
The Chicago Medical School
North Chicago, Illinois

WITH EDITORIAL CONSULTATION BY
Michael A. Lieberman, Ph.D.
Dean, Instructional and Research Computing, UCit
Distinguished Teaching Professor
University of Cincinnati
Cincinnati, OH

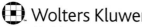

Wolters Kluwer | Lippincott Williams & Wilkins
Health

Philadelphia · Baltimore · New York · London
Buenos Aires · Hong Kong · Sydney · Tokyo

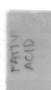

Acquisitions Editor: Charles W. Mitchell
Product Manager: Stacey L. Sebring
Marketing Manager: Jennifer Kuklinski
Designer: Holly Reid McLaughlin
Compositor: Cadmus Communications
Printer: C & C Offset Printing

First Edition, 1990
Second Edition, 1994
Third Edition, 1999
Fourth Edition, 2007

Library of Congress Cataloging-in-Publication Data

Swanson, Todd A.
   Biochemistry, molecular biology, and genetics / Todd A. Swanson, Sandra I. Kim, Marc J. Glucksman ; with editorial consultation by Michael A. Lieberman. — 5th ed.
       p. ;cm. — (Board review series)
   Rev. ed. of: Biochemistry and molecular biology / Todd A. Swanson, Sandra I. Kim, Marc J. Glucksman. 4th ed. c2007.
   Includes bibliographical references and index.
   ISBN 978-0-7817-9875-4 (hardcopy : alk. paper) 1. Biochemistry—Examinations, questions, etc. 2. Molecular biology—Examinations, questions, etc. I. Kim, Sandra I. II. Glucksman, Marc J. III. Lieberman, Michael, 1950- IV. Swanson, Todd A. Biochemistry and molecular biology. V. Title. VI. Series: Board review series.
   [DNLM: 1. Biochemical Phenomena—Examination Questions. 2. Biochemical Phenomena—Outlines. 3. Genetic Processes—Examination Questions. 4. Genetic Processes—Outlines. QU 18.2 S972b 2010]
   QP518.3.S93 2010
   572.8076—dc22

                              2009029693

For
Olga, Maxwell, Anneliese, and the eagerly awaited
new addition to the Swanson clan.
If not for you, all my efforts would be in vain.

Preface

This revision of *BRS Biochemistry, Molecular Biology, and Genetics* includes additional high-yield material to help the reader master clinical principles of medical biochemistry as they prepare for the revamped Step 1 USMLE. Our goal is to offer a review book that both lays the foundations of biochemistry and introduces clinically relevant correlates. In doing so, we have de-emphasized some of the rote memorization of structures and formulas that often obscure the big picture of medical biochemistry. Clinical Correlates in each chapter provide additional clinical insight, distilling numerous clinical correlations into a format that offers the highest yield in review. We hope that these correlations will help answer a commonly asked question: "Why do we have to know this for the boards?"

This revised edition also includes a new chapter on genetics as related to medical biochemistry. We hope this chapter will augment other review texts on genetics that students may consult in preparation for Step 1.

Many of the questions at the end of each chapter have been revised to maximize their value for the student preparing for the exam. A comprehensive exam at the end of this volume reinforces the concepts of the text. Our objective has been to provide the student with clinically relevant questions in a format similar to that encountered on the USMLE Step 1 Boards. The breadth of questions is one of the many features of Lippincott's *Board Review Series* titles.

We hope that the new edition of *BRS Biochemistry, Molecular Biology, and Genetics* becomes a valuable tool for students seeking high-yield resources as they prepare for the USMLE Step 1. We recognize the changing nature of science and medicine, however, and encourage readers to send suggestions for improvement for this text or for our companion flash cards, to us via e-mail at LWW.com.

Todd Swanson
Sandra Kim
Marc Glucksman

Publisher's Preface

The Publisher acknowledges the editorial consultation of Michael A. Lieberman, Ph.D., to this fifth edition. In addition to his role as editorial consultant on every chapter, Dr. Lieberman reviewed the entire manuscript to help ensure the accuracy, consistency, and timeliness of its content.

Acknowledgments

We (T.A.S. and S.I.K.) acknowledge, first and foremost, the support and encouragement of Arthur Schneider, M.D. His help has been instrumental in paving the way for us to become medical educators. As well, T.A.S. thanks Dr. Inga Grills, residency program director, and Dr. Alvaro Martinez, chair, Department of Radiation Oncology, William Beaumont Hospital, for their support in this endeavor.

M.J.G. thanks his family and colleagues for suggestions during this endeavor in medical education. This tome could not have been accomplished without the thousands of students taught in classes and mentored over the last 20 years at three of the finest medical schools. For asking for my participation, I especially thank two of my recent and most brilliant students ... my coauthors.

Last, but not least, we thank the editors at various levels at Lippincott Williams & Wilkins, including Charles W. Mitchell, Acquisitions Editor, and Stacey Sebring, Product Manager.

Contents

Introduction: Organic Chemistry Review

Biomolecules: Life's Building Blocks

I. BRIEF REVIEW OF ORGANIC CHEMISTRY

- Biochemical reactions involve the functional groups of molecules.

A. Identification of carbon atoms (Figure I-1)

- Carbon atoms are either **numbered** or given **Greek letters**.

B. Functional groups in biochemistry

- Types of functional groups include alcohols, aldehydes, ketones, carboxyl groups, anhydrides, sulfhydryl groups, amines, esters, and amides. All these are important components of biochemical compounds (Figure I-2).

C. Biochemical reactions
1. Reactions are classified according to the functional groups that react (e.g., esterifications, hydroxylations, carboxylations, and decarboxylations).
2. Oxidations of sulfhydryl groups to disulfides, of alcohols to aldehydes and ketones, and of aldehydes to carboxylic acids frequently occur.
   a. Many of these oxidations are reversed by **reductions**.
   b. In **oxidation** reactions, electrons are lost.
   c. In **reduction** reactions, electrons are gained.

II. ACIDS, BASES, AND BUFFERS

A. Water
1. Water (H_2O) is the **solvent of life**. It dissociates into hydrogen ions (H^+) and hydroxide ions (OH^-)

$$H_2O \rightleftarrows H^+ + O H^-$$

with an equilibrium constant of

$$K = [H^+][OH^-]/[H_2O]$$

$$CH_3 - \underset{\underset{\gamma}{4}}{C}H - \underset{\underset{\beta}{3}}{\overset{\overset{OH}{|}}{C}}H - \underset{\underset{\alpha}{2}}{C}H_2 - \underset{1}{\overset{\overset{O}{||}}{C}}O^-$$

FIGURE I-1 Identification of carbon atoms in an organic compound. Carbons are numbered starting from the most oxidized carbon-containing group, or they are assigned Greek letters, with the carbon next to the most oxidized group designated as the α-carbon. This compound is 3-hydroxybutyrate or β-hydroxybutyrate. It is a ketone body.

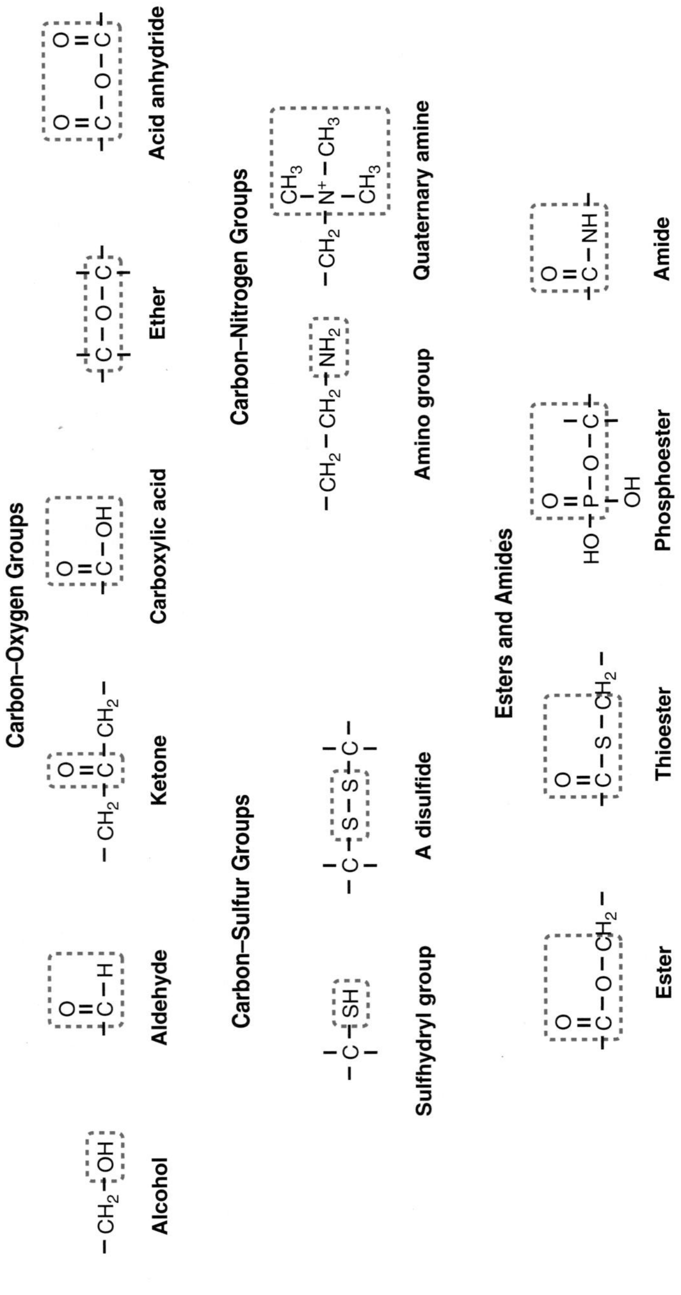

FIGURE I-2 A brief review of organic chemistry: major functional groups in biochemistry.

2. Because the extent of dissociation is not appreciable, $[H_2O]$ remains constant at 55.5 M, and the ion product of H_2O is

$$K_w = [H^+][OH^-] = 1 \times 10^{-14}$$

3. The pH of a solution is the negative $\log_{10}$ of its hydrogen ion concentration $[H^+]$:

$$pH = -\log_{10} [H^+]$$

- For pure water, the concentrations of $[H^+]$ and $[OH^-]$ are equal, as shown below:

$$[H^+] = [OH^-] = 1 \times 10^{-7}$$

- Therefore, **the pH of pure water is 7**, also referred to as **neutral pH**.

B. Acids and bases

- Acids are compounds that donate protons, and bases are compounds that accept protons.

1. Acids dissociate
   a. Strong acids, such as hydrochloric acid (HCl), dissociate completely.

CLINICAL CORRELATES HCl is produced by the **parietal cells** of the stomach. The **H⁺-K⁺ ATPase (the proton pump)** in the cell membrane is responsible for producing as much as 2 L of **acidic gastric fluid** per day. Some individuals have a condition known as **gastroesophageal reflux disease (GERD)**, which results from reflux of HCl back into the esophagus. This condition creates a **burning sensation in the chest**, along with cough and even shortness of breath. The proton pump can be inhibited by **proton pump inhibitors (PPIs)** such as **omeprazole**.

   b. Weak acids, such as acetic acid, dissociate only to a limited extent:

$$HA \rightleftharpoons H^+ + A^-$$

   where HA is the acid, and A^- is its conjugate base.
   c. The **dissociation constant** for a weak acid is

$$K = [H^+][A^-]/[HA]$$

2. The **Henderson-Hasselbalch equation** was derived from the equation for the dissociation constant of a weak acid or base:

$$pH = pK + \log_{10} [A^-]/[HA]$$

where pK is the negative $\log_{10}$ of K, the dissociation constant.

3. The **major acids** produced by the body include **phosphoric acid, sulfuric acid, lactic acid, hydrochloric acid**, and the ketone bodies, acetoacetic acid and β-hydroxybutyric acid. CO_2 is also produced, which combines with H_2O to form **carbonic acid** in a reaction catalyzed by carbonic anhydrase:

$$CO_2 + H_2O \rightleftharpoons H_2CO_3 \rightleftharpoons H^+ + HCO_3^-$$

CLINICAL CORRELATES The **carbonic anhydrase inhibitor, acetazolamide**, blocks the above reaction and is used for the **treatment of glaucoma** as well as altitude sickness.

C. Buffers

1. Buffers consist of **solutions of acid-base conjugate pairs**, such as acetic acid and acetate.
   a. Near its pK, a buffer maintains the pH of a solution, resisting changes due to addition of acids or bases (Figure I-3). For a weak acid, the pK is often designated pK_a.
   b. At the pK_a, $[A^-]$ and $[HA]$ are equal, and the buffer has its maximal capacity.

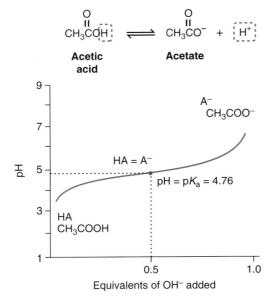

FIGURE I-3 The titration curve of acetic acid. The molecular species that predominate at low pH (acetic acid) and high pH (acetate) are shown. At low pH (high [H⁺]), the molecule is protonated and has zero charge. As alkali is added, [H⁺] decreases (H⁺ + OH⁻ → H₂O), acetic acid dissociates and loses its proton, and the carboxyl group becomes negatively charged.

2. Buffering mechanisms in the body

■ The **normal pH range** of arterial blood is **7.37 to 7.43**.

    a. The major buffers of blood are **bicarbonate** (HCO_3^-/H_2CO_3) and **hemoglobin** (Hb/HHb).

    b. These buffers act in conjunction with mechanisms in the kidneys for excreting protons and mechanisms in the lungs for exhaling CO_2 to maintain the pH within the normal range.

CLINICAL CORRELATES **Metabolic acidosis** can result from accumulation of metabolic acids (lactic acid or the ketone bodies, β-hydroxybutyric acid, and acetoacetic acid) or ingestion of acids or compounds that are metabolized to acids (e.g., methanol, ethylene glycol).

CLINICAL CORRELATES **Metabolic alkalosis** is due to increased HCO_3^-, which is accompanied by an increased pH. Acid-base disturbances lead to compensatory responses that attempt to restore normal pH. For example, a metabolic acidosis causes hyperventilation and the release of CO_2, which tends to raise the pH. During metabolic acidosis, the kidneys excrete NH_4^+, which contains H⁺ buffered by ammonia:

$$H^+ + NH_3 \rightleftharpoons NH_4^+$$

III. CARBOHYDRATE STRUCTURE

A. Monosaccharides

1. Nomenclature

    a. The simplest monosaccharides have the formula $(CH_2O)_n$. Those with three carbons are called **trioses;** four, **tetroses;** five, **pentoses;** and six, **hexoses.**

    b. They are called **aldoses** or **ketoses**, depending on whether their most oxidized functional group is an aldehyde or a ketone (Figure I-4).

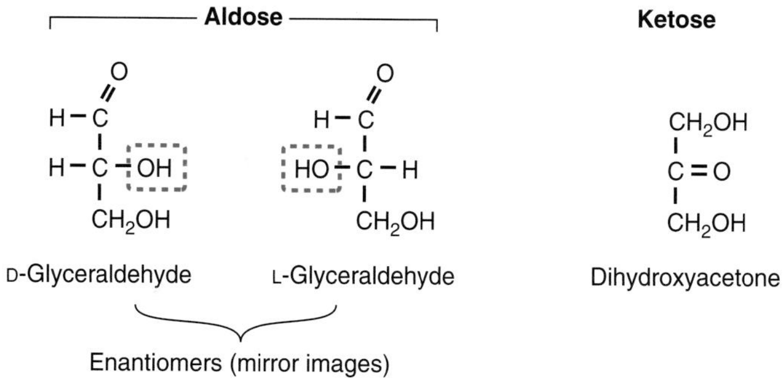

FIGURE I-4 Examples of trioses, the smallest monosaccharides.

2. D **and** L **sugars**

  a. The configuration of the asymmetric carbon atom farthest from the aldehyde or ketone group determines whether a monosaccharide belongs to the D or L series. In the D form, the hydroxyl group is on the right; in the L form, it is on the left (Figure I-4).

  b. An asymmetric carbon atom has four different chemical groups attached to it.

  c. Sugars of the D series, which are related to D-glyceraldehyde, are the most common in nature (Figure I-5).

3. Stereoisomers, enantiomers, and epimers

  a. Stereoisomers have the same chemical formula but differ in the position of the hydroxyl groups on one or more of their asymmetric carbons (Figure I-5).

  b. Enantiomers are stereoisomers that are mirror images of each other (Figure I-4).

  c. Epimers are stereoisomers that differ in the position of the hydroxyl group at only one asymmetric carbon. For example, D-glucose and D-galactose are epimers that differ at carbon 4 (Figure I-5).

4. Ring structures of carbohydrates

  a. Although **monosaccharides** are often drawn as straight chains (Fischer projections), they exist mainly as ring structures in which the aldehyde or ketone group has reacted with a hydroxyl group in the same molecule (Figure I-6).

  b. Furanose and **pyranose** rings contain five and six members, respectively, and are usually drawn as Haworth projections (Figure I-6).

  c. The **hydroxyl group on the anomeric carbon** may be in the α or β configuration.

   (1) In the **α configuration**, the hydroxyl group on the anomeric carbon is on the right in the Fischer projection and below the plane of the ring in the Haworth projection.

   (2) In the **β configuration**, it is on the left in the Fischer projection and above the plane in the Haworth projection (Figure I-7).

  d. In solution, **mutarotation occurs**. The α and β forms equilibrate via the straight-chain aldehyde form (Figure I-7).

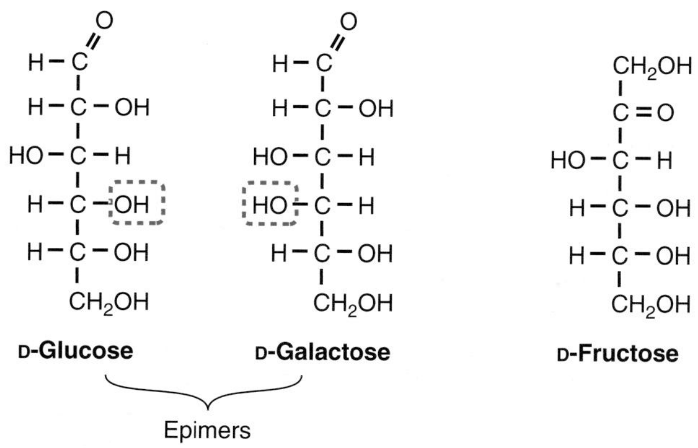

FIGURE I-5 Common hexoses of the D configuration.

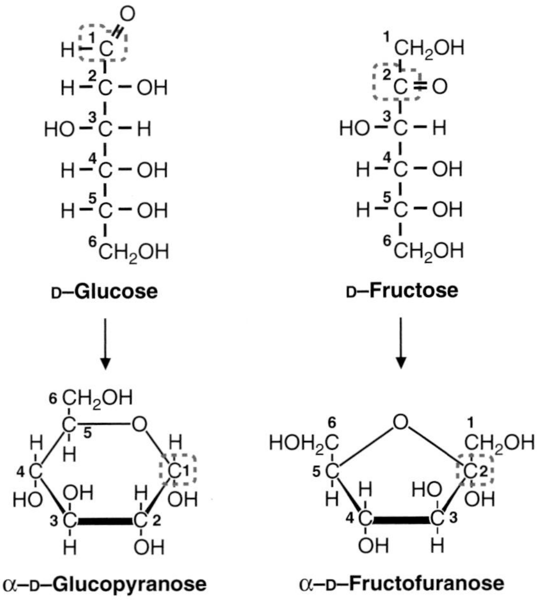

FIGURE I-6 Furanose and pyranose rings formed by glucose and fructose. The anomeric carbons are surrounded by *dashed lines*.

D–Glucose

D–Fructose

α–D–Glucopyranose

α–D–Fructofuranose

B. Glycosides
1. **Formation of glycosides**
   a. Glycosidic bonds form when the **hydroxyl** group on the anomeric carbon of a monosaccharide reacts with an −OH or −NH group of another compound.

CLINICAL CORRELATES The **glycoside digitalis** and its derivatives are of clinical significance because they **inhibit the Na$^+$-K$^+$ ATPase** on cell membranes. Such drugs are used in the treatment of **congestive heart failure**.

   b. **α-Glycosides** or **β-glycosides** are produced depending on the position of the atom attached to the anomeric carbon of the sugar.
2. **O-Glycosides**
   a. **Monosaccharides** can be linked via O-glycosidic bonds to another monosaccharide, forming O-glycosides.
   b. **Disaccharides** contain two monosaccharides. Sucrose, lactose, and maltose are common disaccharides (Figure I-8).
   c. **Oligosaccharides** contain up to about 12 monosaccharides.
   d. **Polysaccharides** contain more than 12 monosaccharides, for example, glycogen, starch, and glycosaminoglycans.

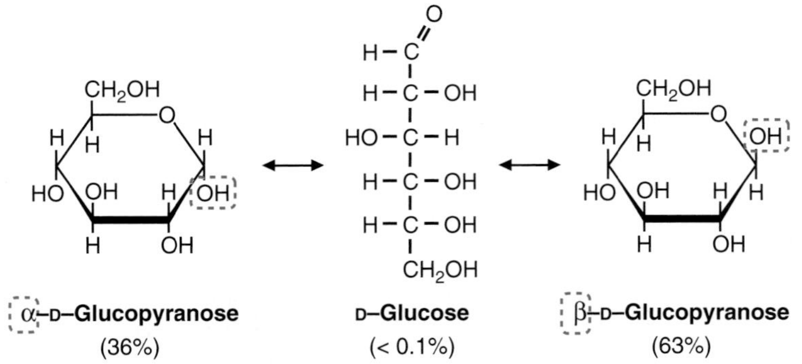

α–D–Glucopyranose (36%) D–Glucose (< 0.1%) β–D–Glucopyranose (63%)

FIGURE I-7 Mutarotation of glucose in solution. The percentage of each form is indicated.

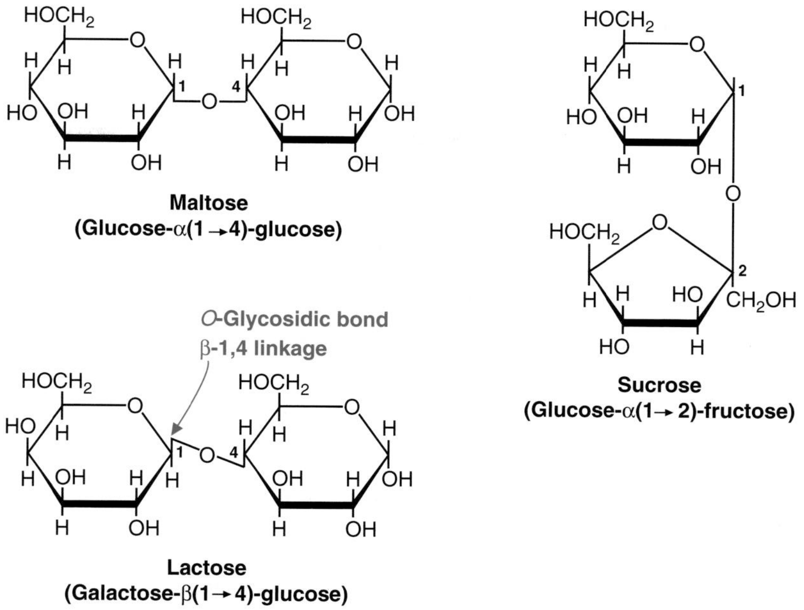

FIGURE I-8 The most common disaccharides.

3. N-Glycosides

- Monosaccharides can be linked via *N*-glycosidic bonds to compounds that are not carbo-hydrates. Nucleotides contain *N*-glycosidic bonds.

C. Derivatives of carbohydrates

1. Phosphate groups can be attached to carbohydrates.
   a. Glucose and fructose can be phosphorylated on carbons 1 and 6.
   b. Phosphate groups can link sugars to nucleotides, as in UDP-glucose.

2. Amino groups, which are often acetylated, can be linked to sugars (e.g., glucosamine and galactosamine).

3. Sulfate groups are often found on sugars (e.g., chondroitin sulfate and other glycosaminogly-cans) (Figure I-9).

D. Oxidation of carbohydrates

1. Oxidized forms
   a. The anomeric carbon of an aldose (C1) can be oxidized to an acid.

   - Glucose forms **gluconic acid** (gluconate). **6-Phosphogluconate** is an intermediate in the pentose phosphate pathway.

CLINICAL CORRELATES   The oxidation of glucose by **glucose oxidase** (a highly specific test for glucose) is used by clinical and other laboratories to measure the amount of **glucose in urine** using a **dipstick**.

---

   b. **Carbon 6 of a hexose** can be oxidized to a uronic acid.
   (1) Uronic acids are found in glycosaminoglycans of proteoglycans (Figure I-9).
   (2) Glucose forms **glucuronic acid**. Conjugation with glucuronic acid makes lipid com-pounds more water soluble (e.g., bilirubin diglucuronide).

CLINICAL CORRELATES   Infants have a **decreased ability to conjugate glucuronic acid** onto drugs such as **chloramphenicol**. Administration of this antibiotic during the neonatal period can result in elevated plasma levels of the drug and a fetal shocklike syndrome referred to as **gray baby syndrome**.

Hyaluronate

Glucuronic   β(1→3)   N–Acetyl-
acid   glucosamine

Chondroitin 6–sulfate

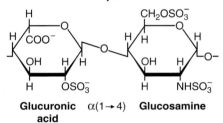

Glucuronic   β(1→3)   N–Acetyl-
acid   galactosamine

Heparin

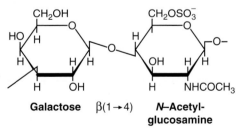

Glucuronic   α(1→4)   Glucosamine
acid

Keratan sulfate

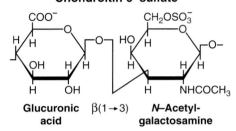

Galactose   β(1→4)   N–Acetyl-
                       glucosamine

Dermatan sulfate

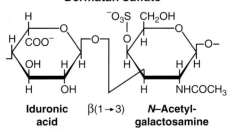

Iduronic   β(1→3)   N–Acetyl-
acid   galactosamine

FIGURE I-9 Examples of repeating disaccharides of glycosaminoglycans.

2. *Test for reducing sugars*

■ Reducing sugars contain a free anomeric carbon that can be oxidized.

    a. When the anomeric carbon is oxidized, another compound is reduced. If the reduced product of this reaction is colored, the intensity of the color can be used to determine the amount of the reducing sugar that has been oxidized.

    b. This reaction is the basis of the reducing-sugar test, which is used by clinical laboratories. The test is not specific. Aldoses such as glucose give a positive test result. Ketoses such as fructose are also reducing sugars because they form aldoses under test conditions.

CLINICAL CORRELATES Because dipsticks only detect glucose, many clinical laboratories use a chemical test for reducing sugars, a modified **Benedict test for reducing sugars**, which also will detect the presence of **sucrose, galactose**, and **fructose**. Most newborn and **infant urine is routinely screened** for reducing sugars to detect **inborn errors in metabolism**.

E. Reduction of carbohydrates

    1. The aldehyde or ketone group of a sugar can be reduced to a hydroxyl group, forming a **polyol** (polyalcohol).

    2. Glucose is reduced to **sorbitol**, and galactose to **galactitol**.

CLINICAL CORRELATES **Sorbitol** does not readily diffuse out of cells. As it accumulates in cells, it causes **osmotic damage** to cells of the nervous system, resulting in **cataracts** and **neuropathy**.

F. Glycosylation of proteins

■ Addition of sugar moieties to proteins can alter proteins in many ways, including modifying their function, protecting them from proteolysis, and directing their intracellular traffic, as well as direct cellular movement.

CLINICAL CORRELATES Patients with **leukocyte adhesion deficiency (LAD) II** have a congenital **deficiency in the ability to glycosylate** ligands for cell surface **selectins**, which mediate immune cell migration. Such patients are prone to **recurrent life-threatening infections**.

IV. PROTEOGLYCANS, GLYCOPROTEINS, AND GLYCOLIPIDS

A. Proteoglycans are found in the extracellular matrix or ground substance of connective tissue, synovial fluid of joints, vitreous humor of the eye, secretions of mucus-producing cells, and cartilage.

    1. Proteoglycans consist of a core protein with long unbranched polysaccharide chains (**glycosaminoglycans**) attached. The overall structure resembles a bottle brush (Figure I-10).

    2. These chains are composed of **repeating disaccharide units**, which usually contain a **uronic acid** and a **hexosamine** (Figure I-9). The uronic acid is generally D-glucuronic or L-iduronic acid.

CLINICAL CORRELATES **Heparin is a glycosaminoglycan**, which is an important **anticoagulant** found in the granules of mast cells. It can be used during the treatment of **myocardial infarction** as well as for the **prevention of deep venous thrombosis** during hospitalizations.

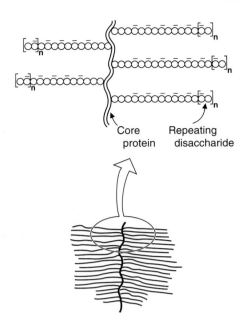

FIGURE I-10 "Bottle brush" structure of a proteoglycan with a magnified segment.

3. The amino group of the hexosamine is usually **acetylated**, and **sulfate** groups are often present on carbons 4 and 6.

4. A xylose and two galactose residues connect the chain of repeating disaccharides to the core protein.

B. **Glycoproteins** serve as enzymes, hormones, antibodies, and structural proteins. They are found in extracellular fluids and in lysosomes and are attached to the cell membrane. They are involved in cell–cell interactions.

　1. The **carbohydrate** portion of glycoproteins differs from that of proteoglycans in that it is **shorter** and often **branched** (Figure I-11).

　　a. Glycoproteins contain mannose, L-fucose, and *N*-acetylneuraminic acid (NANA) in addition to glucose, galactose, and their amino derivatives. NANA is a member of the class of sialic acids.

CLINICAL CORRELATES　　The **influenza virus** infects cells by binding its viral hemagglutinin to **sialic acid** on the surface of epithelial cells.

---

　　b. The antigenic determinants of the ABO and Lewis blood group substances are sugars at the ends of these carbohydrate branches.

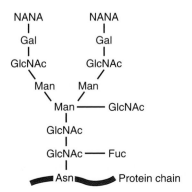

FIGURE I-11 Example of the carbohydrate moiety of a glycoprotein. Note that, in this case, the carbohydrate is attached to an asparagine (*N*-linked). NANA, *N*-acetylneuraminic acid; Gal, galactose; GlcNAc, *N*-acetylglucosamine; Man, mannose; Fuc, fucose.

2. The carbohydrates are attached to the protein via the hydroxyl groups of **serine and threonine** residues or the amide N of **asparagine**.

C. Glycolipids

1. Glycolipids (or sphingolipids) are derived from the lipid ceramide. This class of compounds includes cerebrosides and gangliosides.

   a. Cerebrosides are synthesized from ceramide and UDP-sugars.

   b. Gangliosides have NANA residues (derived from CMP-NANA) branching from the linear oligosaccharide chain.

2. Glycolipids are found in the cell membrane with the carbohydrate portion extending into the extracellular space.

V. AMINO ACIDS

A. Structures of the amino acids (Figure I-12)

1. Most amino acids contain a **carboxyl group**, an **amino group**, and a **side- chain** (R group), all attached to the α-carbon. Exceptions are:

   a. Glycine, which does not have a side chain. Its α-carbon contains two hydrogens.

> **CLINICAL CORRELATES** Glycine functions as an inhibitory neurotransmitter in the brainstem and spinal cord. Its actions are antagonized by the rodenticide strychnine, leading to twitching and muscle spasm.

   b. Proline, in which the nitrogen is part of a ring, is an **imino acid**.

2. All of the 20 amino acids, except glycine, are of the L configuration. Because glycine does not contain an asymmetric carbon atom, it is not optically active, and thus, it is neither D nor L.

3. The **classification** of amino acids is based on the chemistry of their side chains.

   a. Hydrophobic amino acids have side chains that contain **aliphatic** groups (valine, leucine, and isoleucine) or **aromatic groups** (phenylalanine, tyrosine, and tryptophan) that can form hydrophobic interactions.

   - **Tyrosine** has a phenolic group that carries a negative charge above its pK_a ($\approx$10.5), so it is not hydrophobic in this pH range.

   b. Hydroxyl groups found on serine and threonine can form hydrogen bonds.

   c. Sulfur is present in cysteine and methionine.

   - The **oxidation** of the **sulfhydryl groups** of two cysteines can form a **disulfide bond**, producing cystine.

   d. Ionizable groups are present on the side chains of seven amino acids. They can **carry a charge**, depending on the pH. When charged, they can form **electrostatic interactions**.

   e. Amides are present on the side chains of asparagine and glutamine.

   f. The side chain of **proline forms a ring** with the nitrogen attached to the α-carbon.

B. Charges on amino acids (Figure I-13)

1. Charges on α-amino and α-carboxyl groups

   - At physiologic pH, the **α-amino group** is protonated ($pK_a \approx 9$) and carries a **positive charge**, and the **carboxyl group** is dissociated ($pK_a \approx 2$) and carries a **negative charge**.

2. Charges on side chains

   a. Positive charges are present on the side chains of the basic amino acids **arginine, lysine**, and **histidine** at pH 7.

   b. Negative charges are present on the side chains of the acidic amino acids **aspartate and glutamate** at pH 7.

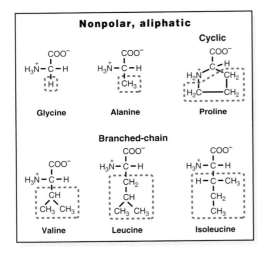

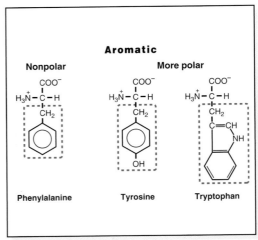

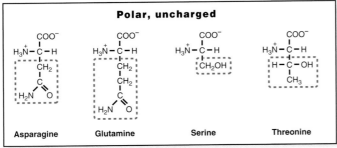

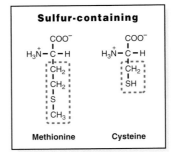

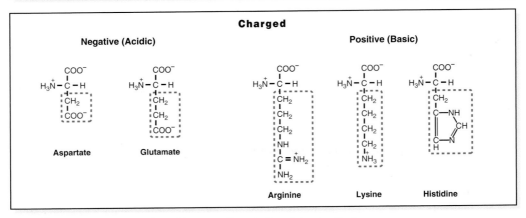

FIGURE I-12 Structures of the amino acids, grouped by polarity and structural features.

CLINICAL CORRELATES Glutamate is the amino acid in the highest concentration in the brain and functions as a neurotransmitter in the brain and spinal cord. Memantine is an antiglutamatergic drug used for treatment of Alzheimer disease. Glutamate antagonism is implicated in schizophrenia, in which drugs of abuse, like ketamine and phencyclidine, affect glutamate binding to its receptor.

   c. The isoelectric point (pI) is the pH at which the number of positive charges equals the number of negative charges such that the molecule has no net charge.

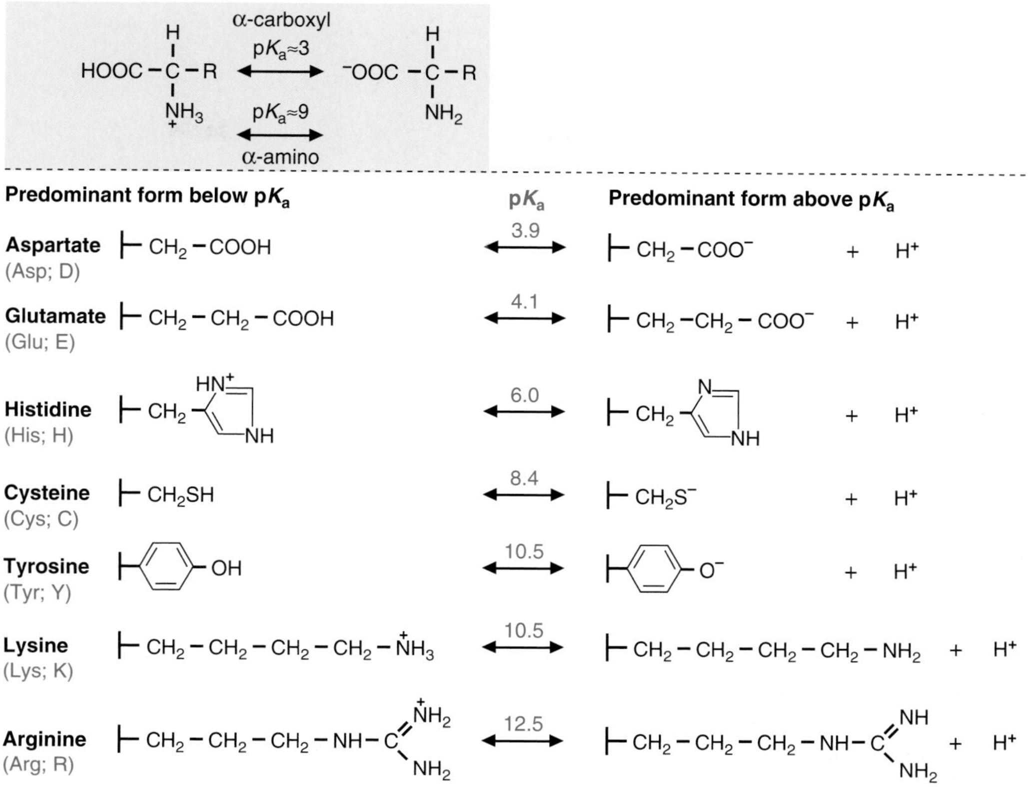

FIGURE I-13 Side chains that are ionizable. For each amino acid, the species that predominates at a pH below the pK_a is shown on the left; the species that predominates at a pH above the pK_a is shown on the right. Note that the charge changes from zero to negative or from positive to zero. At the pK_a, equal amounts of both species are present.

C. Titration of amino acids

- Ionizable groups on amino acids carry protons at low pH (high [H^+]) that dissociate as the pH increases.

1. For an amino acid that does not have an ionizable side chain, **two pK_as** are observed during titration (Figure I-14).
   a. The first (**pK_{a1}**) corresponds to the **α-carboxyl group** ($pK_{a1} \approx 2$). As the proton dissociates, the carboxyl group goes from a zero to a minus charge.
   b. The second (**pK_{a2}**) corresponds to the **α-amino group** ($pK_{a2} \approx 9$). As the proton dissociates, the amino group goes from a positive to a zero charge.
2. For an amino acid with an ionizable side chain, **three pK_as** are observed during titration (Figure I-15).
   a. The α-carboxyl and α-amino groups have pK_as of about 2 and 9, respectively.
   b. The **third pK_a** varies with the amino acid and depends on the pK_a of the side chain (Figure I-15).

D. Peptide bonds

- Peptide bonds covalently join the α-carboxyl group of each amino acid to the α-amino group of the next amino acid in the protein chain (Figure I-16).

1. **Characteristics**
   a. The **atoms** involved in the peptide bond form a **rigid, planar unit**.
   b. Because of its **partial double-bond character**, the planar peptide bond itself has no freedom of rotation.
   c. However, the bonds involving the **α-carbon** can **rotate freely**.

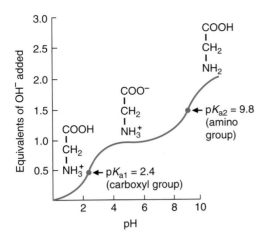

FIGURE I-14 Titration curves for glycine. The molecular species of glycine present at various pHs are indicated by the molecules above the curve.

2. Peptide bonds are extremely stable. Cleavage generally involves the hydrolytic action of proteolytic enzymes.

VI. LIPIDS

A. **Fatty acids** exist "free" or esterified to glycerol (Figure I-17).

1. In humans, fatty acids usually have an even number of carbon atoms, are 16 to 20 carbon atoms in length, and may be saturated or unsaturated (containing double bonds). They are

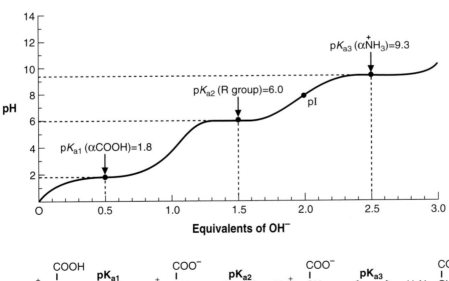

Predominant species

FIGURE I-15 Titration curves for histidine. For histidine, pK_{a2} is the dissociation constant of the imidazole (side chain) group.

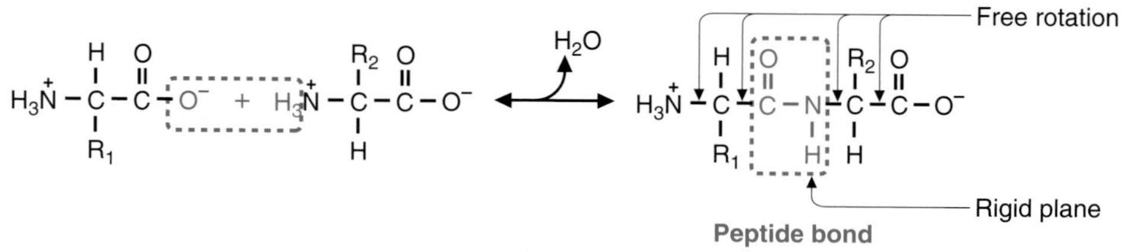

FIGURE I-16 The peptide bond.

described by the number of carbons and the positions of the double bonds (e.g., arachidonic acid, which has 20 carbons and 4 double bonds, is 20:4,$\Delta^{5,8,11,14}$).

2. Polyunsaturated fatty acids are often classified according to the position of the first double bond from the ω-end (the carbon furthest from the carboxyl group; e.g., ω-3 or ω-6).

B. **Monoacylglycerols (monoglycerides), diacylglycerols (diglycerides), and triacylglycerols (triglycerides)** contain one, two, and three fatty acids esterified to glycerol, respectively.

C. **Phosphoglycerides** contain fatty acids esterified to positions 1 and 2 of the glycerol moiety and a phosphoryl group at position 3 (e.g., phosphocholine).

D. **Sphingolipids** contain ceramide with a variety of groups attached.
   1. Sphingomyelin contains phosphocholine.
   2. Cerebrosides contain a sugar residue.
   3. Gangliosides contain a number of sugar residues.

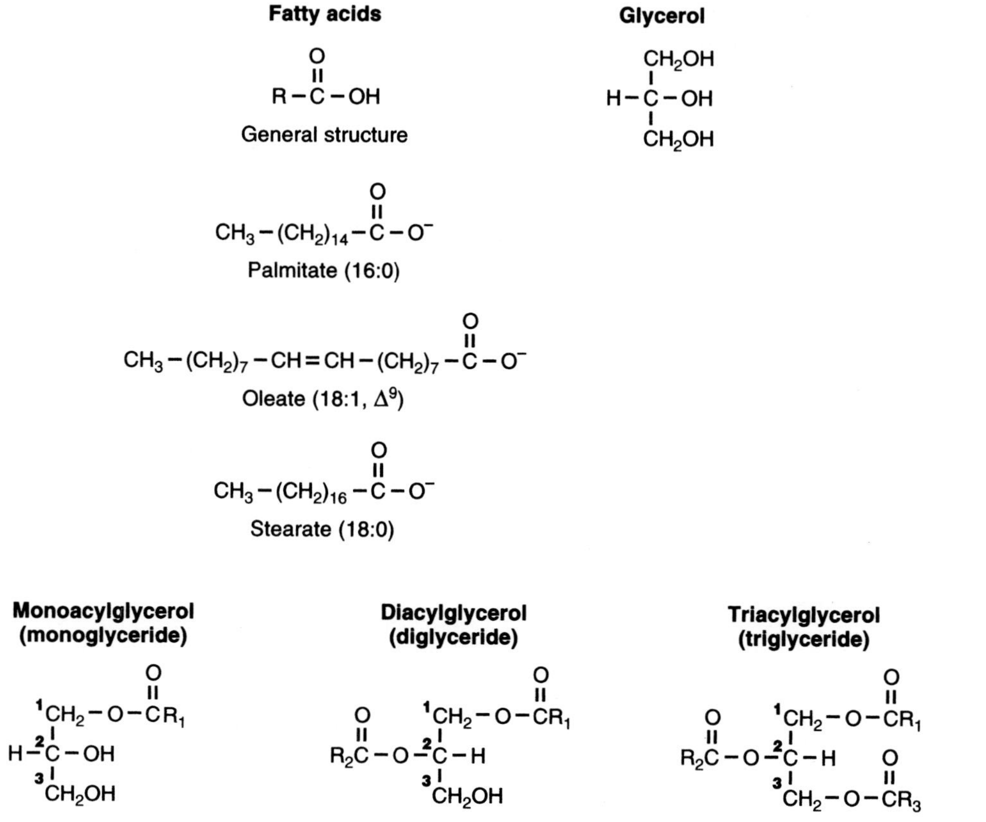

FIGURE I-17 The structures of fatty acids, glycerol, and the acylglycerols. *R* indicates a linear aliphatic chain. Fatty acids are identified by the number of carbons, the number of double bonds, and the positions of the double bonds in the molecule (e.g., 18:1, Δ^9 describes oleic acid as having 18 carbons, 1 double bond, with the double bond between carbons 9 and 10 of the fatty acid).

CLINICAL CORRELATES	Cholera toxin binds to the ganglioside GM_1 receptor on cells and upon entry causes a potentially life-threatening watery diarrhea.

E. **Cholesterol** contains four rings and an aliphatic side chain.

■ Bile salts and steroid hormones are derived from cholesterol.

F. **Prostaglandins and leukotrienes** are derived from polyunsaturated fatty acids such as arachidonic acid.

G. **The fat-soluble vitamins** include vitamins A, D, E, and K.

VII. MEMBRANES

A. **Membrane structure**
   1. **Membranes** are composed mainly of lipids and proteins (Figure I-18).
   2. Phosphoglycerides are the major membrane lipids, but sphingolipids and cholesterol are also present.

      ■ **Phospholipids** form a bilayer, with their hydrophilic head groups interacting with water on both the extracellular and intracellular surfaces and their hydrophobic fatty acyl chains in the central portion of the membrane.

   3. Peripheral proteins are attached at the periphery of the membrane; integral proteins span from one side of the membrane to the other.
   4. Carbohydrates are attached to proteins and lipids on the exterior side of the cell membrane. They extend into the extracellular space.
   5. Lipids and proteins can diffuse laterally within the plane of the membrane. Therefore, the membrane is termed "fluid mosaic."

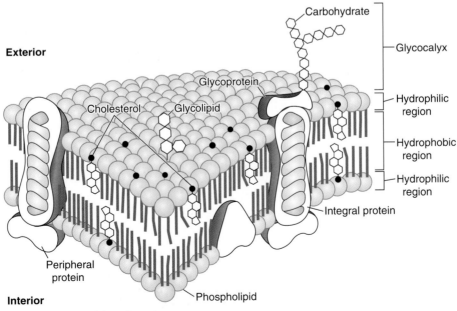

FIGURE I-18 The structure of the cell membrane.

B. Membrane function

1. Membranes serve as **barriers** that separate the contents of a cell from the external environment or the contents of individual organelles from the remainder of the cell.

2. The **proteins** in the cell membrane have many functions.

    a. Some are involved in the **transport** of substances across the membrane.

    b. Some are **enzymes** that catalyze biochemical reactions.

    c. Those on the exterior surface can function as **receptors** that bind external ligands such as hormones or growth factors.

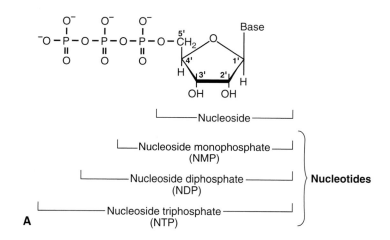

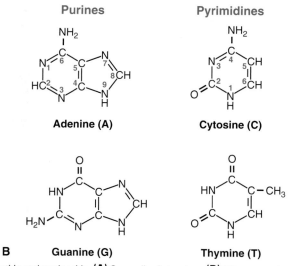

FIGURE I-19 Nucleotide and nucleoside. **(A)** Generalized structure. **(B)** Nitrogenous bases.

   d. Others are **mediators** that aid the ligand–receptor complex in triggering a sequence of events (e.g., G proteins) known as **signal transduction;** as a consequence, **second messengers** (e.g., cyclic adenosine monophosphate [cAMP]) that alter metabolism are produced inside the cell. Therefore, an external agent, such as a hormone, can elicit effects intracellularly without entering the cell.

VIII. NUCLEOTIDES

A. Nucleotide structure
  1. Heterocyclic, basic compounds composed of purines and pyrimidines (Figure I-19)
  2. Derivatives of nucleotides that contain sugars linked to a nitrogenous base are termed **nucleosides**.
    a. Ribonucleosides contain the purine or pyrimidine base linked through a **β-N-glycosidic bond** to either the **N-1 of pyrimidines** or the **N-9 of a purine** to the sugar **D-ribose**.
    b. Deoxyribonucleotides have a similar structure, but instead, the sugar linked to the base is a **2-deoxy-D-ribose**.
    c. Nucleotides are nucleosides with **phosphoryl groups** esterified to a **hydroxyl group of the sugar** (usually at carbon 5 of ribose or deoxyribose). These can contain one (mononucleotides), two (dinucleotides), and three (trinucleotides) phosphodiester bonds, adding additional high-energy phosphate bonds.
    d. Polynucleotides result from polymerization of nucleotides through a **3′ to 5′ phosphodiester** bond between the phosphate of one monomer (attached to the 5′OH) to the 3′OH of the pentose sugar.

B. Nucleotide function
  1. Serves as energy stores (i.e., adenosine triphosphate [ATP]).
  2. Forms portions of several coenzymes (i.e., nicotinamide adenine dinucleotide [NAD$^+$])
  3. Serves as signaling intermediates (i.e., cAMP, cyclic guanosine monophosphate [cGMP])
  4. Is an allosteric modifier of certain regulated enzymes
  5. Conveys genetic information (DNA and RNA)

Review Test

Directions: Each of the numbered questions or incomplete statements in this section is followed by answers or by completions of the statement. Select the **one** lettered answer or completion that is **best** in each case.

1. Acetazolamide is a carbonic anhydrase inhibitor and is used in the treatment of all the following conditions except which one?

(A) Dehydration
(B) Glaucoma
(C) Epilepsy
(D) Altitude sickness
(E) Congestive heart failure

2. Sickle cell disease results in abnormal hemoglobin formation because of a point mutation in DNA that leads to the insertion of which amino acid into β-globin?

(A) Glutatmate
(B) Glutamic acid
(C) Tyrosine
(D) Serine
(E) Valine

3. A 67-year-old man suffers from congestive heart failure. He is taking digoxin, an effective chronotrope and inotrope, which is an ether that contains a sugar component (glycol) and a nonsugar (aglycone) component attached via oxygen. Digoxin would be best classified as which of the following?

(A) Glycoprotein
(B) Glycoside
(C) Oligosaccharide
(D) Glucosteroid
(E) Thioester

4. Which amino acid is a major neurotransmitter in the brain?

(A) Tyrosine
(B) Glutamate
(C) Trytophan
(D) Serine
(E) Hisitidine

5. Influenza virus results in more than 500,000 deaths worldwide annually. Influenza A contains an eight-piece segmented negative-sense RNA genome. Two important proteins encoded by this genome are HA (hemagglutinin) and NA (neuraminidase). The HA protein directly binds to which host cell epithelial component?

(A) Sialic acid
(B) Cerebrosides
(C) Cytokine receptors
(D) Serine-threonine kinase receptors
(E) Uronic acid subgroups

6. A young infant, who was nourished with a synthetic formula, was found to have a serum and urine sugar compound that yielded a positive reducing-sugar test but was negative when measured with glucose oxidase. Treatment of the urine and serum with acid to cleave glycosidic bonds did not increase the amount of reducing sugar measured. Which of the following compounds is most likely to be present in this infant's urine and serum?

(A) Glucose
(B) Fructose
(C) Sorbitol
(D) Maltose
(E) Lactose

7. A medical student is assigned to a patient in the intensive care unit. A review of the patient's medications shows that he is taking a proton pump inhibitor (PPI). This class of drugs inhibits the production of which of the following major acids produced by the body?

(A) Phosphoric acid
(B) Sulfuric acid
(C) Lactic acid
(D) β-Hydroxybutyric acid
(E) Hydrochloric acid

8. Proton pump inhibitors are a mainstay in the treatment of peptic ulcer disease and inhibit the gastric hydrogen ATPase. ATPases are in a class of enzymes that catalyze the hydrolysis of a high energy bond in adenosine triphosphate (ATP) to form adenosine diphosphate (ADP) and a free phosphate ion. The hydrogen ATPase in the gastric mucosal parietal cell utilizes this energy to exchange one hydrogen ion from the cytoplasm for one extracellular potassium ion. What type of transport is this enzyme catalyzing?

(A) Antiport coupled transport
(B) Symport coupled transport
(C) Facilitated diffusion
(D) Simple diffusion
(E) Osmosis

9. A 76-year-old bedridden nursing home resident begins to develop swelling of her left leg. A venous Doppler ultrasound is ordered and shows an obstructive deep vein thrombosis extending from her left common femoral vein to her popliteal vein with limited blood flow. The patient is immediately started on heparin to further prevent the clot from enlarging. Heparin is an example of which of the following?

(A) Sphingolipid
(B) Cerebroside
(C) Ganglioside
(D) Glycosaminoglycan
(E) Prostaglandin

10. A 43-year-old alcoholic man has been taking the drug cimetidine for gastric reflux. His primary care physician warns that this is not a good idea given his poor liver function and decreased ability for glucuronidation. Glucuronidation involves the addition of a carbohydrate molecule that has been derived from glucose, by which of the following mechanisms?

(A) Oxidation
(B) Sulfation
(C) Reduction
(D) Phosphorylation
(E) Mutarotation

11. In a patient with severe chronic obstructive pulmonary disease (COPD), COPD "flares" are common and result in an inability to ventilate and the accumulation of carbon dioxide in the body, leading to a primary respiratory acidosis. Of the following mechanisms, which is the most important for the management of acid-base status?

(A) $CO_2 + H_2O \iff H_2CO_3 \iff H^+ + HCO_3^-$
(B) $H^+ + NH_3 \iff NH_4^+$
(C) $CH_3COOH \iff CH_3COO^- + H^+$
(D) $H_2O \iff H^+ + HO^-$
(E) $CH_3CHOHCH_2COOH \iff CH_3CHOHCH_2COO^- + H^+$

12. A newborn girl is delivered after her mother had an uncomplicated 9-month pregnancy. The family is concerned because their 10-year-old son has been diagnosed with cystic fibrosis and has already developed several severe pulmonary infections requiring hospitalization. They request that their pediatrician order a sodium chloride sweat test to determine whether their newborn daughter has the disease. The disease is due to a defect in which of the following?

(A) A peripheral membrane protein
(B) A transmembrane protein
(C) Increased cholesterol content of the lipid bilayers
(D) An enzyme
(E) The ability to glycosylate ligands for selectins

Answers and Explanations

1. **The answer is A.** Acetazolamide is a potent carbonic anhydrase inhibitor and helps to reduce conditions of volume overload (not volume decrease, which would be brought about by dehydration). In the eye, carbonic anhydrase inhibitors lead to a decrease in the secretion of aqueous humor, which reduces intraocular pressure. In patients with epilepsy, these inhibitors block the activity of the central nervous system neuron carbonic anhydrase, which decreases excessive neuronal discharge. In the treatment of individuals with altitude sickness, the mechanism of the carbonic anhydrase inhibitor appears to be related to the acid-base effects of the drug. Patients with congestive heart failure take these inhibitors, and the effect of the inhibitors is to act as a diuretic, which helps to manage and reduce intravascular volume.

2. **The answer is E.** Sickle cell anemia is caused by a point mutation in DNA, which leads to glutamic acid at position 6 of the β-chain of globin being replaced with the hydrophobic amino acid valine. This mutation of the β-globin gene causes the polymerization of hemoglobin under low oxygen conditions, distorting the red blood cells into an inelastic, sickle shape. The most life-threatening manifestations of sickling, or a "sickle crisis," are aplastic crisis, splenic sequestration, vaso-occlusive crisis, and acute chest syndrome.

3. **The answer is B.** Digoxin is a medication that can improve the contraction of the heart. It is a drug that has been around for centuries and is made from the foxglove plant. A glycoside is an ether containing a sugar component (glycol) and a nonsugar (aglycone) component attached via oxygen or nitrogen bond; hydrolysis of a glycoside yields one or more sugars. A glycoprotein contains sugars attached via glycosidic linkage to amino acid side chains of the protein. An oligosaccharide is the linkage of a number of sugars in glycosidic bonds. A glucosteroid is a type of steroid hormone. A thioester linkage contains a sulfur bonded to a carbon, which has a carbonyl group also attached to it.

4. **The answer is B.** Glutamate functions as the most important and abundant excitatory neurotransmitter in the brain. It is released from the presynaptic membrane and interacts with postsynaptic glutamate receptors such as the NMDA (*N*-methyl-D-aspartate) receptor. Antagonists of NMDA, such as ketamine, are used clinically to provide dissociative anesthesia in children.

5. **The answer is A.** The influenza virus enters the epithelial host cell by binding to sialic acid residues found on the cell surface. Sialic acid is a modified sugar residue. Cerebrosides are glycolipids synthesized from ceramide and a UDP-sugar; a common one is glucocerebroside. Cytokine receptors (which work through the JAK kinase and STAT transcription factors) and serine-threonine kinase receptors are two types of receptors involved in signal transduction, which is initiated after a chemical messenger (e.g., hormone, neurotransmitter, or cytokine) binds to the receptor on the plasma membrane. Uronic acid is an oxidized sugar and is a component of proteoglycans. Uronic acid is not usually found as a part of glycoproteins, as sialic acid is.

6. **The answer is B.** Fructose gives a positive result in a reducing-sugar test and a negative result in a glucose oxidase test. Glucose would yield a positive test result with the enzyme glucose oxidase. Sorbitol has no aldehyde or ketone group and, thus, is not a reducing sugar and cannot be oxidized in the reducing-sugar test. Maltose and lactose are disaccharides that undergo acid hydrolysis, which doubles the amount of reducing sugar. Because fructose is a monosaccharide, acid would have no effect on the amount of reducing sugar present.

7. **The answer is E.** The proton pump inhibitors, such as omeprazole, inhibit the H^+-K^+ ATPase, which is responsible for the production of hydrochloric acid by the gastric parietal cells. Many patients are given these medications in the hospital to prevent the development of gastric ulcers. Phosphoric acid and sulfuric acid are important acids that are byproducts of normal

metabolism. Lactic acid is yet another product of metabolism, primarily anaerobic glycolysis. β-Hydroxybutyric acid is a ketone body that results from lipid metabolism.

8. **The answer is A.** The action of the gastic hydrogen ATPase is in antiport coupled transport: the exchange between hydrogen for potassium is driven by the energy released by the conversion of ATP to ADP. Symport coupled transport, although a form of active transport as well, results in the passage of molecules together across a membrane, such as the glucose-Na^+ cotransporter. Facilitated and simple diffusion are passive mechanisms for the transfer of a molecule across a membrane. The driving force for passive and simple diffusion relies primarily on the concentration gradient of the molecule across the membrane and requires no energy. Facilitated diffusion uses a carrier protein to transfer the molecule across the membrane, whereas simple diffusion does not require a carrier. Osmosis is the diffusion of a solvent (usually water in biologic systems) across a semipermeable membrane in response to a difference in solute concentration across the membrane.

9. **The answer is D.** Heparin is an example of a glycosaminoglycan, a long repeating chain of disaccharide units attached to a core protein. The sugar residues of heparin are sulfated. Cerebrosides and gangliosides are both examples of sphingolipids derived from the lipid ceramide. Prostaglandins are derived from polyunsaturated fatty acids, an example of which is arachidonic acid.

10. **The answer is A.** Glucuronidation makes the drug more water soluble and, therefore, more easily secreted by the kidneys. Glucuronic acid is derived from glucose via oxidation of the oxygen on carbon 6 of glucose. Sulfated sugars are found in glycosaminoglycans. Reduction of glucose at carbon 1 forms sorbitol, whereas phosphorylation of glucose (usually at position 6) traps glucose within the cell and commits it to metabolism. Mutarotation occurs when α-glucose is converted to β-glucose, a process that requires passage through a straight-chain aldehyde.

11. **The answer is A.** The primary conversion of carbon dioxide into a soluble form that can be expired (and thereby removed from the body) is through mechanism A. Mechanism B is seen in metabolic acidosis as the kidney tries to excrete hydrogen protons via NH_4^+. Accumulation of acetic acid during metabolic acidosis (e.g., diabetic ketoacidosis, DKA) can result in the reaction seen in mechanism C. Mechanism D is the simple equilibrium reaction of water into its conjugate acid and base. Mechanism E is the ionization of β-hydroxybutyric acid, a "ketone body" product produced during diabetic ketoacidosis.

12. **The answer is B.** The protein involved in cystic fibrosis is the cystic fibrosis transmembrane conductance regulator (CFTR), encoded by the *CRFT* gene. About 90% of cystic fibrosis patients in the American Caucasian population have a particular mutation known as ΔF_{508}. ΔF_{508} refers to the loss of three nucleotides from the *CFTR* gene, at codon 508, which codes for a phenylalanine (F) residue. Thus, the protein produced is missing this critical phenylalanine in the primary structure. Individuals who inherit two copies of this mutation frequently die from respiratory failure secondary to repeat pulmonary infections and buildup of thick, tenacious mucus in the respiratory passages. There are numerous diseases associated with defects in enzymes, particularly those of key metabolic enzymes. An increased cholesterol content of lipid bilayer membranes can result in spur cell anemia. Defects in the ability to glycosylate ligands for selectins are found in the disorder leukocyte adhesion deficiency II.

1 Protein Structure and Function

I. GENERAL ASPECTS OF PROTEIN STRUCTURE (FIGURE 1-1)

A. The linear sequence of amino acid residues in a polypeptide chain determines the three-dimensional configuration of a protein.

B. The structure of a protein determines its function.

1. The **primary structure** is the sequence of amino acids along the polypeptide chain.
   a. By convention, the **sequence** is written from left to right, starting with the **N-terminal** amino acid and ending with its C-terminal amino acid.
   b. Because there are no dissociable protons in peptide bonds, the **charges** on a polypeptide chain are due only to the N-terminal amino group, the C-terminal carboxyl group, and the side chains on amino acid residues.
   c. A protein will **migrate** in an **electric field,** depending on the sum of its charges at a given pH (the net charge).
      (1) **Positively charged** proteins are cations and migrate toward the **cathode (–).**
      (2) **Negatively charged** proteins are anions and migrate toward the **anode (+).**
   d. At the **isoelectric pH** (the pI), the net charge is zero, and the protein does not migrate.

2. **Secondary structure** includes various types of local conformations in which the atoms of the side chains are not involved.
   a. An **α-helix** is generated when each carbonyl of a peptide bond forms a **hydrogen bond** with the –NH of a peptide bond four amino acid residues further along the chain (Figure 1-2).
   b. The side chains of the amino acid residues in an α-helix extend outward from the central axis of the rodlike structure. This allows the formation of high tensile strength fibrillary proteins.
   c. The α-helix is disrupted by proline residues, in which the ring imposes geometric constraints, and by regions in which numerous amino acid residues have charged groups or large, bulky side chains.

> **CLINICAL CORRELATES** **Marfan syndrome** results from mutations in the gene for the highly α-helical fibrillary protein *fibrillin,* which is a major component of microfibrils found in the extracellular matrix. Patients have defective connective tissue, particularly in the ligaments and aorta. They present with **excessively long extremities and fingers, arachnodactyly,** and a predisposition to **dissecting aortic aneurysms** and valvular disease.

3. **β-Sheets** are formed by **hydrogen bonds** between two extended polypeptide chains or between two regions of a single chain that folds back on itself (Figure 1-3).
   a. These **interactions** are between the **carbonyl** of one peptide bond and the **–NH** of another.
   b. The chains may run in the same direction (parallel) or in opposite directions (antiparallel).

Primary

— Ser — Ala — Glu — Val — Leu — Arg — Gly —

Secondary

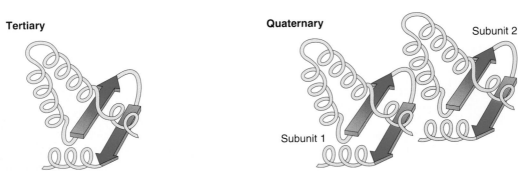

α-helix   β-sheet

Tertiary

Quaternary

Subunit 2

Subunit 1

FIGURE 1-1 Schematic diagram of the primary, secondary, tertiary, and quaternary structure of a protein.

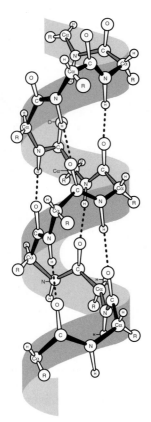

FIGURE 1-2 An α-helix. The *dotted lines* represent the hydrogen bonding that occurs between the carbonyl (C = O) of one peptide bond and the –NH of another peptide bond that is four amino acid residues further along the chain.

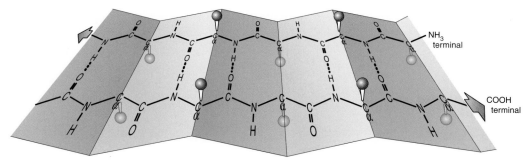

FIGURE 1-3 The structure of an antiparallel β-sheet. The orientation is indicated by *arrows,* and the hydrogen bonds by *dotted lines.*

CLINICAL CORRELATES Prion diseases like **Creutzfeldt-Jakob disease (CJD)** result from the transmission of a proteinaceous agent that is capable of **altering the normal α-helical arrangement** of the prion protein and replacing it with **β-pleated sheets** and smaller α-helices, similar to the pathogenic form. The resulting misfolded protein is resistant to degradation, with death of the affected neurons. Patients suffer pronounced involuntary jerking movements (**startle myoclonus**) and rapidly **deteriorating dementia.**

---

   c. **Supersecondary structures**
     (1) Certain motifs involving a combination of α-helices and β-sheets are frequently found and include the **helix-turn-helix, leucine zipper,** and **zinc finger.** These motifs are often found in **transcription** factors because they help mediate **binding of proteins to DNA.**
     (2) Other types of **helices** or **loops** and **turns** can occur that differ from one protein to another (random coils).

CLINICAL CORRELATES The family of transcription factors known as **homeobox proteins** contains **helix-turn-helix** motifs. They play a significant role in pattern development during development of the limbs and other body parts. Disruption of **protein–DNA** interactions in these proteins may result in congenital malformations.

C. The tertiary structure of a protein refers to its overall three-dimensional **conformation.** It is produced by interactions between disparate amino acid residues that may be located at a considerable distance from each other in the primary sequence of the polypeptide chain (Figure 1-4).
   1. Hydrophobic amino acid residues tend to reside and cluster in the **interior** of globular proteins, where they exclude water, whereas **hydrophilic** residues are usually found on the **surface,** where they interact with water.
   2. The types of **noncovalent** interactions between amino acid residues that produce the **three-dimensional shape** of a protein include hydrophobic interactions, **electrostatic (ionic)** interactions, **hydrogen bonds,** and van der Waals interactions. **Covalent disulfide bonds** also occur in tertiary structure.
   3. All the information required for proteins to correctly assume their tertiary structure is defined by their primary sequence. Sometimes molecules known as "**chaperones**" interact with the polypeptide **to help find the correct tertiary structure.** Such proteins either catalyze the rate of folding or protect the protein from forming "nonproductive" intramolecular tangles during the folding process.

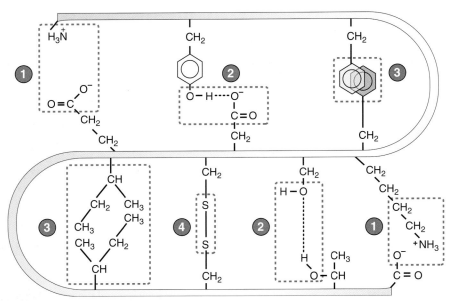

FIGURE 1-4 Interactions between amino acid residues in a polypeptide chain: (1) electrostatic interactions; (2) hydrogen bonds; (3) hydrophobic interactions; and (4) a disulfide bond.

CLINICAL CORRELATES   **Heat shock proteins** (hsps) are a group of **chaperones**. Mutations in such proteins sometimes lead to human disease. Some patients with **Charcot-Marie-Tooth (CMT) disease,** one of the most common inherited **neuromuscular diseases,** have been found to have mutations in hsps.

D. **Quaternary structure** refers to the spatial arrangement of subunits in a protein containing more than one polypeptide chain (Figure 1-1).

- The subunits are joined together by the same types of **noncovalent interactions** within a single polypeptide to form its tertiary structure. In some cases, covalent disulfide bonds are also found in quaternary structure.

E. **Denaturation and renaturation**
1. Proteins can be **denatured** by agents such as **heat** and **urea** that unfold polypeptide chains without causing hydrolysis of peptide bonds.
2. If a denatured protein returns to its native state after the denaturing agent is removed, the process is called **renaturation.**

F. **Protein misfolding**
1. Misfolded proteins can result spontaneously from **mutations in the gene encoding the protein.**
2. Misfolded proteins can aggregate to form insoluble β-pleated fibrils, or amyloid. These fibrils accumulate in tissue, often resulting in worsening pathology as the amyloid accumulates. See Table 1-1 for some clinically relevant **amyloidopathies.**

CLINICAL CORRELATES   Mutations in patients with α_1-antitrypsin (AAT) deficiency result in a misfolded protein that gets trapped within the cell. Patients with decreased levels of this protease inhibitor manifest with **cirrhosis** and **emphysema.**

t a b l e **1-1** Amyloidosis and Human Disease		
Amyloid Protein Component	**Associated Disease**	**Notes**
β-amyloid	Alzheimer disease	The most common cause of **progressive dementia**
β₂-microglobulin	Hemodialysis-associated amyloidosis	Deposition of amyloid in bone joints results in arthritis and cartilage and bone destruction.
Calcitonin	Medullary carcinoma of the thyroid	Deposition of **amyloid around the C cells of the thyroid,** the source of the calcitonin
Immunoglobulin light chain	Multiple myeloma	Patients have renal (**myeloma kidney**) and **heart failure** due to accumulation of protein in these tissues.
Islet amyloid protein	Type 2 diabetes mellitus	Deposition of the islet amyloid protein, normally secreted with insulin, may contribute to further **islet dysfunction.**
Transthyretin	Familial amyloidotic neuropathies	Deposition of amyloid in neurons with axonal degeneration

CLINICAL CORRELATES **Huntington disease** results from the expansion of a region of **polyglutamine repeats** within the *Huntington* **protein.** The protein aggregates and forms intranuclear inclusions, resulting in neuronal cell death. Patients present with **progressive movement disorders and dementia.**

G. **Post-translational modifications** of proteins occur after the protein has been synthesized on the ribosome. A given protein can have many combinations of modifications.
  1. **Post-translational modifications** include phosphorylation, glycosylation, adenosine diphosphate (ADP) ribosylation, hydroxylation, and acetylation.
  2. Such modifications alter the charge on proteins and the interactions between amino acid residues, **altering the three-dimensional configuration** and, thus, the function of the protein.
  3. See Table 1-2 for medically relevant post-translational modifications.

H. **Protein degradation**
  1. Proteins from the intracellular environment may be targeted for degradation by the **ubiquitin–proteasomal pathway** (Figure 1-5).
    a. **Ubiquitin,** a small globular protein, is covalently attached to the target protein to be degraded.
    b. **Further** ubiquitination of the target protein results in **polyubiquitination.**
    c. Polyubiquitinated "tagged" proteins are then recognized by a large multiprotein proteolytic complex, known as the **proteasome.**
    d. The **proteasome** degrades proteins into small peptides, which are then further degraded into amino acid precursors or presented on the surface of cells as small peptides for immune recognition.

CLINICAL CORRELATES The novel anticancer drug **bortezomib (Velcade)** is used for the treatment of **multiple myeloma** and **inhibits the proteasome.** It is believed that cancer cells are more dependent on proteasomal degradation than normal cells for proliferation, metastasis, and survival.

  2. Alternatively, some proteins are degraded in a **PEST sequence**–dependent manner.
    ● Proteins that have **PEST** sequences in their N terminus (proline [**P**], glutamate [**E**], serine [**S**], and threonine [**T**]) are targeted for rapid degradation after synthesis by nonspecific proteases.

t a b l e **1-2**	Various Post-Translational Modifications	
Modification	**Protein Target**	**Clinical Consequence**
Acetylation	Histones	Involved in the regulation of protein–DNA interactions because histone proteins are often acetylated
Acylation	RAS (p21)	RAS is anchored to the inner cytoplasmic membrane by **farnesyl (a fatty acyl moiety)**. Inhibitors of this modification are being developed to **suppress the oncogenicity of RAS.**
ADP ribosylation	Rho (a small GTP protein)	***Clostridium botulinum* toxin** is an enzyme that **ADP-ribosylates Rho,** leading to **inhibition of the release of acetylcholine** and a subsequent **flaccid paralysis.**
Carboxylation	Clotting factors	Carboxylation of **factors VII, IX, X, fibrinogen, and proteins C and S** are required for coagulation. This process is inhibited by the drug **warfarin.**
Disulfide bond formation	Antibodies	Antibodies are complex immune molecules whose function requires numerous intramolecular as well as intermolecular disulfide bonds.
Glycation	Hemoglobin	**Nonenzymatic addition of sugar** to proteins contributes to disease complications. **Glycated hemoglobin, HBA$_{1c}$,** is normally 6% of the total hemoglobin but increases when red blood cells are exposed to high levels of blood glucose and is a measure of **long-term glucose control** in diabetic patients.
Glycosylation	Red blood cell proteins	Different **sugars added to red blood cell proteins** determine an individual's **blood type. Transfusions** of blood products and successful **transplantation** require correct blood type matching.
Glycosyl phosphatidyl inositol (GPI)	Complement regulatory proteins	Patients with **paroxysmal nocturnal hemoglobin** (PNH) lack the ability to form **GPI linkage.** Such patients cannot produce cell surface complement regulatory proteins, causing **red blood cell destruction** and subsequent **anemia**.
Phosphorylation	Growth factor receptors	**Phosphorylation of proteins usually results in growth-promoting signals.** A number of newly developed anticancer drugs seek to prevent phosphorylation.
Ubiquitination	Proteins targeted for degradation	Improper ubiquitination and degradation of various proteins can lead to abnormalities in protein folding. Aberrant protein folding can lead to diseases such as Alzheimer disease.

3. Proteins from the extracellular environment are degraded within lysosomes.
   a. Material enters the cell by endocytosis.
   b. The endocytic vesicle fuses with the lysosome to form the phagolysosome.
   c. The proteolytic enzymes within the lysosome digest the endocytosed material into peptides.
   d. These peptides can then be completely degraded or, in some cases, presented to cells of the immune system.

CLINICAL CORRELATES   Patients with **Chédiak-Higashi syndrome** have a defect in the ability to **transfer enzymes from lysosomes to phagocytic vesicles.** They have **recurrent infections** owing to a lack of microbial killing, anemia, and thrombocytopenia.

II. EXAMPLES OF MEDICALLY IMPORTANT PROTEINS

A. **Hemoglobin** (Figure 1-6) is a globular oxygen transport protein necessary for human life, whose biochemistry is well studied.

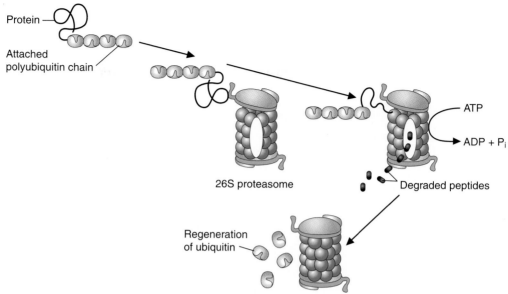

FIGURE 1-5 Protein degradation of ubiquitinated proteins by the proteasome.

1. **Structure of hemoglobin**
   - Adult hemoglobin (HbA) consists of **four polypeptide chains** (two α and two β chains), each containing a molecule of **heme.**

   a. The **α and β chains** of HbA are **similar** in three-dimensional configuration to each other and to the single chain of muscle myoglobin, although their amino acid sequences differ.
   b. Eight α-helices occur in each chain.
   c. **Heme,** a complex of a **porphyrin ring** and a **ferrous (Fe^{2+})** ion, fits into a crevice in each globin chain and interacts with two histidine residues.

CLINICAL CORRELATES Many types of **mutations** produce alterations in the structure of hemoglobin. One common mutation results in **sickle cell anemia,** in which the β chain of hemoglobin contains a **valine rather than a glutamate at position 6.** Thus, in the mutant hemoglobin (HbS), a hydrophobic amino acid replaces an amino acid with a negative charge. This change allows **deoxygenated molecules of HbS to polymerize.** Red blood cells that contain large complexes of HbS molecules can assume a sickle shape. These cells undergo **hemolysis,** and an **anemia** results. Painful **vaso-occlusive crises** also occur, and **end-organ damage** may result.

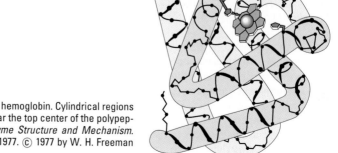

FIGURE 1-6 The structure of the β chain of hemoglobin. Cylindrical regions contain α-helices. The planar structure near the top center of the polypeptide chain is heme. (From Fersht, A. *Enzyme Structure and Mechanism.* Reading, UK: WH Freeman and Company, 1977. © 1977 by W. H. Freeman and Company. Used with permission.)

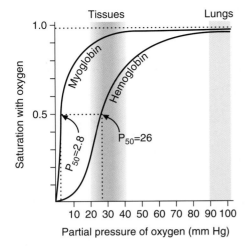

FIGURE 1-7 Oxygen saturation curves for myoglobin and adult hemoglobin (HbA). Myoglobin has a hyperbolic saturation curve. HbA has a sigmoidal curve. The HbA curve shifts to the right at lower pH, with higher concentrations of 2,3-biphosphoglycerate (BPG), or as CO_2 binds to HbA in the tissues. Under these conditions, O_2 is released more readily. P_{50} is the partial pressure of O_2 at which half-saturation with O_2 occurs on the proteins.

2. **Function of hemoglobin**
   a. The oxygen saturation curve for hemoglobin is sigmoidal (Figure 1-7).
      (1) **The iron of each heme** binds **one O_2** molecule, for a total of four O_2 molecules per HbA molecule. HbA changes from the taut or tense **(T) form** to the relaxed **(R) form** when oxygen binds.
      (2) Binding of O_2 to one heme group in hemoglobin increases the affinity for O_2 of its other heme groups. This allosteric effect produces the sigmoidal oxygen saturation curve.

CLINICAL CORRELATES   **Hemoglobin has about 250 times the affinity for carbon monoxide** than it does for oxygen. Prolonged or heavy exposure to carbon monoxide results in disorientation, headache, and **potentially fatal asphyxiation.** Patients may have "**cherry-red mucous membranes**" due to the accumulation of **carboxyhemoglobin.**

   b. The binding of **protons** to HbA stimulates the release of O_2, a manifestation of the **Bohr effect**.
      (1) Thus, O_2 is readily released in the tissues where $[H^+]$ is high due to the production of CO_2 by metabolic processes:

$$CO_2 + H_2O \rightleftarrows H_2CO_3 \rightleftarrows H^+ + HCO_3^-$$
$$\text{Lungs}$$
$$H^+ + HbAO_2 \rightleftarrows HHbA + O_2$$
$$\text{Tissues}$$

      (2) These reactions are reversed in the lung. O_2 binds to HbA, and CO_2 is exhaled.
   c. Covalent binding of **CO_2** to HbA in the tissues also causes O_2 release.
   d. Binding of **2,3-bisphosphoglycerate (BPG)** (formerly known as 2,3-diphosphoglycerate [DPG]), a side product of glycolysis in red blood cells, decreases the affinity of HbA for O_2. Consequently, O_2 is more readily released in tissues when BPG is bound to HbA.

B. **Collagen** refers to a group of very similar structural proteins that are found in the **extracellular matrix,** the **vitreous humor** of the eye, and **bone and cartilage.** Numerous other structural proteins are important in human disease; for other select examples, see Table 1-3.
   1. **Structure of collagen**
      a. Collagen consists of three chains that intertwine to form a triple helix (Figure 1-8).
      b. Collagen contains about 1000 amino acids, one third of which are **glycine.** The sequence Gly-X-Y frequently occurs, in which X is often **proline** and Y is **hydroxyproline** or **hydroxylysine.**

table **1-3**	Structural Proteins and Disease	
Protein	**Disease**	**Disease Characteristics**
Spectrin	Hereditary spherocytosis	**Hereditary anemia** and splenomegaly; treatment sometimes involves **splenectomy.**
Dystrophin	Muscular dystrophy	**Progressive motor weakness,** eventual respiratory failure, and cardiac decompensation; **X-linked inheritance.**
β-Myosin heavy chain	Familial hypertrophic cardiomyopathy	Enlargement of the heart with outlet obstruction. **Most common cause of sudden, otherwise unexplainable death in young athletes.**
Collagen (α₅ chain of type IV collagen)	Alport syndrome	**X-linked syndrome** characterized by **renal failure, nerve deafness,** and **cataracts.**

CLINICAL CORRELATES
Osteogenesis imperfecta is a group of related disorders in the **synthesis of type I collagen.** Such defects have a wide spectrum of clinical consequence, although they all share bone fragility (with a predisposition to **multiple childhood fractures**), hearing loss, and a **distinctive blue sclera.**

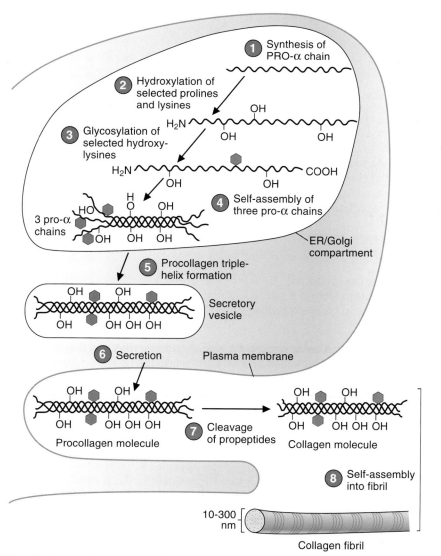

FIGURE 1-8 Steps in the formation of mature collagen fibrils.

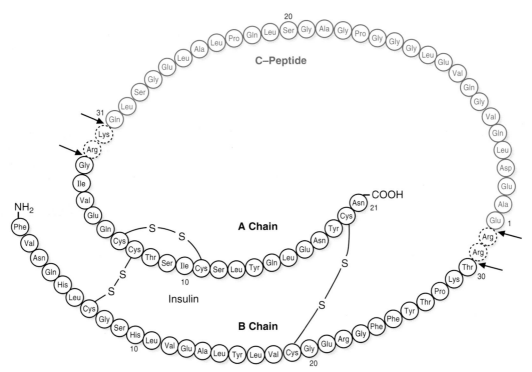

FIGURE 1-9 The cleavage of proinsulin to form insulin. Cleavage occurs at the *arrows*, which release the C-peptide. The A and B chains of insulin are joined by disulfide bonds. (From Murray RK, et al. *Harper's Biochemistry*, 23rd ed. Stamford, CT: Appleton & Lange, 1993:500.)

2. **Synthesis of collagen**
   a. The polypeptide chains of **preprocollagen** are synthesized on the **rough endoplasmic reticulum,** and the signal (pre) sequence is cleaved.
   b. **Proline** and **lysine** residues are **hydroxylated** by a reaction that requires O_2 and **vitamin C.**
   c. **Galactose** and **glucose** are added to hydroxylysine residues.
   d. The **triple helix** forms, and procollagen is secreted from the cell and cleaved to form collagen.
   e. **Cross-links** are produced. The side chains of lysine and hydroxylysine residues are oxidized to form aldehydes, which can undergo aldol condensation or form Schiff bases with the amino groups of lysine residues.

CLINICAL CORRELATES   **Ehlers-Danlos syndrome** is a group of disorders characterized by a defect in the synthesis or structure of collagen. One of the subtypes, **Ehlers-Danlos type VI,** results from a **defect in the enzyme lysyl hydroxylase.** Defects in collagen synthesis are characterized by **hyperextensible skin,** laxity of joints, and defects in large blood vessels.

C. **Insulin**
   1. **Structure of insulin** (Figure 1-9)

   ● Insulin is a polypeptide hormone that is produced by the **β cells** of the **pancreas.** The mature form has 51 amino acids in **two polypeptide chains (A and B),** which are linked by two **disulfide bridges.**

2. **Synthesis of insulin** (Figure 1-9)
   a. **Preproinsulin,** consisting of the A and B chains joined by a C-peptide, is synthesized on the rough endoplasmic reticulum and the pre- (signal) sequence is removed to form proinsulin.
   b. In secretory granules, **proinsulin** is cleaved, and the **C-peptide** is released. The remainder of the molecule forms the active hormone.

CLINICAL CORRELATES   **C-peptide levels are used to differentiate the causes of high insulin in patients.** In cases of low blood glucose due to increased levels of circulating insulin via endogenous production, as in **tumors of pancreatic β cells,** serum levels of **C-peptide will also be elevated.** However, in cases of **surreptitious insulin administration** (purposeful injection of insulin), **C-peptide is not elevated** because commercial insulin preparations have purified away this contaminate.

Review Test

Directions: Each of the numbered questions or incomplete statements in this section is followed by answers or by completions of the statement. Select the **one** lettered answer or completion that is **best** in each case.

1. Which of the following statements is correct concerning prion disease?

(A) It is a disease process in which proteins appear to be the sole pathophysiologic entity
(B) It is a disease process in which a messenger RNA secondary structure appears to be the sole pathophysiologic entity
(C) The disease is only found in humans
(D) Effective treatments are available for the disease
(E) The disease process is readily reversible

2. The mutation associated with Marfan syndrome is with the fibrillary protein fibrillin. What aspect of protein structure is affected in this disorder?

(A) β-turn
(B) β-sheet
(C) Primary structure
(D) Tertiary structure
(E) Quaternary structure

3. A 65-year-old man with a history of type 2 diabetes is complaining of blurred vision and numbness in his toes. Laboratory results were significant for increased blood urea nitrogen (BUN) and creatinine, indicative of renal failure. Laboratory work also revealed an HbA_{1C} of 9.0. One of the mechanisms for the damage responsible for the man's symptoms is the nonenzymatic covalent bonds formed between glucose and structural proteins. How would this reaction best be classified?

(A) Acylation
(B) Carboxylation
(C) Glycation
(D) Hydroxylation
(E) Esterification

4. A 24-year-old man presents to your clinic with several concerning symptoms. He states that he has uncontrollable movements called *chorea*, occasional stiffness, slurring of speech, difficulty planning his day and balancing his checkbook, and bouts of anxiety and crying spells. He also professes that this has been noted in some relatives on his mother's side. What is true about the nature of the molecular mutation of this disorder?

(A) A point mutation in a single gene
(B) A nucleotide deletion in a single gene
(C) A triplet repeat expansion within a gene
(D) A frameshift mutation within a gene, creating a truncated protein
(E) A chromosomal deletion of many bases that covers many genes

5. A 2-week-old infant presents to your rural family medicine clinic and appears ill; he is febrile and jaundiced and has extensive, reddened skin. According to his mother, it appears that since the delivery of the baby at home he has always "carried a fever." You are able to send off some laboratory tests and are surprised to see that he has significant neutropenia and hypergammaglobulinemia. What is the most likely diagnosis?

(A) DiGeorge syndrome
(B) Severe combined immunodeficiency disease
(C) Chédiak-Higashi syndrome
(D) Wiskott-Aldrich syndrome
(E) Myeloperoxidase deficiency

6. In the figure below, four bonds are indicated by numbers. Match the bonds with their correct description below.

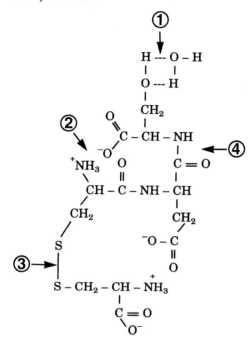

(A) (1) Electrostatic interaction; (2) hydrogen bond; (3) disulfide bond; (4) peptide bond
(B) (1) Hydrogen bond; (2) peptide bond; (3) disulfide bond; (4) electrostatic interaction
(C) (1) Hydrogen bond; (2) disulfide bond; (3) electrostatic interaction; (4) peptide bond
(D) (1) Hydrogen bond; (2) electrostatic interaction; (3) disulfide bond; (4) peptide bond
(E) (1) Hydrogen bond; (2) electrostatic interaction; (3) peptide bond; (4) disulfide bond

7. A 27-year-old firefighter is brought to the emergency room after being exposed to smoke during a training exercise. He looks ill and has labored breathing. He is clutching his head and exhibits an altered mental status. On examination, you note that he appears red, and his pulse oximetry reads 100%. You suspect carbon monoxide toxicity. What is true of the oxygen saturation curve during carbon monoxide toxicity?

(A) The oxygen saturation curve is shifted to the left.
(B) The oxygen saturation curve is shifted to the right.
(C) The effect of carbon monoxide on hemoglobin is similar to that of having increased levels of 2,3 bisphosphoglycerate.
(D) The effect of carbon monoxide on hemoglobin is similar to that of a low pH state.
(E) The effect of carbon monoxide on hemoglobin is similar to that of an increased temperature state.

8. A 59-year-old man presents with nephrotic syndrome. Immunoelectrophoresis detects a monoclonal immunoglobulin G (IgG) λ subtype in his serum and free λ light chains in his urine. A renal biopsy shows amyloidosis. Although several different proteins are precursors to amyloid deposition, all amyloid fibrils share an identical secondary structure that is which of the following?

(A) α-Helix
(B) β-Pleated sheet
(C) Triple helix
(D) Helix-turn-helix
(E) Leucine zipper

9. The patient described in question 8, who has multiple myeloma, has not responded to numerous treatments, and his disease is progressing. He sees his oncologist, who wants to start him on the drug bortezomib. Bortezomib inhibits the proteasome from degrading proteins. Which class of intracellular proteins will not be specifically degraded as a result of taking this drug?

(A) Proteins with PEST sequences
(B) Amyloid proteins
(C) Polyubiquitinated proteins
(D) Immunoglobulin light chains
(E) Immunoglobulin heavy chains

Answers and Explanations

1. **The answer is A.** Prion diseases include a handful of diseases that affect animals (e.g., bovine spongiform encephalopathy is "mad cow disease") and humans (Creutzfeldt-Jakob disease). The pathogenesis is mediated primarily by a protein that can exist in two conformations: one normal, the other leading to disease. The abnormally folded proteins are resistant to degradation by the host and affect the central nervous system. The change in protein structure is not reversible. The messenger RNA in the disease state is not altered compared with the normal state. There is no effective treatment, and patients develop rapidly progressive dementia.

2. **The answer is C.** The fibrillin mutation found in Marfan syndrome results in a defective α-helix due to an alteration in the sequence of amino acids in the protein, an altered primary structure. The tertiary and quaternary structures are not altered, nor are β-sheets or turns. Additionally, it is important to note that the main organ systems affected are the musculoskeletal system (arachnodactyly, dolichostenomelia, scoliosis), cardiovascular system (acute aortic dissection, mitral valve prolapse), pulmonary system (spontaneous pneumothorax), and eyes (lens subluxation, decreased nighttime vision).

3. **The answer is C.** Glycation refers to the reaction of the aldehyde group of glucose reacting with the amino groups of protein, forming an amide linkage. The increased rate of glycation of collagen during hyperglycemia is implicated in the development of complications of diabetes, such as blindness and renal and vascular disease. Clotting factors are often carboxylated; histones can be acylated. Collagen is a prominent example of a protein that is hydroxylated during its production.

4. **The answer is C.** This patient has all the classic signs and symptoms of Huntington disease. Huntington disease is an autosomal dominant disorder that involves the *huntington* gene. This gene encodes a sequence of repeating trinucleotides, which gives rise to a polyglutamine stretch in the protein. In certain individuals, those that express Huntington disease, this trinucleotide repeat is greatly expanded, and the stretch of polyglutamine in the protein is enlarged, leading to a dysfunctional protein that, over time, leads to altered neuronal function. Other diseases that result from trinucleotide repeat expansion include spinobulbar muscular atrophy, spinocerebellar ataxia, fragile X syndrome, Friedreich ataxia, and myotonic dystrophy. Huntington disease is not due to a single nucleotide change, a frameshift mutation, or a deletion event within the gene.

5. **The answer is C.** This patient has Chédiak-Higashi syndrome, a primary immunodeficiency disorder of phagocytic vesicles in which the lysosomes are unable to destroy bacteria. Primary immunodeficiency disorders are grouped into humoral/antibody/B-cell disorders (e.g., hypogammaglobulinemia, common variable immunodeficiency, leukocyte adhesion deficiency), cell-mediated/T-cell disorders (e.g., DiGeorge syndrome), combined humoral and cell-mediated deficiencies (e.g., severe combined immunodeficiency, Wiskott-Aldrich syndrome), complement deficiencies (e.g., angioedema), and phagocyte dysfunction (e.g., Chédiak-Higashi syndrome). All these disorders affect children early in life and are associated with significant morbidity and mortality.

6. **The answer is D.** Bond 1: The hydroxyl group of serine forms hydrogen bonds with water. Bond 2: A positively charged amino group and a negatively charged carboxyl group form an electrostatic interaction. Bond 3: Two sulfur residues are covalently joined by a disulfide bond. Bond 4: In peptides, adjacent amino acids are joined covalently by peptide bonds.

7. **The answer is A.** Oxygen saturation curves relate the saturation of hemoglobin with oxygen for a given partial pressure of oxygen. If carbon monoxide binds to one of the subunits of hemoglobin, the affinity of the other subunits for oxygen is increased (due to the cooperative nature of oxygen binding to hemoglobin). This shifts the oxygen binding curve to the left. Because the oxygen now has a higher affinity for hemoglobin, it is more difficult for hemoglobin to release oxygen to the

tissues, leading to hypoxia despite oxygen being bound to hemoglobin. Conditions that shift the curve to the right allow oxygen to be released more readily: low pH, increased PCO_2, increased temperature, presence of 2,3-bisphosphoglycerate, and absence of carbon monoxide. In other words, hemoglobin will release oxygen in states that allow for normal binding of oxygen and increased oxygen demands by tissues.

8. **The answer is B.** Regardless of the type of amyloid disease, the pathogenesis is related to the accumulation of β-pleated protein. In the case of multiple myeloma, it is the accumulation of immunoglobulin light chains in the kidney and heart. α-Helical proteins include native fibrillary proteins. The triple helix is a unique structure found in collagen. Helix-turn-helix and leucine zippers are supersecondary structures that are often found in transcription factors, like homeo-box proteins (helix-turn-helix).

9. **The answer is C.** The proteasome normally degrades proteins that have been polyubiquitinated. As such, in the presence of bortezomib, polyubiquitinlated proteins will accumulate within cells, leading to a selective adverse effect on the cancer cells (myeloma cells) because these are the cells growing most rapidly. Proteins with PEST sequences are rapidly degraded by nonspecific intra-cellular proteases. Although the immunoglobulin light chains are forming the amyloid proteins in this disease, these structures are difficult to degrade, such that inhibiting the proteasome has no effect on the degradation of the amyloid proteins. Immunoglobulin heavy chains are not accu-mulating in this disorder.

2 Enzymes

I. GENERAL PROPERTIES OF ENZYMES

A. **Naming enzymes**
   1. Names most often describe the reaction catalyzed with the suffix **"-ase"** to indicate the protein is an enzyme.
   2. Common names of enzymes may have no apparent logical basis (e.g., trypsin) with respect to function. A systematic classification system based on function has been introduced.

B. **The reactions of the cell** would not occur rapidly enough to sustain life if enzyme catalysts were not present. Enzymes **"speed up" reactions** by 10^6 to 10^{11} times.

C. **At the active sites** of enzymes, **substrates (reactants) bind** "tightly" to the enzyme, and the enzyme then **catalyzes** their conversion to products, which are released. **The transition state is a high-energy reactive conformation of reactants** with enzyme and has a very high probability of a **structural rearrangement of bonds** producing the products of the reaction.

D. **Enzymes are highly specific** for their substrates and products.

CLINICAL CORRELATES The nucleoside analogs **valacyclovir** and **valganciclovir** are valine ester **prodrugs** of the antiviral **acyclovir** (treating herpes simplex virus types 1 and 2 and varicella-zoster infections) and **ganciclovir** (treating cytomegalovirus retinitis in patients with acquired immunodeficiency syndrome [AIDS]), **respectively.** This new therapeutic approach involves a **"prodrug"** that is activated and converted by hepatic and intestinal enzymes to an active drug with higher bioavailability and efficacy. **Famciclovir** is another acyclovir compound used for shingles and recurrent outbreaks of herpes simplex virus type 2.

   1. Many enzymes recognize only a single compound as a substrate.
   2. Some enzymes (e.g., proteases that hydrolyze proteins to peptides), such as those involved in digestion, are less specific.
   3. **Enzymes as drug targets account for about 30% of pharmacotherapeutic agents.** Many newer agents are designed with the aid of protein structure information, allowing researchers to create enzyme-specific drugs based on such approaches. This strategy is known as **rational drug design.**

E. **Many enzymes require** small organic molecules, or **cofactors** (often called **coenzymes**), to catalyze their reactions. The cofactors are frequently derivatives of **vitamins or metal ions**.

F. **Enzymes decrease the energy of activation (Ea)** for a reaction and hence speed up the rate of **reactions**.

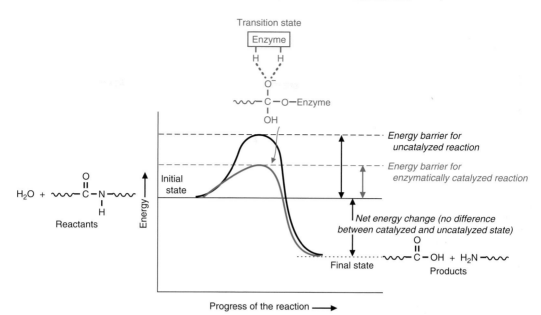

FIGURE 2-1 Free energy of activation (Ea) and the action of catalysts for a typical enzyme. Enzymes decrease the energy of activation for a reaction; however, they do not change the energy level of the substrates or products.

1. Enzymes **do not** affect the thermodynamics (ΔG) of the reaction (net free energy change for the reaction or equilibrium concentrations of the substrates and products).
2. The **thermodynamics of the reaction remain UNCHANGED** (Figure 2-1).
3. The transition state is at the apex (the top) of the energy diagram between reactants and products.
4. The difference in the average free energy of the reactants and the average free energy of the transition state is the **activation energy barrier (free energy of activation; Ea).**

II. DEPENDENCE OF VELOCITY ON ENZYME AND SUBSTRATE CONCENTRATIONS, TEMPERATURE, AND PH

A. The **velocity** of a reaction, **v, increases with the enzyme concentration, [E]**, if the **substrate concentration, [S]**, is constant.
   1. If [E] is constant, v increases with [S] until the **maximum velocity, V_{max}** (a measure of the maximum enzyme activity), is attained.
   2. At V_{max}, all the **active sites** of the enzyme are **saturated** with substrate.

B. The **velocity** of a reaction **increases with temperature** until a maximum ($37°$ C in humans) is reached, after which the velocity decreases owing to denaturation of the enzyme (Figure 2-2A).

C. **Each enzyme-catalyzed reaction** has an **optimal pH** (not always physiologic pH).
   1. The optimal pH is the pH at which the enzyme and substrate exhibit the most efficient interaction and the velocity is at a maximum.

CLINICAL CORRELATES The **optimal pH for pepsin is 2**, reflecting its need as a digestive enzyme in the acidic gastric juice of the **stomach. The optimal pH for alkaline phosphatase is 9**, reflecting the basic pH environment in **bone.**

   2. Changes in the pH can alter the interaction between enzyme and substrate such that the reaction proceeds at a slower rate. If the pH is too high or too low, the enzyme can also undergo **denaturation** (Figure 2-2B).

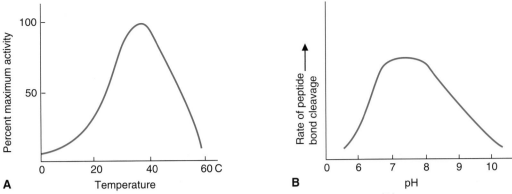

FIGURE 2-2 The effects of varying reaction conditions on enzyme-catalyzed reactions. **(A)** Effects of temperature are illustrated. **(B)** Example of how pH changes the reaction rate. The exact shape of the curve is determined by the ionization states (pK_a) of the amino acids in the active site. The descending portion of the curve in panel A reflects the loss of catalytic activity, as proteins are denatured at high temperatures.

III. THE MICHAELIS-MENTEN EQUATION

A. If, during a reaction, an **enzyme–substrate complex** is formed that **dissociates** (becoming free enzyme and substrate) or **reacts** (to release the product and regenerate the free enzyme), then:

$$\begin{array}{cc} k_1 & k_3 \\ E + S \rightleftharpoons ES \rightarrow E + P \\ k_2 \end{array}$$

where E is the enzyme; S the substrate; ES the enzyme–substrate complex; P the product; and k_1, k_2, and k_3 are rate constants.

B. From this concept, the **Michaelis-Menten equation** was derived:

$$v = \frac{V_{max}[S]}{K_m + S}$$

where $K_m = (k_2 + k_3)/k_1$ and **V_{max} is the maximum velocity,** or how fast the enzyme can go at full "speed." **V_{max} is reached when all of the enzyme is in the enzyme–substrate complex.**

CLINICAL CORRELATES The drug **isoniazid**, used in the treatment of tuberculosis, is acetylated by an **N-acetyltransferase.** A polymorphism of the enzyme exists, and individuals are classified into two groups: in the first group, the fast acetylators/metabolizers clear the drug from blood about 300% faster than in the second group of individuals, the slow acetylators/poor metabolizers, in whom the presence of drug is prolonged, causing hepatotoxicity and neuropathy. The **K_m** (affinity of isoniazid substrate) is **normal**, but the **V_{max}** of "fast" N-acetyltransferase, is **three times normal.**

C. K_m is the **substrate concentration** at which **v = $\frac{1}{2}$ V_{max}.**
   1. K_m approximately describes the **affinity** of the substrate for the enzyme. The lower the value of K_m, the higher the apparent affinity for substrate.
   2. When $[S] = K_m$, the Michaelis-Menten equation yields $v = \frac{1}{2} V_{max}$.

CLINICAL CORRELATES **Hypersensitivity to alcohol** exists when drinking small amounts of alcohol causes facial flushing and tachycardia (rapid heartbeat). Alcohol dehydrogenase generates acetaldehyde, which is converted to acetate by **aldehyde dehydrogenase.** The latter enzyme exists in two forms, a high-affinity (low K_m) form and a low-affinity (high K_m) form. Those **sensitive to alcohol lack the high-affinity form**, resulting in excess acetaldehyde and, hence, vasodilation.

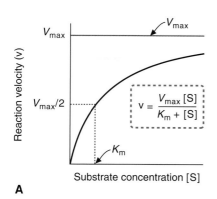
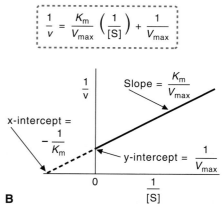

FIGURE 2-3 The velocity of an enzyme-catalyzed reaction that exhibits Michaelis-Menten kinetics. **(A)** Velocity (v) versus substrate concentration ([S]). **(B)** Lineweaver-Burk plot. Note the points on each plot from which V_{max} and K_m can be determined. V_{max}, maximum velocity; K_m, the substrate concentration at $1/2$ V_{max}.

D. When the velocity is plotted versus [S], a hyperbolic curve is produced (Figure 2-3A).
   1. **At low substrate** concentration (left part of the curve, below K_m), the reaction rate increases sharply with increasing substrate concentration because there is abundant free enzyme available (E) to bind added substrate.
   2. **At high substrate** concentration, the reaction rate reaches a plateau (V_{max}) as the enzyme active sites are saturated with substrate (ES complex), and there is no free enzyme to bind the added substrate.

IV. THE LINEWEAVER-BURK PLOT (FIGURE 2-3B)

A. Because of the difficulty of exactly determining V_{max} from a hyperbolic curve, the Michaelis-Menten equation was transformed by Lineweaver and Burk into an equation for a straight line.

B. This is a double reciprocal plot of 1/V versus 1/[S].

V. INHIBITORS

Inhibitors are molecules that interact with enzymes, **decreasing the rate of enzymatic reactions**. Inhibitors can be substrate analogs, toxins, drugs, or metals.

A. **Competitive inhibitors** compete with the substrate for binding at the active site of the enzyme and form an enzyme–inhibitor complex, EI, with the free enzyme only (Figure 2-4A). Structurally, these inhibitors are similar to substrate because they compete for the same site.
   1. Competitive inhibition is reversed by increasing substrate [S].
   2. **V_{max}** remains the same, but the **apparent K_m (K'_m) is increased.**
   3. For Lineweaver-Burk plots, **lines** for the inhibited reaction **intersect** on the **Y-axis** with those for the uninhibited reaction.

CLINICAL CORRELATES Drugs such as **physostigmine, a competitive reversible inhibitor of acetylcholinesterase**, are used to treat a variety of diseases such as glaucoma (increased intraocular pressure) and myasthenia gravis (an autoimmune disease acting at the neuromuscular junction).

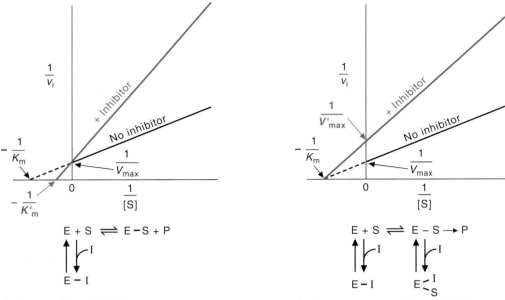

FIGURE 2-4 Effect of inhibitors on Lineweaver-Burk plots. **(A)** Competitive inhibition. **(B)** Pure noncompetitive inhibition (in which the inhibitor binds to E and ES with the same affinity). If the affinities differ, the lines will not intersect on the X-axis, and the apparent K_m (K'_m) will differ from K_m. V'_{max}, the apparent V_{max}.

B. **Noncompetitive inhibitors** bind to the enzyme or the enzyme–substrate complex at a site distinct from the active site, decreasing the activity of the enzyme (Figure 2-4B). Thus, **V_{max} is decreased.** Inhibition **cannot** be overcome by increasing substrate. Structurally, these inhibitors are **not** similar to substrate.

C. **Irreversible inhibitors** are enzyme **inactivators** that bind covalently to the enzyme and **inactivate** it. Their kinetics appear exactly like noncompetitive inhibition—an increase in inhibition with length of exposure and the inability to remove by dilution (because they are covalently bound).

D. A high yield summary of various forms of inhibition (graphic representations) is presented in Figure 2-5.

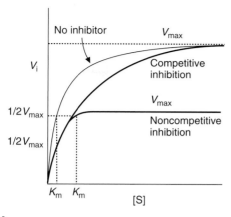

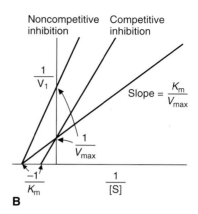

FIGURE 2-5 Summary of effects of competitive and noncompetitive inhibitors on **(A)** Michaelis-Menten plots, **(B)** Line-weaver-Burk plots, and **(C)** physical interpretation.

Inhibitor type	Binding site on enzyme	Kinetic effect
COMPETITIVE	Specifically at the catalytic site, where it competes with substrate for binding in a dynamic equilibrium-like process. Inhibition is reversible by substrate.	Vmax is unchanged. Km, as defined by [S] required for 1/2 maximal activity, is increased.
NONCOMPETITIVE	Binds E or ES complex other than at the catalytic site. Substrate binding unaltered, but ESI complex cannot form products, inhibition cannot be reversed by substrate.	Vmax is decreased proportionately to inhibitor concentration. Km appears unaltered.

C

VI. ALLOSTERIC ENZYMES

A. Virtually every metabolic pathway is subject to feedback control, and allosteric enzymes are used. This is a component of **feedback inhibition, whereby the concentration of the end product** of a pathway is **"monitored" to shut off the first (usually an allosteric) enzyme in a pathway** to prevent unwanted and wasted production of intermediate compounds.

B. Allosteric enzymes are oligomeric (multiple subunits) and, through conformational changes, **bind activators or inhibitors** at sites other than (but interacting with) the active substrate binding sites (Figure 2-6).

C. **Sigmoidal curves** are generated by plots of v versus [S]. Allosteric enzymes do **not** obey Michaelis-Menten kinetics, and a Lineweaver-Burk plot is not interpretable.
   1. An allosteric enzyme has two or more subunits, each with **substrate-binding sites** that exhibit **cooperativity.** Binding of a substrate molecule at one site facilitates binding of other substrate molecules at other sites.
      a. **Allosteric activators** cause the enzyme to bind substrate more readily.
      b. **Allosteric inhibitors** cause the enzyme to bind substrate less readily.
   2. Similar effects occur during O_2 binding to **hemoglobin** (see Figure 1-7).

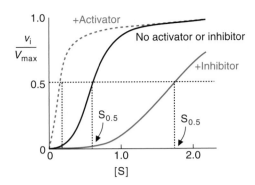

FIGURE 2-6 Effect of activators and inhibitors on an allosteric enzyme.

VII. REGULATION OF ENZYME ACTIVITY BY POST-TRANSLATIONAL (COVALENT) MODIFICATION

A. **Enzyme activity** may increase or decrease after the covalent addition of a chemical group.

B. **Phosphorylation** affects many enzymes.
   1. Pyruvate dehydrogenase and glycogen synthase are inhibited by phosphorylation, whereas glycogen phosphorylase is activated.
   2. Phosphatases that remove phosphate groups alter the activities of these enzymes.

C. **Proenzyme**
   1. An inactive, precursor protein (also called **zymogen**) with an additional peptide attached

---

CLINICAL CORRELATES   **C-peptide** links the insulin A and B chains in proinsulin. The peptide is removed by proteolytic processing via **carboxypeptidase E, yielding active insulin.** Mutations in carboxypeptidase E rendering it inactive or lowering its activity may cause **hyperproinsulinemia and diabetes** in the homozygous state.

VIII. REGULATION BY PROTEIN–PROTEIN INTERACTIONS

A. Proteins can bind to enzymes, altering their activity. For example, regulatory subunits inhibit the activity of protein kinase A. When these regulatory subunits bind cyclic adenosine monophosphate (cAMP) and are released from the enzyme, the catalytic subunits become active.

B. Enzymes can be arranged as **enzyme cascades**, exponentially amplifying the availability/activity of products in the pathway (e.g., hormone activation, blood clotting).

CLINICAL CORRELATES   **Hemostasis and thrombosis** are mediated by enzymes along cascading steps of the blood coagulation pathways. Inherited **deficiencies of clotting factors result in uncontrolled bleeding. Factor VIII deficiency** causes **hemophilia A**, an X-linked disease rife in some European royal families.

IX. ISOENZYMES

A. Isoenzymes (or isozymes) are enzymes composed of different amino acid sequences that catalyze the same reaction. Isozymes also differ in many of their physical properties.

B. Tissues contain characteristic isozymes or mixtures of isozymes. Enzymes such as creatine kinase (CK) differ from one tissue to another. Knowing which isozyme is elevated can be indicative of specific tissue damage.
  1. **Creatine kinase** contains two subunits. Each subunit may be either of the muscle (M) or the brain (B) type. Three isozymes exist (MM, MB, and BB). The MB fraction is most prevalent in heart muscle.

CLINICAL CORRELATES With regard to isozyme distribution, CK-MM makes up 99% of skeletal muscle and about 75% of myocardium. CK-MB makes up about 25% of myocardium, but it is **not found in any other tissues**, so **CK-MB is a significant marker for a myocardial infarction (heart attack, MI)**. CK-MB levels begin to rise **within a few hours of an MI** and remain elevated for up to 3 days. This is used in conjunction with another protein marker, **troponin**.

Review Test

Directions: Each of the numbered questions or incomplete statements in this section is followed by answers or by completions of the statement. Select the **one** lettered answer or completion that is **best** in each case.

1. Allopurinol is used in the treatment of gout because of its ability to inhibit xanthine oxidase. This inhibition makes it impossible for the enzyme to degrade xanthine and hypoxanthine, which reduces the synthesis of urate, the culprit of gout. Allopurinol works through which one of the following mechanisms?

(A) Suicide inhibition
(B) Noncompetitive inhibition
(C) Allosteric interaction with the enzyme that increases V_{max}
(D) Feedback inhibition
(E) Subunit cooperativity

2. A 10-year-old boy presents with vomiting, sweating, drooling, and a decreased heart rate. His friends state that he was in a corn field when it was sprayed by a crop duster. The chemical being sprayed was an organophosphate derivitive that covalently binds to acetylcholinesterase and inactivates the enzyme. What type of inhibition is being displayed?

(A) Competitive
(B) Noncompetitive
(C) Irreversible
(D) Feedback
(E) Allosteric

3. Nerve agents are toxic substances used in chemical warfare that add covalently to the enzyme acetylcholinesterase, thereby preventing the enzyme from hydrolyzing acetylcholine. This results in persistent acetylcholine in the synapse and continual muscle contractions. Which of the following substances can directly reactivate acetylcholinesterase after exposure to such a toxin?

(A) Pralidoxime chloride
(B) Atropine
(C) Scopolamine
(D) Ipratropium
(E) Diphenhydramine

4. You are called to the emergency room (ER) to admit a patient to the medicine service. The patient appears malnourished and suffers from alcoholism. These are chronic issues, but there is an acute change that resulted in him being brought to the ER by the life squad. The patient is exhibiting some ataxia and increased confusion, and has new-onset short-term memory loss. Besides eliciting the above on examination, you note that he also has a lateral rectus muscle palsy. Which one of the following statements is correct concerning this patient's condition?

(A) It is the result of irreversible inhibition.
(B) It cannot be effectively treated.
(C) It is the result of noncompetitive inhibition.
(D) It is the result of competitive inhibition.
(E) It is due to the lack of a fundamental coenzyme.

5. A competitive reversible inhibitor such as physostigmine is used to treat glaucoma and myasthenia gravis and to reverse anticholinergic syndrome. Based on this, which one of the following statements is true concerning the clinical implications of using physostigmine?

(A) Use of the drug will decrease the K_m of the targeted enzyme.
(B) An overdose of physostigmine can typically be reversed.
(C) Physostigmine will increase the V_{max} of the targeted enzyme.
(D) Physostigmine will decrease the V_{max} of the targeted enzyme.
(E) Physostigmine is unable to cross the blood-brain barrier.

6. A 64-year-old man complains of an acute onset of unilateral eye pain and reduction in visual acuity. On physical examination, you notice conjunctival injection (eye redness) and a mid-dilated and nonreactive pupil. Funduscopic examination reveals cupping of the optic disc. Recognizing the signs and symptoms as glaucoma, you administer the medication acetazolamide to decrease the production of aqueous fluid and lower the intraocular pressure. Acetazolamide is a noncompetitive inhibitor of carbonic anhydrase and, therefore, will lead to which of the following concerning the kinetic constants of carbonic anhydrase?

(A) An increase in the apparent K_m

(B) A decrease in the apparent K_m

(C) An increase in V_{max}

(D) A decrease in V_{max}

(E) A decrease in both the apparent K_m and V_{max}

7. Which one of the following ailments, seen by an emergency room physician, is most likely caused by enzyme denaturation?

(A) A 34-year-old man diagnosed with a gastrinoma complaining of diarrhea for 2 weeks

(B) A 58-year-old man with chest pain and shortness of breath with increased activity

(C) An 18-year-old boy presenting with a sore throat and fever of 101° F; he has small minimally tender anterior cervical lymph nodes and a red pharynx

(D) An 18-month-old boy with a 4-day history of symptoms of an upper respiratory infection presenting with fever, irritability, and pulling at his left ear for the past 24 hours

(E) A 48-year-old woman complaining of knee pain after twisting her leg playing tennis

8. A 3-year-old boy in good health began having generalized seizures consisting of a sudden turning of the head to the left, tonic posturing of the left arm, and loss of awareness for 1 to 2 minutes. The patient was successfully treated with the anticonvulsant phenytoin (dilantin). Dilantin is a substrate that binds to and is metabolized by an enzyme in the liver. Which one of the following statements best describes the relationship between an enzyme, substrate, and product?

(A) Enzyme–product complexes enhance substrate binding.

(B) All the active sites of the enzyme are saturated with substrate at high substrate concentrations.

(C) At high substrate concentrations, substrate–substrate interactions interfere with enzyme activity.

(D) At low substrate concentrations, none of the enzyme is found in the ES complex.

(E) Significant product formation results in activation of the reaction.

Answers and Explanations

1. **The answer is A.** Allopurinol is a substrate for xanthine oxidase, which converts allopurinol to oxypurinol, and which binds tightly to the enzyme and is not released from the enzyme. This blocks substrate binding and further activity of the enzyme. This is an example of irreversible suicide inhibition. Such inhibition leads to a decrease of V_{max}. Noncompetitive inhibition occurs when inhibitors bind to a site other than the active site, which is not the case with allopurinol. Additionally, noncompetitive inhibitors are not substrates for the enzyme, as are suicide inhibitors. There is no end-product regulation of xanthine oxidase by allopurinol, thereby ruling out feedback inhibition. Cooperativity exists when there are two or more sites for substrate binding (and in positive cooperativity it is easier for substrate to bind as the concentration of substrate is increased), but this is not observed with xanthine oxidase.

2. **The answer is C.** This is an example of irreversible inhibition because a covalent bond has been formed between the inhibitor and the required serine at the active site of the enzyme. This enzyme can only be reactivated if that covalent bond is hydrolyzed, which is unlikely. Both competitive and noncompetitive binding are reversible because the inhibitor is not covalently linked to the enzyme. Allosteric inhibitors also bind to enzymes via noncovalent forces, and feedback inhibition refers to the normal regulation of a pathway by an end product of the pathway.

3. **The answer is A.** Pralidoxime chloride (2-PAM) is the nerve agent antidote that reactivates the poisoned acetylcholinesterase. Nerve agents (e.g., Sarin, VE) inhibit acetylcholinesterase by phosphorylation of the active site serine hydroxyl group of the enzyme. 2-PAM reactivates the cholinesterase by removing the phosphoryl group that is bound to the serine hydroxyl side chain and creates inactivated organophosphate and pralidoxime that undergo rapid metabolism and removal from the synapse. Atropine is a competitive antagonist for the muscarinic acetylcholine receptor and decreases the effects of acetylcholine. Although it is used in nerve agent poisoning, it does not directly reactivate the poisoned acetylcholinesterase. Scopolamine is an anticholinergic competitive anatagonist at muscarinic (M1) acetylcholine receptors used to treat nausea and eye conditions that require mydriasis (e.g., iritis, uveitis). Scopolamine does not reactivate inhibited acetylcholinesterase. Ipratropium is a nonselective anticholinergic that blocks muscarinic receptors in the lung and decreases bronchoconstriction and mucus secretion, but has no direct effect on acetylcholinesterase. Diphenhydramine is an antihistamine, which has no effects on acetylcholinesterase.

4. **The answer is E.** This patient has the classic symptoms of Wernicke encephalopathy, which results from an inadequate intake or absorption of thiamine. The patient is thus thiamine deficient. Within the United States, the condition is most often observed in chronic alcoholics with poor diets. Thiamine pyrophosphate is a required coenzyme for the oxidative decarboxylation of pyruvate and α-ketoglutarate during energy metabolism. The absence of thiamine leads to reduced energy production by all organs and tissues. Treatment includes intravenous thiamine, magnesium, and glucose and is reversible in the acute setting. The reduction in neuronal energy metabolism is not based on a type of enzyme inhibition (such as competitive, noncompetitive, or irreversible), but on the lack of a required cofactor for two enzymes.

5. **The answer is B.** Physostigmine is both a naturally occurring substance (Calabar bean) and a chemically synthesized substance that is a competitive reversible inhibitor of acetylcholinesterase. The drug easily crosses the blood-brain barrier. By definition, a competitive reversible inhibitor acts at the catalytic site with the substrate and competes with substrate binding to the enzyme. Thus, the effects of the inhibitor can be overcome by addition of the substrate, leading to an effective reversal of drug overdose. This is a reversible inhibition, so the V_{max} is unchanged because if sufficient substrate is added, the effects of the inhibitor can be overcome. With a competitive inhibitor, the K_m is increased because more substrate is needed to reach $1/2\,V_{max}$.

6. **The answer is D.** A noncompetitive inhibitor binds to the enzyme at a site different than where the substrate binds. Therefore, the number of enzymes capable of catalyzing the reaction is decreased, resulting in a decrease in V_{max}. Because the inhibitor binds at a site distinct from that of the substrate, increasing the substrate concentration cannot overcome the effect of the inhibitor. Consequently, K_m remains unchanged, and the inhibitor does not interfere with substrate binding.

7. **The answer is A.** Factors that cause protein unfolding include heat, chemical denaturants, and changes in pH. A gastrinoma is a neuroendocrine tumor that secretes excessive gastrin, resulting in increased gastric acid secretion. This, in turn, results in a paradoxical acidic environment in the duodenum and denaturation of the pancreatic digestive enzymes. The diarrhea is a result of an osmotic pull owing to the undigested nutrients' inability to be absorbed in the gut. Although a fever (choice C) included an increase in temperature, most proteins are denatured above 50° C, a temperature well above the normal body temperature of 37° C. The other choices (potential heart attack, choice B; an ear infection, choice D; and a sore knee, choice E) are not initially a result of enzyme denaturation.

8. **The answer is B.** The rate of an enzyme-catalyzed reaction will generally increase exponentially with respect to substrate concentration until the substrate concentration exhausts the catalytic sites of the enzyme population. Once this occurs, the rate of reaction remains the same regardless of an increase of substrate because all enzymes are saturated (V_{max} has been achieved). Substrate cannot bind to enzyme–product complexes because the substrate binding sites are occupied by product. Substrate–substrate interactions are the same regardless of concentration of substrate, and such interactions do not affect enzyme activity. An ES complex can form at low substrate concentration as well as at high substrate concentration. Product formation does not stimulate enzyme activity and can slow down the reaction rate.

3 Biochemistry of Digestion

I. DIGESTION OF CARBOHYDRATES

A. **Dietary carbohydrates** (mainly starch, sucrose, and lactose) constitute about 50% of the calories in the average diet in the United States.
1. **Starch,** the storage form of carbohydrates, is similar in structure to glycogen (Figure 3-1).
   a. Starch contains amylose (long, unbranched chains with glucose units linked α-1,4)
   b. Starch also contains amylopectin (α-1,4–linked chains with α-1,6–linked branches). Amylopectin has fewer branches than glycogen.
2. **Sucrose** (a component of table sugar and fruit) contains glucose and fructose residues linked via their anomeric carbons (see Figure I-8).
3. **Lactose** (milk sugar) contains galactose-linked β-1,4 to glucose (see Figure I-8).

B. **Digestion of dietary carbohydrates in the mouth** (Figure 3-2)
1. In the mouth, **salivary α-amylase** cleaves starch by breaking α-1,4 linkages between glucose residues within the chains (Figure 3-1).
2. Dextrins (linear and branched oligosaccharides) are the major products that enter the stomach.

C. **Digestion of carbohydrates in the intestine** (Figure 3-2)
1. The stomach contents pass into the intestine, where **bicarbonate** (HCO_3^-) secreted by the pancreas neutralizes the stomach acid, raising the pH into the optimal range for the action of the intestinal enzymes.
2. Digestion by **pancreatic enzymes** (Figure 3-2)
   a. The pancreas secretes an **α-amylase** that acts in the lumen of the small intestine and, like salivary amylase, cleaves α-1,4 linkages between glucose residues.
   b. The products of pancreatic α-amylase are the disaccharides maltose and isomaltase, trisaccharides, and small oligosaccharides containing α-1,4 and α-1,6 linkages.

CLINICAL CORRELATES Serum **amylase** is elevated in cases of **pancreatitis,** and the test to measure amylase is often ordered in patients to evaluate such a condition. However, serum **lipase** is another marker of **pancreatitis** that demonstrates higher sensitivity and specificity compared with **amylase.**

3. Digestion by **enzymes of intestinal cells**
   a. **Complexes of enzymes,** produced by intestinal epithelial cells and located in their **brush borders,** continue the digestion of carbohydrates (Figure 3-2).
   b. **Glucoamylase** (an α-glucosidase) and other **maltases** cleave glucose residues from the nonreducing ends of oligosaccharides and also cleave the α-1,4 bond of maltose, releasing the two glucose residues.
   c. **Isomaltase** cleaves α-1,6 linkages, releasing glucose residues from branched oligosaccharides.

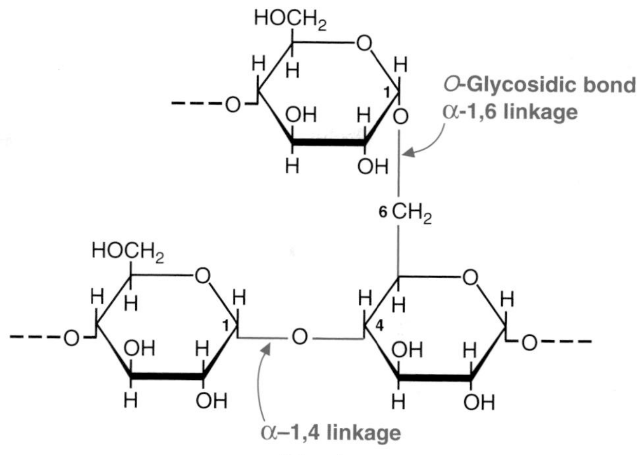

FIGURE 3-1 The α-1,4 and α-1,6 linkages between glucose residues in starch and glycogen.

d. **Sucrase** converts sucrose to glucose and fructose.
e. **Lactase** (a β-galactosidase) converts lactose to glucose and galactose.

CLINICAL CORRELATES **Acarbose, an α-glucosidase inhibitor,** works in the intestine, slowing down digestion of carbohydrates and lengthening the time it takes for carbohydrates to be converted to glucose, which facilitates **better postdigestive blood glucose control.**

CLINICAL CORRELATES **Lactase deficiency** occurs in more than 80% of Native, African, and Asian Americans. Lactose is not digested at a normal rate and accumulates in the gut, where it is metabolized by bacteria. **Bloating, abdominal cramps,** and **watery diarrhea** result.

D. **Carbohydrates that cannot be digested**
1. Indigestible polysaccharides are part of the **dietary fiber** that passes through the intestine into the feces.
2. For example, because enzymes produced by human cells **cannot cleave the β-1,4 bonds of cellulose,** this polysaccharide is indigestible.

E. **Absorption of glucose, fructose, and galactose**
1. **Glucose, fructose, and galactose**—the final products generated by digestion of dietary carbohydrates—can be absorbed by intestinal cells by **two forms of transport:** facilitated transport and active transport.
2. Using **facilitated transport,** monosaccharides bind to transport proteins and are transported into cells moving down a concentration gradient.
3. Glucose also moves into cells by **secondary active transport,** in which sodium ions are carried along with glucose. An Na^+-K^+ ATPase pumps Na^+ into the blood, and Na^+ moves down a concentration gradient from the blood into the cell, bringing glucose with it.

II. DIGESTION OF DIETARY TRIACYLGLYCEROL

A. **Dietary triacylglycerols** are digested in the **small intestine** by a process that requires bile salts and secretions from the pancreas (Figure 3-3). Normally, 95% of lipids are absorbed. Major digestion of all lipids occurs in the lumen of the duodenum and jejunum.

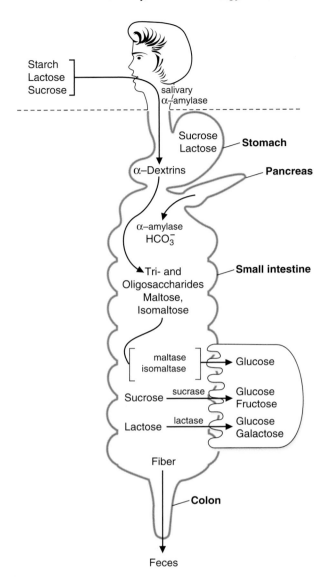

FIGURE 3-2 Digestion of carbohydrates. Starch is digested by salivary and pancreatic α-amylases and intestinal cell maltase and isomaltase. Sucrose and lactose are digested by intestinal enzymes.

CLINICAL CORRELATES   **Steatorrhea** occurs when excess lipids are excreted into the feces because of lipid malabsorption from impaired lipolysis, micelle or chylomicron formation, or chylomicron transport.

---

1. **Bile salts** are synthesized in the liver from cholesterol and are secreted into the bile. Bile is stored in the **gallbladder** and is released in response to hormones. Bile then passes into the intestine, where it **emulsifies the dietary lipids.**

2. The **pancreas** secretes digestive enzymes and bicarbonate, which neutralizes stomach acid, raising the pH into the optimal range for the digestive enzymes.

3. **Pancreatic lipase,** with the aid of colipase, digests the triacylglycerols to 2-monoacylglycerols and free fatty acids, which are packaged into micelles. The micelles, which are tiny microdroplets emulsified by bile salts, also contain other dietary lipids such as cholesterol and the fat-soluble vitamins.

4. The **micelles** travel to the microvilli of the intestinal epithelial cells, which absorb the fatty acids, 2-monoacylglycerols, and other dietary lipids.

5. The **bile salts are resorbed in the terminal ileum,** recycled by the liver, and secreted into the gut during subsequent digestive cycles.

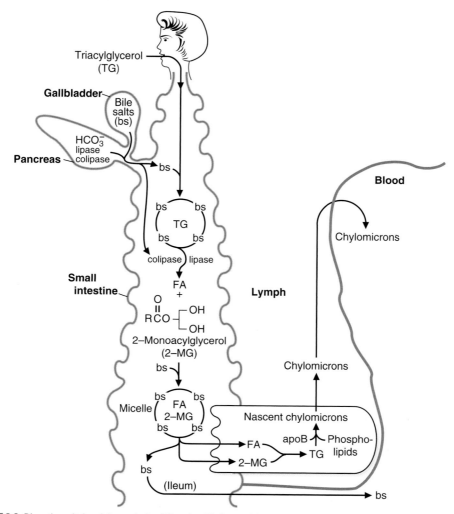

FIGURE 3-3 Digestion of triacylglycerols. bs, Bile salts; FA, fatty acid; 2-MG, 2-monoacylglycerol; TG, triacylglycerols.

CLINICAL CORRELATES The antiobesity drug, **orlistat,** inhibits pancreatic and gastric lipase, resulting in about 30% blockage of dietary fat from digestion and absorption, leading to **reduction in body weight in some patients.**

CLINICAL CORRELATES **Olestra** is an artificial fat composed of a sucrose polyester and fatty acids. It is not degraded by gastric or pancreatic lipases and **passes through the body undigested and unabsorbed.** Excess use in foods may interfere with absorption of fat-soluble vitamins.

B. Synthesis of chylomicrons

1. In intestinal epithelial cells, the **fatty acids** from micelles are **activated** by fatty acyl coenzyme A (CoA) synthetase to form fatty acyl CoA.

2. A **fatty acyl CoA** reacts with a 2-monoacylglycerol to form a **diacylglycerol.** Then another fatty acyl CoA reacts with the diacylglycerol to form a **triacylglycerol.**

3. The triacylglycerols pass into the lymph packaged in **nascent (newborn) chylomicrons,** which eventually enter the blood.

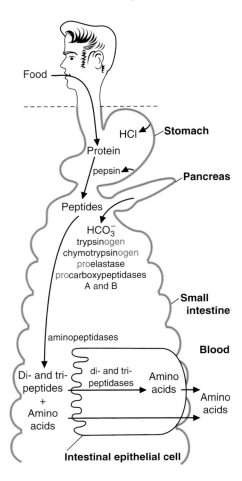

FIGURE 3-4 Digestion of proteins. HCl, hydrochloric acid; HCO_3^-, bicarbonate.

III. PROTEIN DIGESTION AND AMINO ACID ABSORPTION

A. **Digestion of proteins** (Figure 3-4)
1. The 70 to 100 g of **protein consumed** each day and an equal or larger amount of protein that enters the digestive tract as **digestive enzymes** or in **sloughed-off cells** from the intestinal epithelium is converted to amino acids by **digestive enzymes.**

CLINICAL CORRELATES   **Nontropical sprue** (adult **celiac disease**) results from a **reaction to gluten,** a protein found in grains. Intestinal epithelial cells are damaged, and **malabsorption** results. Common symptoms are steatorrhea, diarrhea, and weight loss.

2. In the **stomach,** pepsin is the major proteolytic enzyme. It cleaves proteins to smaller polypeptides (Figure 3-5).
   a. **Pepsin** is produced and secreted by the chief cells of the stomach as the inactive zymogen **pepsinogen.**
   b. **Hydrochloric acid (HCl)** produced by the parietal cells of the stomach causes a conformational change in pepsinogen that enables it to cleave itself (autocatalysis), forming **active pepsin.**
   c. **Pepsin** has a **broad specificity** but tends to cleave peptide bonds in which the carboxyl group is contributed by the acidic amino acids, aromatic amino acids, or leucine.

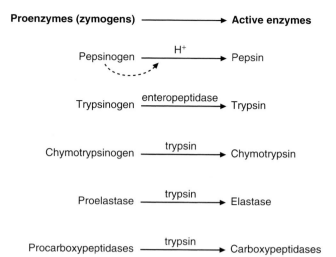

FIGURE 3-5 Activation of gastric and pancreatic zymogens. Pepsin can catalyze its own cleavage. Trypsin is required for the activation of pancreatic zymogens.

CLINICAL CORRELATES   Patients with **achlorhydria,** which is the lack of ability to produce HCl (usually due to autoimmune destruction of gastric parietal cells), have **deficiencies in protein digestion and absorption.**

---

3. In the **intestine,** the partially digested material from the stomach encounters **pancreatic secretions,** which include bicarbonate and a group of proteolytic enzymes.
   a. **Bicarbonate** neutralizes the stomach acid, raising the pH of the contents of the intestinal lumen into the optimal range for the digestive enzymes to act.
   b. **Endopeptidases** from the pancreas cleave peptide bonds within protein chains (Figure 3-5).
      (1) Trypsin cleaves peptide bonds in which the carboxyl group is contributed by **arginine** or **lysine.**
      (i) Trypsin is secreted as the inactive zymogen trypsinogen. Trypsinogen is cleaved to form trypsin by the enzyme **enteropeptidase (enterokinase)**, which is produced by intestinal cells. Trypsinogen may also undergo autocatalysis by trypsin.

CLINICAL CORRELATES   **Bicarbonate is released** from the pancreas in response to the hormone **secretin,** which is synthesized by the cells lining the duodenum. Failure to fully neutralize the acidic gastric contents results in **peptic ulcers** in the duodenum.

CLINICAL CORRELATES   Hereditary **deficiency of enterokinase** has been reported. Deficiency of this important zymogen activator results in diarrhea, failure to thrive, and hypoproteinemia and is managed during infancy with pancreatic enzyme supplementation. When patients become adults, they no longer need such supplementation, owing to the decreased anabolic demands and the autocatalysis of digestive enzymes.

---

   (2) Chymotrypsin usually cleaves peptide bonds at the carboxyl group of **aromatic amino acids** or **leucine. Chymotrypsinogen,** the inactive zymogen, is cleaved to form active chymotrypsin by trypsin (Figure 3-5).
   (3) Elastase cleaves at the carboxyl end of amino acid residues with small, uncharged side chains such as alanine, glycine, or serine. **Proelastase,** the inactive zymogen, is cleaved to active elastase by trypsin (Figure 3-5).

   c. **Exopeptidases** in the pancreas (carboxypeptidases A and B) cleave one amino acid pro-
      gressively from the C-terminal end of the peptide.
      (1) The carboxypeptidases are produced as inactive **procarboxypeptidases,** which are
         cleaved to their active form by trypsin.
      (2) **Carboxypeptidase A** cleaves **aromatic** amino acids from the C terminus.
      (3) **Carboxypeptidase B** cleaves the **basic** amino acids, lysine and arginine, from the C
         terminus.
   d. **Proteases** produced by **intestinal epithelial cells** complete the conversion of dietary
      proteins to peptides and finally to amino acids.
      (1) **Aminopeptidases** are exopeptidases produced by intestinal cells, cleaving one amino
         acid at a time from the N terminus of peptides.
      (2) **Dipeptidases** and **tripeptidases** associated with the intestinal cells produce amino acids
         from dipeptides and tripeptides.

B. **Transport of amino acids from the intestinal lumen into the blood**
   1. Amino acids are absorbed by intestinal epithelial cells and released into the blood by two types
      of transport systems.
   2. At least seven distinct carrier proteins transport different groups of amino acids.
   3. **Sodium-amino acid carrier system**
      a. The major transport system involves cellular uptake by the cell of a **sodium ion** and an
         amino acid by the same carrier protein on the luminal surface.
      b. The **sodium ion** is pumped out of the cell into the blood by the Na^+-K^+ ATPase, whereas
         the **amino acid** travels down its concentration gradient into the blood.
      c. Thus, amino acid transport from the intestinal lumen to the blood is driven by hydroly-
         sis of adenosine triphosphate (ATP) (**secondary active transport**).

CLINICAL CORRELATES   In **cystinuria,** transport of cysteine and basic amino acids is defective in both
the intestine and kidney. Cysteine cannot be resorbed from the glomerular
filtrate and concentrates in the urine. Within the urine, the cysteine is oxidized to cystine, which can
crystallize, forming kidney stones.

CLINICAL CORRELATES   In **Hartnup disease,** transport of neutral amino acids is defective, resulting in
potential **deficiencies of essential amino acids** because they are not absorbed
from the diet.

---

   4. **γ-Glutamyl cycle**
      a. An amino acid in the lumen reacts with **glutathione** (γ-glutamyl-cysteinyl-glycine) in the
         cell membrane, forming a γ-glutamyl amino acid and the dipeptide cysteinyl-glycine.
      b. The amino acid is carried across the cell membrane attached to γ-**glutamate** and
         released into the cytoplasm. The γ-glutamyl moiety is used in the resynthesis of
         glutathione.

CLINICAL CORRELATES   Translocation of amino acids in the γ-glutamyl cycle is mediated **by γ-glutamyl
transferase (GGT). Elevated serum levels** of GGT often occur in intrahepatic and
posthepatic **biliary obstructions,** indicating cholestasis, in some primary neoplasms, and in
pancreatic cancer and alcohol-induced liver disease.

Review Test

Directions: Each of the numbered questions or incomplete statements in this section is followed by answers or by completions of the statement. Select the **one** lettered answer or completion that is **best** in each case.

1. Which condition can lead to life-threatening autodigestion of lipids and proteins?

(A) Peptic ulcer disease
(B) Pancreatitis
(C) Celiac sprue
(D) Crohn disease
(E) Ulcerative colitis

2. A 38-year-old man gets bloated and has episodes of diarrhea after eating his favorite ice cream. It also occurs when he consumes yogurt, cheese, and other milk-containing products. The patient lacks the ability to cleave which one of the following glycosidic bonds?

(A) Glucose-α ($1\rightarrow4$) glucose
(B) Glucose-α ($1\rightarrow2$) fructose
(C) Galactose-β ($1\rightarrow4$) glucose
(D) Glucose-α ($1\rightarrow6$) glucose
(E) Glucose-β ($1\rightarrow4$) glucose

3. A child is brought to your clinic who appears malnourished. Obtaining a history is difficult from the non–English-speaking parents. You obtain basic blood work and the following radiograph. Based on your observations and the radiograph, what is the most likely diagnosis?

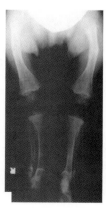

(From Becker KL, Bilezikian JP, Brenner WJ, et al. *Principles and Practice of Endocrinology and Metabolism*, 3rd Ed. Philadelphia: Lippincott Williams & Wilkins, 2001.)

(A) Rickets
(B) Scurvy
(C) Pellegra
(D) Beriberi
(E) Lead poisoning

4. Which statement is true concerning the intestinal brush border membrane?

(A) Amylase is only found in the brush border.
(B) Disaccharides cross the brush border.
(C) Insulin is required for the uptake of glucose.
(D) Fructose requires a sodium-independent monosaccharide transporter.
(E) Minimal carbohydrate digestion occurs here because most occurs in the mouth and stomach.

5. A 31-year-old Asian woman presents with a chief complaint of "difficulty eating dairy products." The patient clarifies her symptoms and states that she develops bloating, abdominal pain, diarrhea, and excessive flatulence. Which one of the following statements is true about this patient's condition?

(A) She lacks $\beta_{1\rightarrow4}$ endoglucosidase activity.
(B) She cannot obtain galactose and glucose from a disaccharide.
(C) She has an inability to emulsify dietary lipids.
(D) She is exhibiting an autosomal dominant condition.
(E) Her associated diarrhea is of an infectious etiology.

6. A 55-year-old man has been attempting to lose weight using a low-carbohydrate diet. After 2 months of little success, he confides to his son that he adds sugar to his coffee in the morning and after dinner. He tells him that only some of the sugar will be absorbed and should not be the cause of his limited success. The son, a medical student, states that glucose is almost completely absorbed from the gut. What type of

transport mechanism does glucose utilize for gastrointestinal absorption?

(A) Passive
(B) Facilitated
(C) Active
(D) Passive and facilitated
(E) Active and facilitated

7. A 63-year-old man presents to the emergency room with lower gastrointestinal bleeding, bloating, and cramping. He states that this has happened before and resolves in a day or two. On examination, he has a low-grade fever, left lower quadrant tenderness to palpation, and guaiac-positive stools. Blood work reveals leukocytosis and a normal hematocrit. A computed tomography scan is ordered with oral and intravenous contrast and reveals numerous out-pouchings in his distal colon. Which of the following is true about this condition?

(A) Polysaccharides rich in $\beta_{1,4}$ bonds of cellulose are a mainstay of treatment.
(B) This patient has a digestive enzyme deficiency.
(C) A biopsy of the lesions would reveal a malignant process.
(D) This patient has gastroenteritis from a heat-stable protein.
(E) These signs and symptoms are consistent with *Clostridium difficile* colitis

8. As an experiment, a high school professor convinces each of his students to put a soda cracker in their mouth and not swallow it. After several minutes, some of the students report a sweet taste. Which of the following enzymes is responsible for this phenomenon?

(A) Amylase
(B) Sucrase
(C) Lactase
(D) Maltase
(E) Isomaltase

9. A morbidly obese woman decides to see her physician to begin a weight loss program. He tells her that diet and exercise play an essential role in her program. She is concerned that she does not have the time to devote to exercise and wants to know if there is any pharmacologic treatment for her. The physician decides to start her on orlistat, which will directly inhibit which one of the following steps in fat digestion?

(A) Bile salt formation
(B) Micelle formation

(C) Pancreatic and gastric lipase
(D) Absorption of free fatty acids
(E) Chylomicron formation

10. An 18-year-old man is involved in a severe motor vehicle crash. He is rushed to surgery for an emergent laparotomy. Unfortunately, he undergoes a complete pancreatectomy, which will have all of the following consequences except for which one?

(A) Failure to convert pepsinogen into pepsin
(B) Diabetes
(C) Increased likelihood of duodenal ulcer formation
(D) Decreased synthesis of trypsinogen and chymotrypsinogen
(E) Steatorrhea

11. A 65-year-old man expresses his concern about developing colon cancer to his physician. He states that his father and grandmother died of colon cancer. After a normal physical examination, negative Hemoccult tests, and unremarkable colonoscopy, the physician recommends a diet low in fat and high in fiber. The doctor explains that studies have shown a decreased risk for colon cancer with insoluble fiber consumption. Which of the following glycosidic bonds prevents humans from completely digesting fiber?

(A) Glucose α (1→4) glucose
(B) Glucose α (1→6) glucose
(C) Glucose β (1→4) glucose
(D) Glucose α (1→ β 2) fructose
(E) Galactose β (1→4) glucose

12. A newborn is seen by a neonatologist for failure to thrive. The nurses in the pediatric intensive care unit note that the child has diarrhea every time he feeds. In addition, laboratory studies suggest severe hypoproteinemia. The neonatologist sends for a panel of tests, which indicate a congenital deficiency of enterokinase. This enzyme normally activates which zymogen?

(A) Procolipase
(B) Procarboxypeptidase
(C) Trypsinogen
(D) Proelastase
(E) Chymotrypsinogen

13. A 65-year-old woman is evaluated by a gastroenterologist for progressive signs and symptoms of malnutrition. Throughout her workup, she is found to have significantly decreased stomach acid. She is also found to have antibodies to gastric parietal cells, which are normally responsible for the production of acid. Why is hydrochloric acid secretion within the stomach important in digestion?

(A) It stimulates the cleavage of trypsinogen to trypsin.

(B) It is required for the activity of α-amylase.

(C) It drives secondary active transport of amino acids.

(D) It converts pepsinogen to pepsin.

(E) It is required for lipid digestion.

Answers and Explanations

1. **The answer is B.** Pancreatitis is an inflammatory process commonly caused by gallstones or alcoholism that results in pancreatic autodigestion by lipase. In advanced cases, life-threatening hypocalcemia can occur from fat saponification by lipase. Peptic ulcer disease may rarely lead to perforation of a viscous (gastric ulcer), but is not commonly seen in industrialized countries. Peptic ulcer disease affects the stomach. Celiac sprue is an autoimmune disorder in response to gluten, which leads to destruction of the villi on the intestinal epithelial cells. Crohn disease is another autoimmune disorder that affects various parts of the gastrointestinal system, but does not affect the pancreas. Ulcerative colitis results from ulcers in the colon, without pancreatic involvement.

2. **The answer is C.** The vignette is a classic presentation of lactase deficiency. Lactase is an intestinal enzyme that cleaves the β $(1\rightarrow4)$ linkage of lactose, releasing galactose and glucose. Sucrase cleaves the glucose-α $(1\rightarrow2)$ fructose bond. Maltase cleaves glucose-α $(1\rightarrow4)$ glucose bonds, whereas isomaltase cleaves glucose-α $(1\rightarrow6)$ glucose bonds. Humans lack the enzymes necessary to cleave glucose β $(1\rightarrow4)$ glucose bonds, a predominant glycosidic bond found in fiber.

3. **The answer is A.** This child has clear bowing of the legs secondary to vitamin D deficiency and has rickets. A blood calcium level may reveal hypocalcemia, and treatment includes vitamin D and calcium supplementation and increased exposure to the sun. Scurvy, which is caused by inadequate vitamin C intake, presents with painful thighs, with the infant assuming a frog-leg posture for comfort, purple or hemorrhagic oral mucosa, and subperiosteal hemorrhage of the femur and tibia. Pellegra, caused by severe vitamin B_3 (niacin) deficiency, presents with diarrhea, dermatitis, and dementia. Beriberi, caused by severe vitamin B_1 (thiamin) deficiency, presents in adults and infants. Infantile beriberi presents in three forms: (1) cardiologic form with high-output heart failure, (2) aphonic form with loss of voice due to paralysis of the vocal cords, and (3) pseudomeningitic form with clinical signs of meningitis but absence of infection in the cerebrospinal fluid. Lead poisoning is seen in children, especially if they live in older homes with lead-painted walls. Diagnosis of lead poisoning is done by whole blood lead levels, but radiographs of long bones may show growth arrest lines.

4. **The answer is D.** The brush border of the jejunum is one of the main sites of carbohydrate digestion through the action of maltase, pancreatic amylase, lactase, and other disaccharidases and oligosaccharidases. Initial digestion of carbohydrate occurs in the mouth (using salivary amylase), but once the food enters the stomach, the reduction in pH inactivates salivary amylase. Once digested into monosaccharides in the intestine, absorption occurs through specific transporters that are sodium dependent (SGLT-1 for the transport of glucose) and independent (GLUT-5 for the transport of fructose). GLUT-4, the insulin-responsive transporter, is not expressed in the intestinal epithelial cells. Once galactose, glucose, and fructose are in the intestinal mucosal cells, GLUT-2 transports these monosaccharides into the portal circulation. Disaccharides are not transported across the intestinal epithelial cell membrane.

5. **The answer is B.** This patient has lactose intolerance, which is a reduced ability to metabolize lactose (a disaccharide) into galactose and glucose. This problem usually manifests after adulthood. The loss of lactase activity is not due to an autosomal dominant disorder; in fact, lactase persistence (high levels of lactase throughout life) is inherited in an autosomal dominant fashion. Absence of $\beta_{1\rightarrow4}$ endoglucosidases is innate to all humans, making digestion of dietary fiber (i.e., cellulose) not possible. An inability to emulsify dietary lipids will lead to steatorrhea, which may have some overlap with this patient's symptoms, but is not the unifying diagnosis given her

chief complaint. Diarrhea in patients with lactose intolerance is an osmotic diarrhea from the remnant colonic lactose that is not entirely fermented by normal gut flora.

6. **The answer is E.** Glucose absorption in the small intestine occurs via two types of transport. The first is facilitated transport (a form of passive transport in which molecules move down a concentration gradient with the assistance of transport proteins). The second is active transport (requires energy, usually in the form of ATP, to allow the substrate to move against a concentration gradient), in which sodium ions are carried along with glucose into cells. An Na^+-K^+ ATPase pumps Na^+ into the blood, which drives the active transport of glucose into the intestinal epithelial cell. Glucose moves down a concentration gradient to enter the blood from the intestinal epithelial cell.

7. **The answer is A.** This patient has diverticulosis, which is out-pouchings on the colonic wall secondary to weakness of the muscle layers that are most often found in the sigmoid colon. Sometimes these out-pouchings can harbor stool and become infected, resulting in diverticulitis. Colonoscopy confirms the diagnosis, although computed tomographic scanning is the most available modality in the acute setting. Although the out-pouchings are not malignant, colonoscopy may identify malignant lesions. These symptoms are not consistent with gastroenteritis, and in the absence of diarrhea, recent antibiotic use, or hospitalization, *Clostridium difficile* infection is quite unlikely. Consuming fiber (such as foods containing cellulose) will increase stool bulk and moisture, which will reduce travel time through the colon, reducing the risk for diverticulitis.

8. **The answer is A.** Carbohydrate digestion is initiated in the mouth through the action of salivary α-amylase. This enzyme will digest starch, releasing glucose residues. The salivary amylase is rendered inactive in the stomach because of the acidic environment, being replaced by pancreatic α-amylase, which is secreted into the duodenum. The enzyme specifically cleaves the α-1,4 bonds between the glucosyl residues of starch, resulting in glucose polysaccharides of varying numbers of residues. The other glycosidases (sucrase, lactase, maltase, and isomaltase) are associated with enzyme complexes on the brush border of enterocytes of the intestine and would not lead to glucose production in the mouth.

9. **The answer is C.** Orlistat inhibits pancreatic and gastric lipase, thereby preventing the release of free fatty acids from triacylglycerol in the intestinal lumen. The absorption of fatty acids by the intestinal epithelial cells is thus blocked because free fatty acids are not being produced from the triacylglycerol of the diet. The normal sequence of triacylglycerol digestion is that triacylglycerols are emulsified by bile salts from the gallbladder. These micelles are then acted on by lipases, leading to the liberation of fatty acids. The fatty acids are absorbed by enterocytes, which then reassemble triacylglcerol for packaging into chylomicrons.

10. **The answer is A.** Patients who undergo a pancreatectomy suffer from many debilitating conditions, including diabetes due to the inability to secrete or produce insulin, increased likelihood of duodenal ulcers from the absence of bicarbonate secretion, and decreased ability to absorb fats (due to the lack of pancreatic lipase), resulting in steatorrhea. Trypsinogen and chymotrypsinogen are secreted by the pancreas and will not be present in this patient, resulting in poor protein digestion. Pepsinogen is activated to pepsin in the stomach by the release of HCl by the parietal cells, which is not affected by the removal of the pancreas.

11. **The answer is C.** The glucose β $(1\rightarrow4)$ glucose glycosidic bond, found in cellulose, a major component of fiber, cannot be digested by human enzymes. Humans can, however, digest glucose α $(1\rightarrow4)$ glucose (starch, glycogen, maltose) bonds, galactose β $(1\rightarrow4)$ glucose (lactose) bonds, glucose (α $1\rightarrow2$) fructose (sucrose) bonds, and glucose α $(1\rightarrow6)$ glucose (glycogen, isomaltose) bonds.

12. **The answer is C.** Enterokinase (also called *enteropeptidase*) cleaves the zymogen trypsinogen to the active enzyme trypsin. Trypsinogen is also capable of autoactivation. Trypsin, in turn, cleaves the zymogens proelastase to elastase, chymotrypsinogen to chymotrypsin, procarboxypeptidase to carboxypeptidase, and procolipase to colipase.

13. **The answer is D.** The acidic environment of the stomach stimulates the conversion of pepsinogen to pepsin, the major proteolytic enzyme of the stomach. Patients with achlorhydria, as in this case, have deficiencies in protein digestion as well as vitamin B_{12} absorption (as the parietal cells, in addition to secreting HCl, also synthesize intrinsic factor). Amylase is inactivated by acid, as are lipases and other proteases. When the acidic stomach contents enter the duodenum, the pancreas is stimulated to relase bicarbonate, which aids in neutralizing the stomach acid so that the intestinal and pancreatic digestive enzymes will be active. The conversion of trypsinogen to trypsin is catalyzed by the enzyme enterokinase.

4 Glycolysis

I. GENERAL OVERVIEW

A. Glycolysis is the **principal route of metabolism for glucose** as well as fructose, galactose, and other dietary carbohydrates.

B. The enzymes and transporters of the pathway **demonstrate stereospecificity** for naturally occurring **D-isomers.**

C. The reactions of glycolysis take place within the **cytoplasm.**

D. Glycolysis can provide adenosine triphosphate (ATP) in the **absence of oxygen.**

> **CLINICAL CORRELATES** **Red blood cells (RBCs),** which **lack mitochondria,** are nearly **completely reliant on glycolysis** as a source of energy. As such, many of the deficiencies of glycolytic enzymes have a profound effect on RBC function.

II. TRANSPORT OF GLUCOSE INTO CELLS

A. Glucose travels across the cell membrane on a **transport protein.**

B. Insulin stimulates glucose transport into muscle and adipose cells by causing glucose transport proteins (GLUT-4) within cells to move to the cell membrane.

C. Insulin does not significantly stimulate the transport of glucose into tissues such as liver, brain, and RBCs.

> **CLINICAL CORRELATES** **Hereditary deficiency of GLUT-1, an insulin-independent transporter,** results in decreased glucose in the **cerebrospinal fluid.** Patients manifest with intractable seizures in infancy and developmental delay.

III. REACTIONS OF GLYCOLYSIS (FIGURE 4-1)

A. **Overall reaction of glycolysis:**

$$\text{Glucose} + 2\ P_i + 2\ \text{ADP} + 2\ \text{NAD}^+ \rightarrow 2\ \text{Pyruvate} + 2\ \text{ATP} + 2\ \text{NADH} + 2\ \text{H}^+ + 2\ \text{H}_2\text{O}$$

B. **Glucose** is converted to glucose 6-phosphate in a reaction that uses ATP and produces adenosine diphosphate (ADP).

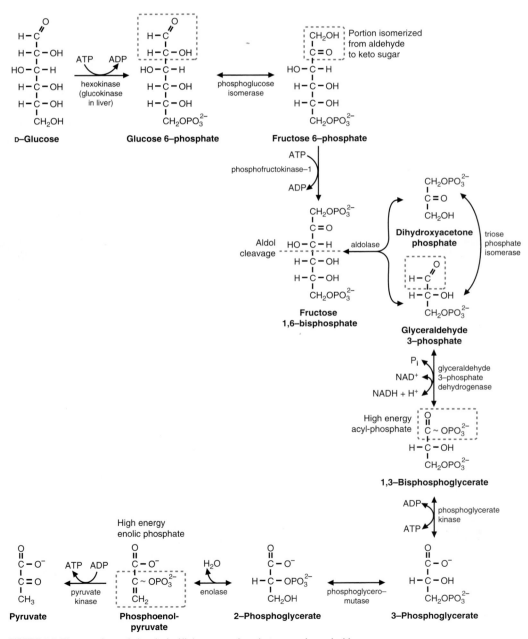

FIGURE 4-1 The reactions of glycolysis. High-energy phosphates are shown in *blue*.

1. Enzymes: **hexokinase** in all tissues and, in the liver, **glucokinase.** Both enzymes are subject to regulatory mechanisms.
2. Unlike glucose, which can diffuse through the transporters on the cell membranes, **glucose 6-phosphate is obligated to the intracellular compartment.**

C. **Glucose 6-phosphate** is isomerized to fructose 6-phosphate.
   - Enzyme: phosphoglucose isomerase

D. **Fructose 6-phosphate** is phosphorylated by ATP, forming fructose 1,6-bisphosphate and ADP.
   1. Enzyme: **phosphofructokinase-1 (PFK-1)**
   2. The first committed step of glycolysis.

E. **Fructose 1,6-bisphosphate** is cleaved—with the enzyme **aldolase**—to form the triose phosphates, glyceraldehyde 3-phosphate and dihydroxyacetone phosphate (DHAP).

> **CLINICAL CORRELATES** Absence of the A isoform of **aldolase** (found in RBCs and muscle) has been reported. The disorder presents with a nonspherocytic **hemolytic anemia.** Patients also have episodes of **rhabdomyolysis** (destruction of muscle cells) following febrile illness.

F. **Dihydroxyacetone phosphate** is isomerized—by the enzyme **triose phosphate isomerase**—to glyceraldehyde 3-phosphate.
   - **Note:** Two moles of glyceraldehyde 3-phosphate are formed from 1 mole of glucose.

> **CLINICAL CORRELATES** Patients with **triose phosphate isomerase (TPI)** deficiency have neonatal-onset **hemolytic anemia** as well as progressive **neurologic involvement.** Children have progressive hypotonia with eventual diaphragm paralysis that requires ventilation, as well as **cardiomyopathy.**

G. **Glyceraldehyde 3-phosphate** is oxidized by NAD^+ and reacts with inorganic phosphate (P_i) to form 1,3-bisphosphoglycerate and $NADH + H^+$.
   1. Enzyme: **glyceraldehyde 3-phosphate dehydrogenase**
   2. The aldehyde group of glyceraldehyde 3-phosphate is oxidized to a carboxylic acid, which forms a high-energy anhydride with P_i.

H. **1,3-Bisphosphoglycerate** reacts with ADP—using the enzyme **phosphoglycerate kinase**—to produce 3-phosphoglycerate and **ATP.**

I. **3-Phosphoglycerate** is converted—via the enzyme **phosphoglyceromutase**—to 2-phosphoglycerate in a reaction requiring catalytic amounts of 2,3-bisphosphoglycerate.

J. **2-Phosphoglycerate** is dehydrated—using the enzyme **enolase**—to phosphoenolpyruvate (PEP), which contains a high-energy enol phosphate.

> **CLINICAL CORRELATES** The enzyme **enolase** is inhibited by **fluoride.** To prevent ongoing glycolysis in a patient's blood samples collected for sensitive **glucose tolerance tests,** blood is collected in tubes containing fluoride.

K. **Phosphoenolpyruvate** reacts with ADP to form **pyruvate** and **ATP** in the last reaction of glycolysis.
   1. Enzyme: **pyruvate kinase**
   2. Pyruvate kinase is more active in the fed state than in the fasting state.

IV. SPECIAL REACTIONS IN RED BLOOD CELLS

A. In RBCs, 1,3-bisphosphoglycerate can be converted to **2,3-bisphosphoglycerate** (BPG), a compound that decreases the affinity of hemoglobin for oxygen.

B. BPG is dephosphorylated to form inorganic phosphate and 3-phosphoglycerate, an intermediate that reenters the glycolytic pathway.

> **CLINICAL CORRELATES**   **Fetal hemoglobin (HbF),** composed of two α subunits and two γ subunits, has a lower affinity for BPG than does HbA, and therefore, HbF has a higher affinity for O_2. This difference in maternal and fetal hemoglobin facilitates the unloading of O_2 at the maternal–fetal interface (i.e., the placenta).

V. REGULATORY ENZYMES OF GLYCOLYSIS (FIGURE 4-2)

A. Hexokinase is found in most tissues and is geared to provide glucose 6-phosphate for ATP production even when blood glucose is low.
  1. Hexokinase has a **low K_m** (Michaelis constant) for glucose (about 0.1 mM). Therefore, it is working near its maximum rate (V_{max}), even at fasting blood glucose levels (about 5 mM).
  2. Hexokinase is **inhibited** by its product, **glucose 6-phosphate.** Therefore, it is most active when glucose 6-phosphate is being rapidly used.

B. Glucokinase is found in the **liver** and actively functions at a significant rate only after a meal (when blood glucose is high).
  1. Glucokinase has a **high K_m** for glucose (about 6 mM). Therefore, it is very **active after a meal,** when glucose levels in the hepatic portal vein are high, and it is inactive during the postabsorptive state or fasting, when glucose levels are low.
  2. Glucokinase is **induced** when insulin levels are high.
  3. Glucokinase is not inhibited by its product, glucose 6-phosphate, at physiologic concentrations.

> **CLINICAL CORRELATES**   **Maturity-onset diabetes of the young (MODY)** type 2 is an autosomal dominant disorder involving mutations in the **glucokinase (GCK) gene.** Patients have **nonprogressive hyperglycemia** that is usually asymptomatic at diagnosis and is usually managed with diet alone.

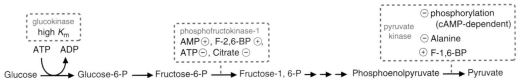

FIGURE 4-2 Regulation of glycolysis. In muscle, phosphofructokinase-1 (PFK-1) is the key enzyme. It is activated (⊕) by AMP and inhibited (⊖) by ATP and citrate. In liver, glucokinase, PFK-1 (activated by fructose 2,6-bisphosphate [F-2,6-BP]), and pyruvate kinase are the key enzymes. cAMP, cyclic adenosine monophosphate.

C. PFK-1 is an allosteric enzyme regulated by several factors. It functions at a rapid rate in the liver when blood glucose is high or in cells such as muscle when there is a need for ATP.

CLINICAL CORRELATES **Phosphofructokinase deficiency** (a form of **glycogen storage disease** [type VII] in which glycogen accumulates in muscles) results in inefficient use of glucose stores by RBCs and muscles. Patients experience **hemolytic anemia** as well as **muscle cramping**.

---

1. PFK-1 is **activated by fructose 2,6-bisphosphate** (F-2,6-BP), an important regulatory mechanism in the liver (Figure 4-3).
   a. After a meal, F-2,6-BP is formed from fructose 6-phosphate by **PFK-2.** (Step 1)
   b. F-2,6-BP activates PFK-1, and **glycolysis is stimulated.** The liver is using glycolysis to produce fatty acids for triacylglycerol synthesis. (Step 2)
   c. **In the fasting state** (when glucagon is elevated), **PFK-2** is phosphorylated by **protein kinase A,** which is activated by cyclic adenosine monophosphate (cAMP). (Step 3)
   d. Phosphorylated PFK-2 converts F-2,6-BP to fructose 6-phosphate. F-2,6-BP levels fall, and **PFK-1 is less active.** (Step 4)
   e. **In the fed state, insulin** causes **phosphatases** to be stimulated. A phosphatase dephosphorylates PFK-2, causing it to become more active in forming F-2,6-BP from fructose 6-phosphate. F-2,6-BP levels rise, and **PFK-1 is more active.** (Step 5)
   f. Thus, **PFK-2** acts as a **kinase** (in the **fed state** when it is dephosphorylated) and as a **phosphatase** (in the **fasting state** when it is phosphorylated). PFK-2 catalyzes two different reactions.
2. PFK-1 is **activated by adenosine monophosphate (AMP),** an important regulatory mechanism in **muscle** (Figure 4-2).
   a. In muscle during **exercise,** AMP levels are high, and ATP levels are low.
   b. Glycolysis is promoted by a more active PFK-1, and ATP is generated.
3. PFK-1 is **inhibited** by **ATP** and **citrate,** which are important regulatory mechanisms in **muscle.**
   a. When ATP is high, the cell does not need ATP, and glycolysis is inhibited.
   b. High levels of citrate indicate that adequate amounts of substrate are entering the tricarboxylic acid (TCA) cycle. Therefore, glycolysis slows down.

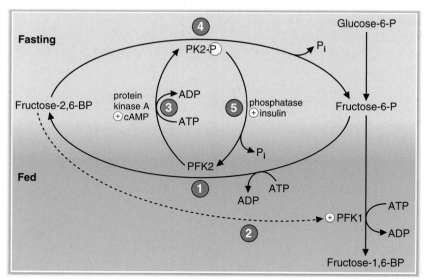

FIGURE 4-3 Regulation of fructose 2,6-bisphosphate (F-2,6-BP) levels in the liver. F-2,6-BP is an activator of phosphofructokinase-1 (PFK1), which converts fructose 6-phosphate to fructose 1,6-bisphosphate. Phosphofructokinase-2 (PFK2) acts as a kinase in the fed state and as a phosphatase during fasting. It regulates the cellular levels of fructose 2,6-bisphosphate. The *circled numbers* correspond with steps 1 to 5 in section V.C.1.a–e in the text. ADP, adenosine diphosphate; ATP, adenosine triphosphate; cAMP, cyclic adenosine monophosphate; P$_i$, inorganic phosphate; PK, pyruvate kinase.

D. Pyruvate kinase
   1. Pyruvate kinase is **activated** by **fructose 1,6-bisphosphate** and **inhibited** by **alanine** and by **phosphorylation** in the liver **during fasting** when glucagon levels are high (Figure 4-2).
      a. Glucagon, via cAMP, activates **protein kinase A,** which phosphorylates and inactivates pyruvate kinase in the liver (but not the muscle).
      b. The inhibition of pyruvate kinase promotes gluconeogenesis in the liver.
   2. Pyruvate kinase is **activated in the fed state.** Insulin stimulates phosphatases that dephosphorylate and activate pyruvate kinase in the liver.

CLINICAL CORRELATES   Deficiency of **pyruvate kinase** causes decreased production of ATP from glycolysis. RBCs have insufficient ATP for their membrane pumps, and a **hemolytic anemia** results.

VI. THE FATE OF PYRUVATE (FIGURE 4-4)

A. Conversion to lactate
   1. Pyruvate can be reduced in the cytosol by NADH, forming **lactate** and regenerating NAD^+.
   2. NADH, which is produced by glycolysis, must be reconverted to NAD^+ so that carbons of glucose can continue to flow through glycolysis.
   3. **Lactate dehydrogenase (LDH)** converts pyruvate to lactate. LDH consists of four subunits that can be either of the muscle (M) or the heart (H) type.
      a. Five isozymes occur (MMMM, MMMH, MMHH, MHHH, and HHHH), which can be separated by electrophoresis.
      b. Different tissues have different mixtures of these isozymes.
   4. Lactate is released by tissues (e.g., RBCs or **exercising muscle**) and is used by the liver for gluconeogenesis or by tissues such as the heart and kidney, where it is converted to pyruvate and oxidized for energy.
   5. The **LDH reaction** is **reversible.**

B. Conversion to acetyl coenzyme A (CoA)
   1. Pyruvate can enter mitochondria.
   2. There it can be converted by **pyruvate dehydrogenase** to acetyl CoA, which can enter the TCA cycle.

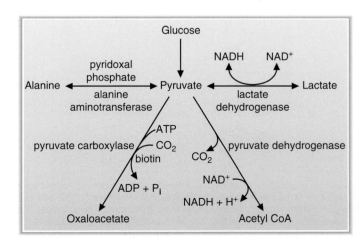

FIGURE 4-4 The fate of pyruvate. ADP, adenosine diphosphate; ATP, adenosine triphosphate; P_i, inorganic phosphate.

C. Conversion to oxaloacetate (OAA)

1. Pyruvate can be converted to OAA by **pyruvate carboxylase.**
2. This reaction serves to **replenish intermediates of the TCA cycle** as well as **provide substrates for gluconeogenesis.**
3. The enzyme is activated by acetyl CoA.

D. Conversion to alanine

1. Pyruvate can be transaminated to form the amino acid **alanine.**
2. The enzyme involved is alanine aminotransferase, which requires pyridoxal phosphate as a cofactor.

VII. GENERATION OF ADENOSINE TRIPHOSPHATE BY GLYCOLYSIS

A. Production of ATP and NADH in the glycolytic pathway

1. One mole of glucose yields 2 moles of pyruvate.
2. Two moles of ATP are used in this pathway, and 4 moles of ATP are produced, for a **net yield of 2 moles of ATP.**
3. In addition, 2 moles of cytosolic NADH are generated.

B. Energy generated by conversion of glucose to lactate (Figure 4-5)

● If the NADH generated by glycolysis is used to reduce pyruvate to lactate, the net yield is 2 moles of ATP per mole of glucose converted to lactate.

C. Energy generated by conversion of glucose to CO_2 and H_2O (Figure 4-6)

1. When glucose is oxidized completely to CO_2 and H_2O, about 30 or 32 moles of ATP are generated.
2. Two moles of ATP and 2 moles of NADH are generated from the conversion of 1 mole of glucose to 2 moles of pyruvate.
3. The 2 moles of pyruvate enter the mitochondria and are converted to 2 moles of acetyl CoA, producing 2 moles of NADH, which generate about 5 moles of ATP by oxidative phosphorylation.
4. The 2 moles of acetyl CoA are oxidized in the TCA cycle, generating about 20 moles of ATP.
5. NADH, produced in the cytosol by glycolysis, cannot directly cross the mitochondrial membrane. Therefore, the electrons are passed to the mitochondrial electron transport chain by two shuttle systems.

   a. **Glycerol phosphate shuttle** (Figure 4-7, *left side*)

      (1) Cytosolic DHAP is reduced to glycerol 3-phosphate by NADH.

      (2) Glycerol 3-phosphate reacts with a flavin adenine dinucleotide (FAD)–linked dehydrogenase in the inner mitochondrial membrane. DHAP is regenerated and reenters the cytosol.

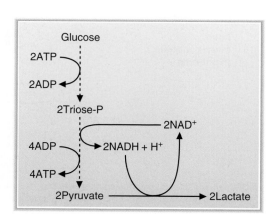

FIGURE 4-5 Conversion of 1 mole of glucose to lactate produces 2 moles of adenosine triphosphate (ATP) (net). The NADH produced by glycolysis is used to convert pyruvate to lactate.

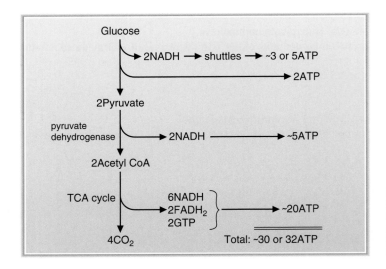

FIGURE 4-6 Adenosine triphosphate (ATP) produced by conversion of glucose to CO_2. The ATP produced by oxidative phosphorylation is approximate (indicated by ~). CoA, coenzyme A.

(3) Each mole of $FADH_2$ that is produced generates about 1.5 moles of ATP via oxidative phosphorylation.

(4) Because glycolysis produces 2 moles of NADH per mole of glucose, about **3 moles of ATP are produced by this shuttle.**

b. Malate-aspartate shuttle (Figure 4-7, *right side*)

(1) Cytosolic OAA is reduced to malate by NADH. The reaction is catalyzed by cytosolic malate dehydrogenase.

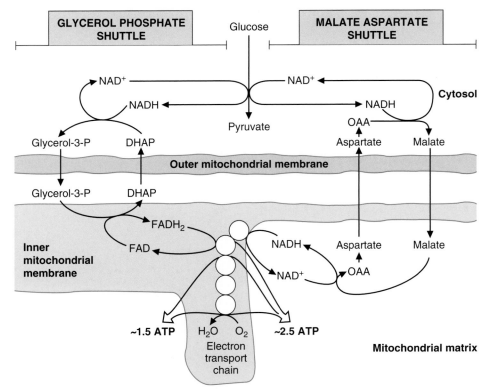

FIGURE 4-7 The glycerol phosphate and malate-aspartate shuttles. *Left,* the glycerol phosphate shuttle produces $FADH_2$, each of which generates about 1.5 moles of ATP by oxidative phosphorylation. *Right,* the malate-aspartate shuttle produces NADH, each of which generates approximately 2.5 moles of ATP. DHAP, dihydroxyacetone phosphate; OAA, oxaloacetate.

(2) Malate enters the mitochondrion and is reoxidized to OAA by the mitochondrial malate dehydrogenase, generating NADH in the matrix.

(3) OAA cannot cross the mitochondrial membrane. To return carbon to the cytosol, OAA is transaminated to aspartate, which can be transported into the cytosol and reconverted to OAA by another transamination reaction.

(4) In the mitochondrial matrix, each mole of NADH generates about 2.5 moles of ATP via oxidative phosphorylation.

(5) Because glycolysis produces 2 moles of NADH per mole of glucose, about **5 moles of ATP are produced by this shuttle.**

6. **Maximal ATP production**

    a. Overall, when 1 mole of glucose is oxidized to CO_2 and H_2O, about **30 moles of ATP** are produced if the **glycerol phosphate shuttle** is used.

    b. If the **malate-aspartate shuttle** is used, **32 moles** of ATP are produced.

Review Test

Directions: Each of the numbered questions or incomplete statements in this section is followed by answers or by completions of the statement. Select the **one** lettered answer or completion that is **best** in each case.

1. A teenager comes to the emergency room looking quite ill. Emergency medical services report that this appears to be a suicide attempt using rat poison. The patient is in hypovolemic shock from profuse vomiting and diarrhea. You note the strong smell of garlic from the patient. Which one of the following correctly describes an action of this toxin?

(A) It inhibits pyruvate dehydrogenase.
(B) It activates pyruvate dehydrogenase.
(C) It reduces the concentration of pyruvate.
(D) It increases glutathione production.
(E) It enables gluconeogenesis to proceed.

2. A 47-year-old obese man complains of having to get out of bed three times a night to urinate (polyuria), being constantly thirsty (polydipsia), and eating more often (polyphagia). The patient is diagnosed with insulin-resistant diabetes mellitus (type 2). If the patient's symptoms are due to a problem at the level of the glucose transporter, which one of the tissues indicated below will be most affected?

(A) RBCs
(B) Small intestine
(C) Muscle
(D) Brain
(E) Liver

3. In which one of the following scenarios would one expect to observe an increase in liver fructose 2,6-bisphosphate levels?

(A) After the release of epinephrine
(B) In an individual who had just finished running a marathon
(C) In a patient exhibiting diabetic ketoacidosis
(D) After the consumption of a large bowl of ice cream
(E) In a patient with kwashiorkor

4. A 58-year-old woman with breast cancer presents with confusion, headaches, and persistent nausea. To evaluate for metastases to the brain, the oncologist orders a positron emission tomography (PET) scan, which covalently links a radioactive isotope to glucose and reveals highly active areas in the body (e.g., a tumor). Which of the following proteins enables the tracer to remain in the cell?

(A) Insulin
(B) GLUT-4
(C) GLUT-1
(D) Hexokinase
(E) PFK-1

5. An 8-year-old girl presents with polydipsia, polyuria, and fatigue. A urinalysis is significant for glucose. To differentiate between type 1 diabetes mellitus and maturity-onset diabetes of the young (MODY), an assay is run to identify one of the six proteins responsible for MODY. Results reveal a missense mutation in exon 7 of the glucokinase gene establishing MODY2. Which of the following is a significant characteristic of glucokinase?

(A) The K_m is above the fasting concentration of glucose in the blood
(B) It is expressed in many tissues
(C) Its activity is stimulated in response to fructose 2,6-bisphosphate
(D) Its activity is inhibited by glucose 6-phosphate
(E) It is expressed only in muscle

6. Which one of the following statements is correct concerning the formation of muscle lactate during exercise?

(A) Lactate formation occurs when the NADH/NAD^+ ratio is high.
(B) The liver preferentially converts lactate into carbon dioxide and water.
(C) The heart preferentially converts lactate into glucose.
(D) Lactate formation is less likely to be found in the eye, testes, and RBCs than in other tissues.
(E) The intracellular pH is typically increased when lactate is produced.

7. A 36-year-old woman is training for her first marathon, and her coach has her keeping a pace that allows her to stay below her anaerobic threshold. By avoiding anaerobic muscle glycolysis, the pyruvate produced in the muscle does not accumulate because it is converted to which one of the following?

(A) Ethanol
(B) Lactic acid
(C) Acetyl CoA
(D) Alanine
(E) OAA

8. A patient presents with dizziness, fatigue, and tremors. A fingerstick test indicates a blood glucose of 36 mmol/L. Of the allosteric activators of glycolysis in the liver, which one of the following is the most important in allowing the liver to maintain a normal blood glucose level?

(A) Citrate
(B) ATP
(C) Fructose 2,6-bisphosphate
(D) Glucose 6-phosphate
(E) Acetyl CoA

9. A 24-year-old woman complains of intermittent right upper quadrant pain that extends to the inferior tip of her scapula. An ultrasound confirms your suspicion of cholelithiasis, and the patient undergoes cholecystectomy. Analysis indicates gallstones containing bilirubin. Measurement of metabolic intermediates, such as 2,3-bisphosphoglycerate and glucose 6-phosphate, are elevated in her serum. A deficiency of which of the following enzymes most likely led to her pigmented gallstones and release of these metabolites into the blood?

(A) Glucose 6-phosphate dehydrogenase
(B) PFK-1
(C) Pyruvate kinase
(D) Pyruvate dehydrogenase
(E) Pyruvate carboxylase

10. Emergency medical services are called to the scene of a diabetic patient who has collapsed and is in a confused state. The patient uses an insulin pump, which appears to have malfunctioned. The patient's blood sugar is found to be 12 mg/dL, and the squad is having difficulty getting intravenous access to administer intravenous glucose. On the way to the hospital, the squad administers an intramuscular injection of glucagon. Which one of the following statements is true regarding the use of glucagon?

(A) It is synthesized in the liver.
(B) It inhibits gluconeogenesis.
(C) It is secreted in the presence of somatostatin.
(D) It is secreted in the presence of insulin.
(E) It inhibits pyruvate formation and is also used in the treatment of β-blocker overdose.

11. A 33-year-old triathlete is admitted to the hospital after he spent the whole day training. He looks ill and complains of diffuse weakness, fatigue, and myalgia. Laboratory tests are sent for analysis, and his lactate level is elevated, creatinine is elevated (suggesting acute renal failure), creatine kinase is 76,000, and urine tests positive for myoglobin. You determine he has rhabdomyolysis and treat him with aggressive intravenous hydration. The basis for the elevated lactate is which one of the following?

(A) An increase in ATP due to the lack of oxygen for the muscle
(B) An increase in NADH due to the lack of oxygen for the muscle
(C) A defect in the M form of lactate dehydrogenase
(D) A defect in the H form of lactate dehydrogenase
(E) A defect in the B form of muscle aldolase

12. A pediatric hematologist sees an 18-month-old patient with jaundice, splenomegaly, and hemolytic anemia. A blood smear indicates RBCs that are more rigid in appearance than normal, and a diagnosis of pyruvate kinase deficiency is made. Because pyruvate kinase catalyzes the last step in the glycolytic pathway, products before this step of the pathway will accumulate. Which one of the following products associated with the pathway will be made in abnormal amounts?

(A) Acetyl CoA
(B) Glucose
(C) 2,3-Bisphosphoglycerate
(D) OAA
(E) Pyruvate

13. A 4-year-old girl is referred to a neurologist because of progressive neurologic deficits, including increased spasticity. On further workup, a peripheral blood smear indicates nonspherocytic hemolytic anemia of Dacie type II (in vitro autohemolysis not corrected by glucose addition). A diagnosis of triose phosphate isomerase deficiency is made. On examination of muscle cells, in the initial phases of the disease, it was found there was an elevated amount of which one of the following?

(A) 6-Carbon glycolytic products
(B) Many 3-carbon glycolytic products
(C) A component of the glycerol phosphate shuttle
(D) A component of the malate-aspartate shuttle
(E) Pyruvate

Answers and Explanations

1. **The answer is A.** Arsenic poisoning is a major public health hazard. Arsenic is an element found in rodenticides, herbicides, industrial chemicals, and improperly made alcohol (e.g., moonshine). Its main toxic effects are to inhibit the enzymes of glycolysis, especially pyruvate dehydrogenase. This results in a reduced flux of carbon through the TCA cycle via the inhibition of the conversion of pyruvate to acetyl CoA. The reduced citric acid cycle activity leads to a reduction in the production of reduced cofactors and a decrease in the production of cellular ATP via oxidative phosphorylation. The lack of ATP leads to a decrease in glutathione production. The lack of ATP also blocks gluconeogenesis from occuring. Because pyruvate dehydrogenase is inhibited, pyruvate will increase, not decrease, in concentration.

2. **The answer is C.** Both muscle and adipose tissue rely primarily on the glucose transporter GLUT-4, which requires insulin for optimal expression on the cell surface. The other glucose transporters are found on the cell surface in the absence of insulin secretion. These include GLUT-1, -2, -3, and -5. GLUT-1 is ubiquitously distributed in various tissues. GLUT-2 is present in liver and pancreatic β cells. GLUT-3 is also found in the intestine with GLUT-1. Finally, GLUT-5 functions primarily as a fructose transporter.

3. **The answer is D.** F-2,6-BP serves an intracellular signal that indicates glucose is abundant. It is a potent activator of PFK-1, the major regulated step of glycolysis. Its levels are increased in the liver when insulin is released; the levels drop when glucagon or epinephrine is released. A marathon runner would have high epinephrine levels and low F-2,6-BP in the liver. A patient in diabetic ketoacidosis lacks insulin. A patient with kwashiorkor also exhibits reduced insulin levels.

4. **The answer is D.** The conversion of glucose to glucose 6-phosphate by glucokinase and hexokinase traps the labeled glucose within the cell. Glucose is transported into the brain through either the insulin-sensitive GLUT-4 transporter or the insulin-independent GLUT-1 transporter. However, until the molecule is phosphorylated, it can be transported out of the cell and down its concentration gradient. Insulin accelerates the rate of glucose transport into cells via GLUT-4 transporters, but does not phosphorylate the glucose molecule to trap it in the cell. PFK-1 is the first committed step of glycolysis, but the conversion to glucose 6-phosphate, and trapping of glucose, occurs before the PFK-1 step.

5. **The answer is A.** Glucokinase and hexokinase catalyze the same reactions; however, they differ in their kinetic properties. Glucokinase has a low-affinity, high K_m, allowing substantial catalytic activity only at high glucose concentration, such as after a meal, whereas hexokinase has a high-affinity, low K_m, and is active at very low glucose concentrations. The K_m of glucokinase is above that of the fasting concentration of glucose in the blood. Glucokinase also escapes any local regulation, although regulation at the level of transcription is influenced via the hormones insulin and glucagon. Glucose 6-phosphate and fructose 2,6-bisphosphate do not regulate glucokinase activity, although glucose 6-phosphate is an allosteric inhibitor of hexokinase activity. Glucokinase is only found in the liver and pancreas and to a small extent in the brain. It is not found in muscle.

6. **The answer is A.** Lactate formation occurs in a high NADH/NAD$^+$ state. The NADH has been generated by the glyceraldehyde 3-phosphate dehydrogenase reaction, and NAD$^+$ needs to be regenerated, under anaerobic conditions, for glycolysis to continue. The formation of lactate, an acid, results in a drop in pH. Lactate formation commonly occurs in poorly vascularized tissues (e.g., eye, renal medulla, testes) or tissues without mitochondria (e.g., RBCs). Lactate, once formed in muscle, diffuses into the bloodstream and is used by other tissues. In the liver, lacate is converted to glucose, whereas in the heart, lactate is preferentially oxidized to provide energy.

7. **The answer is C.** Glycolysis is dependent on NAD^+ (for the glyceraldehyde 3-phosphate dehydrogenase reaction) as a substrate for the pathway to continue to metabolize glucose. Under aerobic conditions, NAD^+ is generated via the electron transport chain. Under anaerobic conditions, an oxygen deficit limits the electron transport chain, and NAD^+ is generated by the conversion of pyruvate to lactate in mammals and to ethanol in yeast and some microorganisms. When oxygen is not limiting, the pyruvate is converted to acetyl CoA to generate energy via the TCA cycle and oxidative phosphorylation. Because acetyl CoA levels are low during exercise, pyruvate carboxylase is not active, and OAA will not be formed.

8. **The answer is C.** The major regulated step of glycolysis is the conversion of fructose 6-phosphate to fructose 1,6-bisphosphate, catalyzed by the enzyme PFK-1. PFK1 is activated by both F-2,6-BP and AMP and inhibited by ATP and citrate. The modulation of F-2,6-BP levels in the liver is controlled by the insulin-to-glucagon ratio in the blood, which is tied to the regulation of PFK-2, the enzyme that both produces and degrades F-2,6-BP. Glucose 6-phosphate acts by negative feedback inhibition on hexokinase (an enzyme not present in liver), whereas acetyl CoA is an inhibitor of the pyruvate dehydrogenase reaction.

9. **The answer is C.** Pyruvate kinase deficiency is an autosomal recessive disease that causes hemolytic anemia of varying degrees depending on the amount of pyruvate kinase activity lost. The RBCs of affected individuals have a significantly reduced ability to make ATP. The lack of ATP impairs the cells' ability to achieve osmotic balance via ion pumping. Because of the loss of osmotic balance, the cells lyse readily. The heme released is converted to bilirubin in excess, which accumulates in the gallbladder, leading to gallstone formation. The presence of 2,3-bisphosphoglycerate and glucose 6-phosphate indicates a pyruvate kinase deficiency as opposed to the more prevalent glucose 6-phosphate dehydrogenase deficiency. The defect in pyruvate kinase leads to PEP accumulation, which is converted back to 3-phosphoglycerate, leading to increased 2,3-bisphosphoglycerate production. The RBCs lack mitochondria and thus do not contain pyruvate dehydrogenase or pyruvate carboxylase. A PFK-1 deficiency would not lead to increased 2,3-bisphosphoglycerate in the serum.

10. **The answer is E.** Glucagon is an amino acid hormone that instructs the liver to secrete glucose, obtained via glycogenolysis and gluconeogenesis. Glucagon secretion from the pancreas (the organ that synthesizes glucagon) is inhibited by insulin and somatostatin. Glucagon is used in β-blocker overdose and exerts its beneficial effects by increasing the concentration of cAMP in the myocardium, through activation of adenylate cyclase.

11. **The answer is B.** Because of the intensity of the patient's training, oxygen delivery to the muscle lagged behind the need to produce ATP, so anaerobic glycolysis was providing the majority of energy (ATP) formation. This leads to elevated NADH, which is converted back to NAD^+ by the lactate dehydrogenase reaction. Because the patient was exercising, ATP levels in the muscle are low, and ADP and AMP levels increase. There is no indication for a change either in the muscle (M) or in the heart (H) forms of lactate dehydrogenase. Muscle expresses the A form of aldolase, but not the B form (which is expressed in the liver).

12. **The answer is C.** Pyruvate kinase converts PEP to pyruvate. Because this reaction has reduced activity, PEP accumulates, which leads to a buildup of 2-phosphoglycerate (2-PG), 3-phosphoglycerate (3-PG), and the intermediate required to convert 2-PG to 3-PG, 2,3-bisphosphoglycerate. RBCs contain no mitochondria, so pyruvate cannot be converted to acetyl CoA or OAA (and, in addition, pyruvate levels are low because of the inherited defect in pyruvate kinase). RBCs lack glucose 6-phosphatase and cannot produce glucose from glucose 6-phosphate, even though glucose 6-phosphate does accumulate in this disorder owing to the block in the glycolytic pathway.

13. **The answer is C.** A defect in triose phosphate isomerase would lead to an accumulation of DHAP (the glyceraldehyde 3-phosphate produced via the aldolase reaction would be metabolized normally through the rest of the glycolytic pathway). DHAP is a component of the glycerol phosphate shuttle for transferring reducing equivalents across the mitochondrial membrane. It is not involved in the malate-aspartate shuttle. Pyruvate levels would not accumulate with this deficiency (because both pyruvate dehydrogenase and pyruvate carboxylase are working normally), nor would glucose 6-phosphate or fructose 6-phosphate accumulate in the initial phases of the disorder. Only one three-carbon product is accumulating (DHAP) in this disorder. The others can be metabolized by the active glycolytic enzymes.

5

The Tricarboxylic Acid Cycle, Electron Transport Chain, and Oxidative Metabolism

I. THE TRICARBOXYLIC ACID CYCLE

A. **Overview of the tricarboxylic acid (TCA) cycle (Krebs cycle, citric acid cycle)**
   1. Involves the oxidation of acetyl coenzyme A (CoA) along with the reduction of coenzymes, which are subsequently reoxidized to produce adenosine triphosphate (ATP).
   2. The cycle is **amphibolic**, providing carbon skeletons for **gluconeogenesis, fatty acid synthesis, and the interconversion of amino acids**.
   3. All the enzymes of the TCA cycle are in the **mitochondrial matrix** except succinate dehydrogenase, which is in the inner mitochondrial membrane.

B. **Entry of pyruvate from glycolysis**
   1. In order for carbons from glucose to enter the TCA cycle, glucose is first converted to pyruvate by glycolysis, then pyruvate forms acetyl CoA.
   2. **Reaction sequence**
      a. Pyruvate dehydrogenase (PDH), a multienzyme complex located exclusively in the mitochondrial matrix, catalyzes the oxidative decarboxylation of pyruvate, forming acetyl CoA, carbon dioxide, and NADH.
      b. The reactions catalyzed by the pyruvate dehydrogenase complex (PDHC) are analogous to those catalyzed by the α-ketoglutarate dehydrogenase complex.

CLINICAL CORRELATES   **Arsenic** is an odorless and tasteless heavy metal, which has been used throughout the centuries as a **poison**. It inhibits one of the subunits of the **PDHC**, resulting in **impaired** production of acetyl CoA and subsequent energy production via oxidative phosphorylation.

---

   3. **Regulation of pyruvate dehydrogenase (PDH)** (Figure 5-1)
      a. In contrast to α-ketoglutarate dehydrogenase, PDH exists in a phosphorylated (inactive) form and a dephosphorylated (active) form.
      b. A **kinase** associated with the multienzyme complex phosphorylates the pyruvate decarboxylase subunit, inactivating the PDHC.
         (1) The products of the PDH reaction, **acetyl CoA** and **NADH**, activate the kinase
         (2) The substrates, **CoA** and **NAD$^+$**, inactivate the kinase.
         (3) The kinase is also inactivated by adenosine diphosphate (ADP).
      c. A **phosphatase** dephosphorylates and activates the PDHC.
      d. When the concentration of substrates is high, the dehydrogenase is active, and pyruvate is converted to acetyl CoA. When the concentration of products is high, the dehydrogenase is relatively inactive.

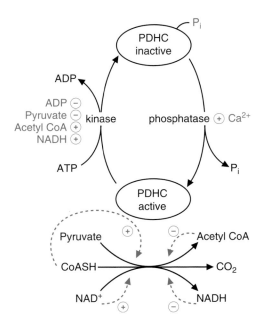

FIGURE 5-1 Regulation of the pyruvate dehydrogenase complex (PDHC). ADP, adenosine diphosphate; ATP, adenosine triphosphate; CoA, coenzyme A; P_i, inorganic phosphate.

CLINICAL CORRELATES **PDHC deficiency** is one of the most common **neurodegenerative disorders** associated with abnormal mitochondrial metabolism. Severe forms of the disease are lethal; mild forms exhibit **ataxia and mild psychomotor delay** and nonspecific symptoms (e.g., severe lethargy, poor feeding, tachypnea) related to **lactate buildup**, especially during times of illness, stress, or high carbohydrate intake.

C. **The reactions of the TCA cycle** (Figure 5-2)
1. **Acetyl CoA** and **oxaloacetate (OAA)** condense, forming citrate.
   a. Enzyme: **citrate synthase**.
   b. Cleavage of the high-energy thioester bond in acetyl CoA provides the energy for this condensation.
   c. Citrate (the product) is an inhibitor of this reaction.
2. **Citrate** is isomerized to isocitrate by a rearrangement of the molecule.
   a. Enzyme: **aconitase**.
   b. Aconitate serves as an enzyme-bound intermediate.

CLINICAL CORRELATES The rat poison **fluoroacetate** reacts with OAA to form fluorocitrate. Fluorocitrate inhibits **aconitase**, leading to the **accumulation of citrate**. Ingestion may result in convulsions, cardiac arrhythmias, and eventually death.

3. **Isocitrate** is oxidized to α-ketoglutarate in the first oxidative decarboxylation reaction. CO_2 is produced, and the electrons are passed to NAD^+ to form $NADH + H^+$.
   a. Enzyme: **isocitrate dehydrogenase**.
   b. This key regulatory enzyme of the TCA cycle is allosterically activated by ADP and inhibited by NADH.
4. **α-Ketoglutarate** is converted to succinyl CoA in a second oxidative decarboxylation reaction. CO_2 is released, and succinyl CoA, NADH, and H^+ are produced.
   a. Enzyme: α-**ketoglutarate dehydrogenase**.
   b. This enzyme requires the same five cofactors as does PDH: thiamine pyrophosphate, lipoic acid, uncombined coenzyme A **(CoASH)**, flavin adenine dinucleotide (FAD), and NAD^+.

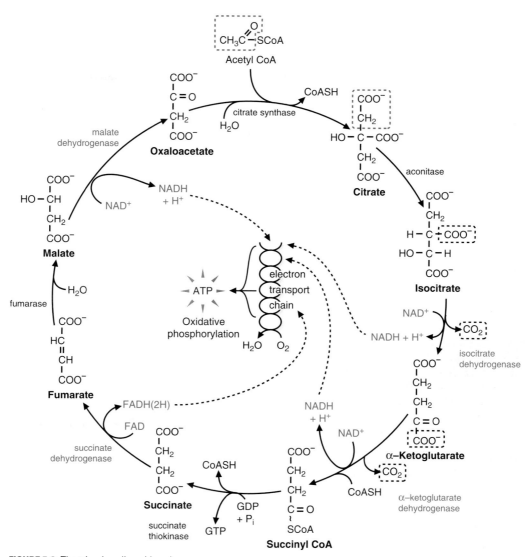

FIGURE 5-2 The tricarboxylic acid cycle.

5. **Succinyl CoA** is cleaved to succinate. Cleavage of the high-energy thioester bond of succinyl CoA provides energy for the **substrate level phosphorylation** of guanosine diphosphate (GDP) to guanosine triphosphate (GTP). Because this does not involve the electron transport chain, it is not an oxidative phosphorylation.
   a. Enzyme: **succinate thiokinase**.
   b. The enzyme is also called succinyl CoA synthetase.
6. **Succinate** is oxidized to fumarate. Succinate transfers two protons together with their electrons to FAD, which forms FADH$_2$.
   a. Enzyme: **succinate dehydrogenase**.
   b. This enzyme is present in the inner mitochondrial membrane. The other enzymes of the cycle are in the matrix.
7. **Fumarate** is converted—by the enzyme **fumarase**—to malate by the addition of water across the double bond.
8. **Malate** is oxidized with the help of the enzyme malate dehydrogenase, regenerating **OAA** and thus completing the cycle. Two protons along with their electrons are passed to NAD$^+$, producing NADH + H$^+$.

D. Energy production by the TCA cycle

1. The NADH and FADH$_2$ (produced by the cycle) donate electrons to the electron transport chain. For each mole of **NADH**, about **2.5 moles of ATP** are generated, and for each mole of **FADH$_2$**, about **1.5 moles of ATP** are generated by the passage of these electrons to O$_2$ (oxidative phosphorylation). In addition, GTP is produced when succinyl CoA is cleaved. **GTP** produces ATP.

$$(GTP + ADP \leftrightarrows ATP + GDP)$$

2. The **total energy** generated by one round of the cycle, starting with one mole of acetyl CoA, is about **10 moles of ATP**.

E. Regulation of the TCA cycle (Figure 5-3)

1. The TCA cycle is regulated by the **cell's need for energy** in the form of ATP. The TCA cycle acts in concert with the electron transport chain and the ATP synthase in the inner mitochondrial membrane to produce ATP.
2. The cell has limited amounts of adenine nucleotides (ATP, ADP, and adenosine monophosphate [AMP]).
3. When ATP is utilized, ADP and inorganic phosphate (P$_i$) are produced.
4. **When ADP levels are high** relative to ATP—that is, when the cell needs energy—the reactions of the electron transport chain are accelerated.
   a. NADH is rapidly oxidized; consequently, the **TCA cycle speeds up**.
   b. ADP allosterically activates isocitrate dehydrogenase.
5. **When the concentration of ATP is high**—the cell has an adequate energy supply—the electron transport chain slows down, NADH builds up, and consequently, **the TCA cycle is inhibited**.
   a. **NADH allosterically inhibits isocitrate dehydrogenase**. Isocitrate accumulates, and because the aconitase equilibrium favors citrate, the concentration of citrate rises. **Citrate inhibits citrate synthase**, the first enzyme of the cycle.

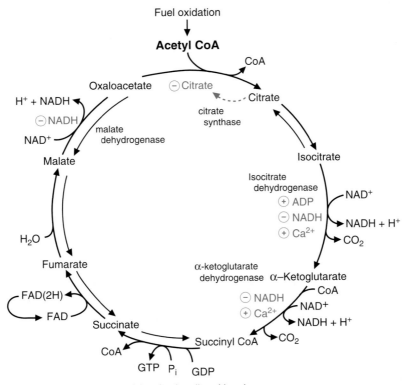

FIGURE 5-3 Major regulatory interactions of the tricarboxylic acid cycle.

b. High NADH (low NAD$^+$) levels also affect the reactions of the cycle that generate NADH, slowing the cycle by mass action.

c. OAA is converted to malate when NADH is high, and therefore, less substrate is available for the citrate synthase reaction.

F. Cofactors and vitamins required for reactions of the TCA cycle

1. NAD$^+$ accepts a hydride ion, which reacts with its nicotinamide ring. NAD$^+$ is reduced; the substrate (RH$_2$) is oxidized; and a proton is released.

$$NAD^+ + RH_2 \leftrightarrows NADH + H^+ + R$$ $NADH \rightarrow NAD^+ + H^+ + 2e^-$

a. NAD$^+$ is frequently involved in oxidizing a hydroxyl group to a ketone.

$$
\begin{array}{ccc}
\text{OH} & & \text{O} \\
| & & \parallel \\
\text{R}-\text{CH}-\text{R}_1 + \text{NAD}^+ & \leftrightarrows & \text{R}-\text{C}-\text{R}_1 + \text{NADH} + \text{H}^+
\end{array}
$$

b. The **nicotinamide ring** of NAD$^+$ is derived from the vitamin **niacin** (nicotinic acid) and, to a limited extent, from the amino acid **tryptophan.**

c. NAD$^+$ is used in the isocitrate dehydrogenase, α-ketoglutarate dehydrogenase, and malate dehydrogenase reactions, as well as the PDH reaction.

2. FAD accepts two hydrogen atoms (with their electrons). FAD is reduced, and the substrate is oxidized.

$$FAD + RH_2 \leftrightarrows FADH_2 + R$$

a. FAD is frequently involved in reactions that produce a double bond.

$$R-CH_2-CH_2-R_1 + FAD \leftrightarrows R-CH=CH-R_1 + FADH_2$$

b. FAD is derived from the vitamin **riboflavin.**

c. **FAD** is the cofactor for **succinate dehydrogenase.** FAD is also required by α-**ketoglutarate dehydrogenase and PDH.**

3. Coenzyme A (Figure 5-4)

a. **CoA** contains a sulfhydryl group that reacts with carboxylic acids to form **thioesters,** such as acetyl CoA, succinyl CoA, and palmityl CoA.

(1) The ΔG° for hydrolysis of the thioester bond is -7.5 kcal/mole (a high-energy bond).

(2) CoA contains the vitamin **pantothenic acid.**

(3) CoA is used in the α-**ketoglutarate dehydrogenase** and PDH complex.

4. Thiamine and lipoic acid, cofactors for α-ketoacid dehydrogenases

a. α-**Ketoacid dehydrogenases** catalyze **oxidative decarboxylations** in a sequence of reactions involving thiamine pyrophosphate, lipoic acid, CoA, FAD, and NAD$^+$.

b. The major α-ketoacid dehydrogenases are as follows:

(1) **PDH**, the enzyme complex that oxidatively decarboxylates pyruvate, forming acetyl CoA

(2) α-**Ketoglutarate dehydrogenase**, which catalyzes the conversion of α-ketoglutarate to succinyl CoA

c. **Thiamine pyrophosphate** (Figure 5-5A) is involved in the **decarboxylation of α-ketoacids.**

(1) The α-carbon of the α-ketoacid becomes covalently attached to thiamine pyrophosphate, and the carboxyl group is released as CO$_2$.

(2) Thiamine pyrophosphate (TPP) is formed from ATP and the vitamin **thiamine.**

d. **Lipoic acid** oxidizes the keto group of the decarboxylated α-ketoacid (Figure 5-6).

(1) After an α-ketoacid is decarboxylated, the remainder of the compound is oxidized as it is transferred from TPP to lipoic acid, which is reduced in the reaction.

(2) The oxidized compound, which forms a thioester with lipoate, is then transferred to the sulfur of CoA.

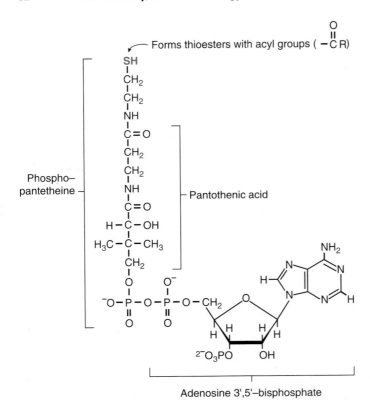

Forms thioesters with acyl groups ($-\overset{\overset{\displaystyle O}{\|}}{C}R$)

FIGURE 5-4 The structure of co-enzyme A. The *arrow* indicates where acyl (e.g., acetyl, succinyl, and fatty acyl) groups bind to form thioesters.

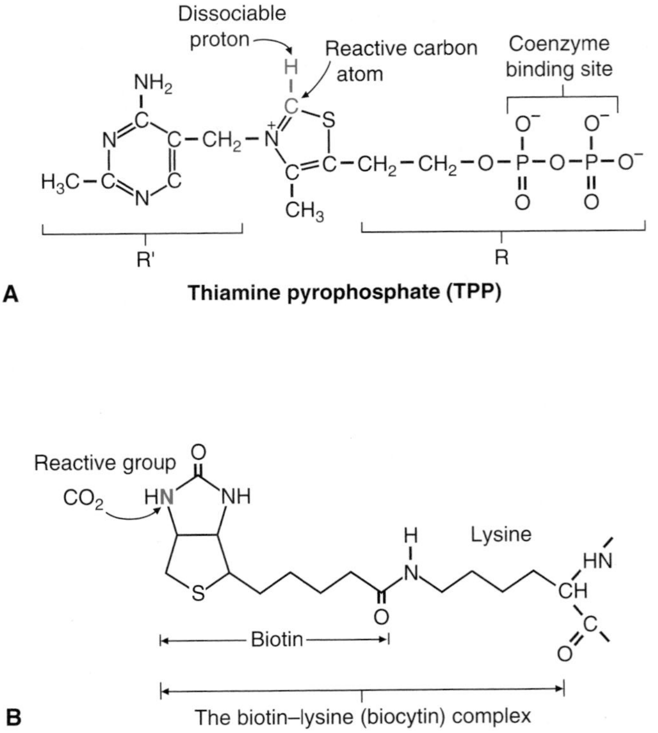

Thiamine pyrophosphate (TPP)

FIGURE 5-5 The structures of (**A**) thia-mine pyrophosphate and (**B**) biotin. The *arrows* indicate the reactive sites. When an α-ketoacid binds to thiamine pyro-phosphate, the keto group attaches, and the carboxyl group is released as CO_2.

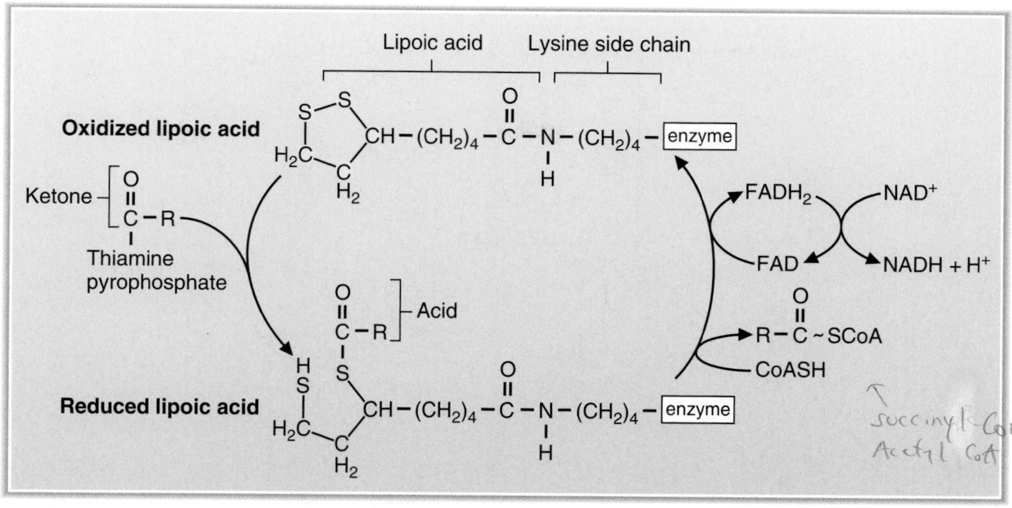

FIGURE 5-6 Role of lipoic acid in oxidative decarboxylation of α-ketoacids.

(3) Because there is a limited amount of lipoate in the cell, reduced lipoate must be reoxidized so that it can be reutilized in these types of reactions. It is reoxidized by FAD, which becomes reduced to $FADH_2$ and is subsequently reoxidized by NAD^+.

(4) Lipoic acid is not derived from a vitamin.

e. **Biotin** is involved in the **carboxylation** of **pyruvate** (which forms OAA), **acetyl CoA** (which forms malonyl CoA), and **propionyl CoA** (which forms methylmalonyl CoA). The vitamin biotin is covalently linked to a lysyl residue of the enzyme (Figure 5-5B).

G. Synthetic functions of the TCA cycle (Figure 5-7)

1. **Intermediates** of the TCA cycle are used in the fasting state in the liver for the production of **glucose** and in the fed state for the synthesis of **fatty acids**. Intermediates of the TCA cycle are also used to synthesize **amino acids** or to convert one amino acid to another.

2. **Anaplerotic reactions** replenish intermediates of the TCA cycle as they are removed for the synthesis of glucose, fatty acids, amino acids, or other compounds.

   a. A key anaplerotic reaction is catalyzed by **pyruvate carboxylase**, which carboxylates pyruvate, forming OAA. (Step 1)

      (1) Pyruvate carboxylase requires **biotin**, a cofactor that is commonly involved in CO_2 fixation reactions.

      (2) Pyruvate carboxylase, found in liver, brain, and adipose tissue (but not in muscle), is **activated by acetyl CoA.**

CLINICAL CORRELATES **Pyruvate carboxylase deficiency** results in accumulation of **lactic acid** in the bloodstream as the conversion of pyruvate to OAA is blocked. The disorder presents early in life with delayed development, muscle weakness (hypotonia), impaired ability to control voluntary movements (ataxia), seizures, and vomiting.

   b. **Amino acids** produce intermediates of the TCA cycle through anaplerotic reactions.

      (1) **Glutamate** is converted to α-ketoglutarate. (Step 2) Amino acids that form glutamate include glutamine, proline, arginine, and histidine.

      (2) **Aspartate** is transaminated to form OAA. Asparagine can produce aspartate.

      (3) **Valine, isoleucine, methionine**, and **threonine** produce propionyl CoA, which is converted to methylmalonyl CoA and, subsequently, to succinyl CoA, an intermediate of the TCA cycle. (Step 3)

      (4) **Phenylalanine, tyrosine**, and **aspartate** form fumarate. (Step 4)

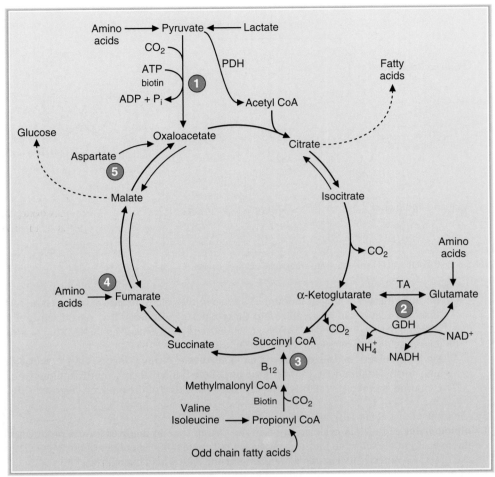

FIGURE 5-7 Anaplerotic and biosynthetic reactions involving the tricarboxylic acid cycle intermediates. Synthetic reactions that form fatty acids and glucose are indicated by *dashed lines*. GDH, glutamate dehydrogenase; PC, pyruvate carboxylase; PDH, pyruvate dehydrogenase; TA, transamination; ① to ⑤, anaplerotic reactions.

3. **Synthesis of glucose**
   a. The synthesis of glucose occurs by the pathway of **gluconeogenesis**, which involves intermediates of the TCA cycle.
   b. As glucose is synthesized, **malate or OAA** is removed from the TCA cycle and replenished by anaplerotic reactions.
      (1) Pyruvate, produced from lactate or alanine, is converted by pyruvate carboxylase to OAA, which forms malate. (Step 5)
      (2) **Various amino acids that supply carbon for gluconeogenesis** are converted to intermediates of the TCA cycle, which form malate and, thus, glucose.
4. **Synthesis of fatty acids**
   a. The pathway for fatty acid synthesis from glucose includes reactions of the TCA cycle.
   b. From glucose, pyruvate is produced and converted to OAA (by pyruvate carboxylase) and to acetyl CoA (by PDH).
   c. OAA and acetyl CoA condense to form **citrate**, which is used for fatty acid synthesis.
   d. Pyruvate carboxylase catalyzes the anaplerotic reaction that replenishes the TCA cycle intermediates.
5. **Synthesis of amino acids**
   a. Synthesis of amino acids from glucose involves intermediates of the TCA cycle.
   b. **Glucose** is converted to pyruvate, which forms OAA, which by transamination forms **aspartate** and, subsequently, **asparagine**.

   c. Glucose is converted to pyruvate, which forms both OAA and acetyl CoA, which condense, forming citrate. Citrate forms isocitrate and then α-ketoglutarate, producing **glutamate, glutamine, proline**, and **arginine**.
6. **Interconversion of amino acids** involves intermediates of the TCA cycle. For example, the carbons of **glutamate** can feed into the TCA cycle at the α-ketoglutarate level and traverse the cycle, forming OAA, which may be transaminated to **aspartate**.

II. ELECTRON TRANSPORT CHAIN AND OXIDATIVE PHOSPHORYLATION

A. Overview of the electron transport chain (ETC) (Figure 5-8)
1. **NADH** (reduced nicotinamide adenine dinucleotide) **and FADH₂** (reduced form of flavin adenine dinucleotide) are produced by glycolysis, β-oxidation of fatty acids, the TCA cycle, and other oxidative reactions. NADH and FADH₂ pass electrons to the components of the ETC, which are located in the inner mitochondrial membrane.
2. **NADH** freely diffuses from the matrix to the membrane, whereas **FADH₂** is tightly bound to enzymes that produce it within the inner mitochondrial membrane.
3. **Mitochondria** are separated from the cytoplasm by two membranes. The soluble interior of a mitochondrion is called the **matrix**. The matrix is surrounded by the inner membrane, which contains vast infoldings to increase surface area, known as **cristae**.
4. The **transfer of electrons** from NADH to oxygen (O_2) occurs in **three stages**, each of which involves a large protein complex in the inner mitochondrial membrane.
5. Some of the genes for the large protein complexes are encoded by **nuclear DNA**, while others are coded for by **mitochondrial DNA (mtDNA)**.

CLINICAL CORRELATES   **Fatal infantile mitochondrial myopathy** involves decreased activity of the **mtDNA-**encoded **respiratory chain complexes (I, III, IV, and V)**. Patients have early progressive **liver failure** and **neurologic abnormalities, hypoglycemia**, and increased lactate in body fluids.

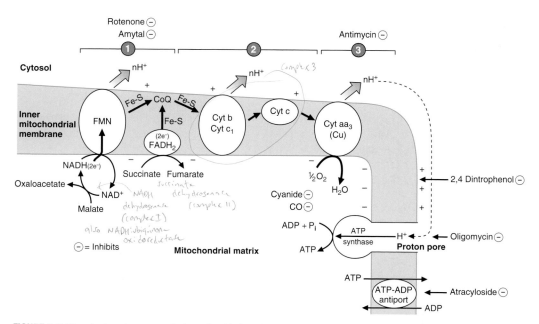

FIGURE 5-8 The electron transport chain and oxidative phosphorylation. *Heavy arrows* indicate the flow of electrons. CoQ, coenzyme Q (ubiquinone); Cyt, cytochrome; Fe-S, iron-sulfur centers; FMN, flavin mononucleotide. nH⁺ indicates that an undetermined number of protons are pumped from the matrix to the cytosolic side. The *numbers* at the top of the figure correspond with the three major stages of electron transfer described in the text (see section I.C).

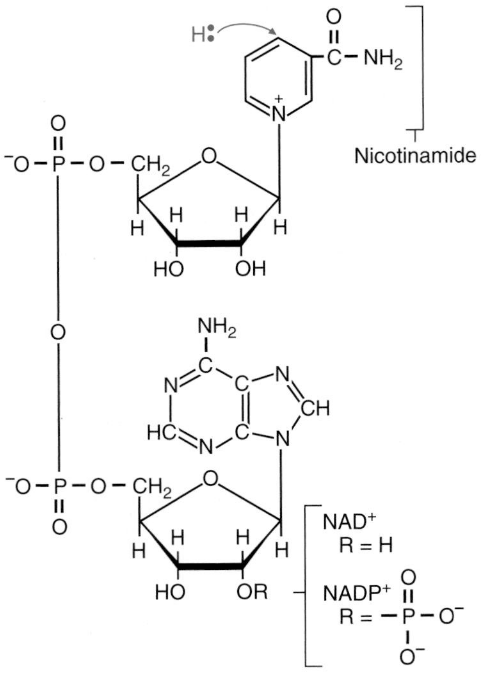

FIGURE 5-9 The structure of NAD^+ and $NADP^+$. R differs for NAD^+ and $NADP^+$ as indicated. The *arrow* shows the position where a hydride ion (H^-; H:) covalently binds when NAD^+ or $NADP^+$ is reduced.

6. Each complex uses the energy from electron transfer to **pump protons** to the cytosolic side of the inner mitochondrial membrane.
7. An **electrochemical potential** or proton-motive force is generated, and ATP is produced as the protons enter back into the matrix through the **ATP synthase** complex.
8. During the transfer of electrons through the ETC, **some** of the **energy is lost as heat**.
9. The electron transport chain has a large negative $\Delta G^{o\prime}$, thus electrons flow from NADH (or $FADH_2$) toward O_2.

B. **Components of the electron transport chain**
1. The reduced cofactors, NADH (Figure 5-9) and $FADH_2$ (Figure 5-10), transfer electrons to the ETC.
2. **Flavin mononucleotide (FMN)** receives electrons from NADH and transfers them through iron-sulfur (Fe-S) centers to coenzyme Q (Figure 5-11). FMN is derived from **riboflavin**.

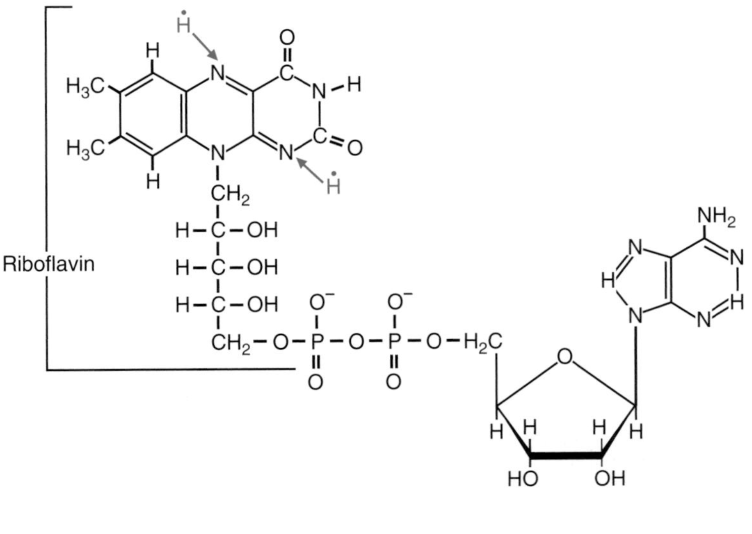

FIGURE 5-10 The structure of flavin adenine dinucleotide (FAD). *Arrows* indicate positions where hydrogens (H·) covalently bind when FAD is reduced to $FADH_2$. Flavin mononucleotide (FMN) consists only of the riboflavin moiety plus one phosphate.

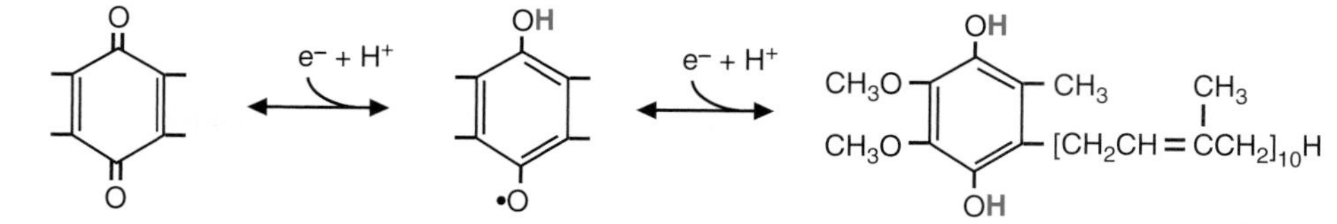

FIGURE 5-11 The structure of coenzyme Q (CoQ), or ubiquinone. Hydrogen atoms can bind, one at a time, as indicated by the *arrows*.

Fully oxidized or quinone form (Q)

Semiquinone form (free radical, Q•)

Reduced or quinol form (dihydroquinol, QH$_2$)

3. **Coenzyme Q** (CoQ) receives electrons from FMN and also through Fe-S centers from FADH$_2$.
   a. FADH$_2$ is not free in solution like NAD$^+$ and NADH; it is tightly bound to enzymes.
   b. CoQ can be synthesized in the body. It is not derived from a vitamin.
4. **Cytochromes** receive electrons from the reduced form of CoQ.
   a. Each cytochrome consists of a **heme** group (Figure 5-12) associated with a protein.
   b. The **iron** of the heme group is reduced when the cytochrome accepts an electron.

$$Fe^{3+} \leftrightarrows Fe^{2+}$$

   c. Heme is synthesized from glycine and succinyl coenzyme A (CoA) in humans. It is not derived from a vitamin.
5. **O$_2$** ultimately receives the electrons at the end of the electron transport chain and is reduced to water (H$_2$O).

C. **The three major stages of electron transport** (Figure 5-8)
   1. **Transfer of electrons from NADH to coenzyme Q (Complex I)**
      a. **NADH** passes electrons via the **NADH dehydrogenase complex** to FMN.
         (1) NADH is produced by the α-ketoglutarate dehydrogenase, isocitrate dehydrogenase, and malate dehydrogenase reactions of the TCA cycle, by the PDH reaction that converts pyruvate to acetyl CoA, by β-oxidation of fatty acids, and by other oxidation reactions.
         (2) NADH produced in the mitochondrial matrix diffuses to the inner mitochondrial membrane where it passes electrons to FMN, which is tightly bound to a protein. (Stage 1)
      b. **FMN** passes the electrons through a series of Fe-S protein complexes to **CoQ**, which accepts electrons one at a time, forming first the semiquinone and then ubiquinol.
      c. The energy produced by these electron transfers is used to pump protons to the cytosolic side of the inner mitochondrial membrane.

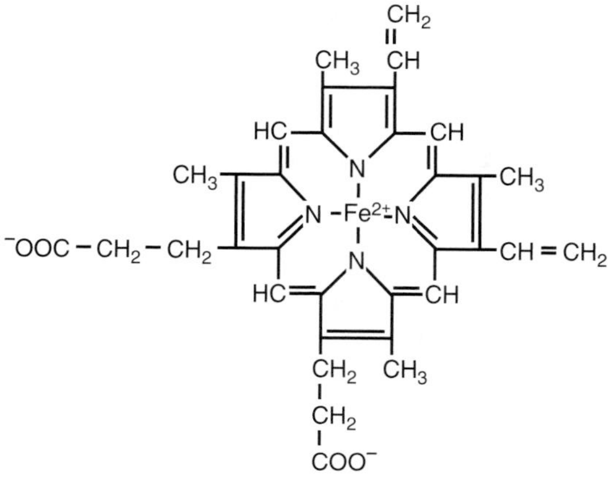

FIGURE 5-12 The general structure of the heme group, which is present in hemoglobin, myoglobin, and the cytochromes b, c, and c$_1$.

CLINICAL CORRELATES Mutations in the mitochondrial encoded gene for **NADH:ubiquinone oxidoreductase (complex I)** results in the disorder **MELAS**. MELAS is an acronym for the clinical manifestations of the disease **mitochondrial encephalopathy, lactic acidosis**, and **stroke**.

2. **Transfer of electrons from CoQ to cytochrome c**
   a. **CoQ** passes electrons through Fe-S centers to **cytochromes b and c_1 (complex III)**, which transfer the electrons to **cytochrome c**. The protein complex involved in these transfers is called **cytochrome c reductase**.
      (1) These cytochromes each contain heme as a prosthetic group but have different apoproteins.
      (2) In the **ferric (Fe^{3+})** state, the heme iron can accept one electron and be reduced to the **ferrous (Fe^{2+})** state.
      (3) Because the cytochromes can only carry one electron at a time, CoQ acts as an adapter between the two electron transfers in complex I, and the one electron transfer in complex III.

CLINICAL CORRELATES Some patients with the **mitochondrial DNA (mtDNA)** disorder known as **Leber's hereditary optic neuropathy (LHON)** have point mutations in the gene for **cytochrome reductase**. Patients are typically males in their 20s to 30s who develop **loss of central vision**.

   b. The energy produced by the transfer of electrons from CoQ to cytochrome c is used to pump protons across the inner mitochondrial membrane. Proton flow back into the mitochondrial matrix, via the ATP synthase, will drive ATP synthesis.
   c. **Electrons from $FADH_2$ (complex II)**, produced by reactions such as the oxidation of succinate to fumarate by succinate dehydrogenase, **enter** the electron transport chain **at the CoQ level** (Figure 5-8).

CLINICAL CORRELATES Some patients with the mtDNA defect known as **Kearns-Sayre syndrome** have mutations in complex II of the ETC. These patients manifest with short stature, complete external **ophthalmoplegia, pigmentary retinopathy**, ataxia, and **cardiac conduction defects**.

3. **Transfer of electrons from cytochrome c to oxygen**
   a. **Cytochrome c** transfers electrons to the **cytochrome aa_3 complex (complex IV)**, which transfers the electrons to molecular O_2, reducing it to H_2O. **Cytochrome c oxidase** catalyzes this transfer of electrons. (Stage 3)

CLINICAL CORRELATES Patients with **Leigh disease**, an **mtDNA** disorder, present with **lactic acidemia, developmental delay**, seizure, **extraocular palsies**, and hypotonia. The disorder is usually **fatal by the age of 2 years**, with some patients exhibiting mutations in **cytochrome oxidase**.

      (1) Cytochromes a and a_3 each contain a heme and two different proteins that each contain **copper**.
      (2) **Two electrons are required to reduce 1 atom of O_2**; therefore, for each mole of NADH that is oxidized, $1/2$ mole of O_2 is converted to H_2O.
   b. The energy produced by the transfer of electrons from cytochrome c to O_2 is used to pump protons across the inner mitochondrial membrane.

$$\tfrac{1}{2}O_2 + 2H^+ \rightarrow H_2O$$

D. ATP production

   1. As elements of the ETC pass electrons from complex I to IV, an **electrochemical potential** or proton-motive force is generated.

   a. The electrochemical potential consists of both a **membrane potential** and a **pH gradient**.

   b. The cytosolic side of the membrane is more acidic (i.e., has a higher $[H^+]$) than the matrix.

   2. The protons can reenter the matrix only through the ATP synthase complex **(complex V, the F_0–F_1/ATPase)**, causing ATP to be generated.

   a. The inner mitochondrial membrane is **impermeable to protons**.

   b. The **(F_0) component forms a channel** in the inner mitochondrial membrane, through which protons can flow.

   c. The **(F_1) is the ATP-synthesizing head**, projecting into the mitochondrial matrix that is connected to the F_0 portion via a **stalk**.

   3. Total ATP production

   a. For every mole of **NADH that is oxidized**, $1/2$ mole of O_2 is reduced to H_2O, and about **2.5 moles of ATP** are produced. Each mole of NADH oxidized leads to 10 moles of protons being extruded from the matrix. Because it requires four moles of protons entering the ATP synthase to generate one mole of ATP, 2.5 moles of ATP can be generated per 10 moles of protons extruded.

   b. For every mole of **$FADH_2$ that is oxidized**, about **1.5 moles of ATP are generated** because the electrons from $FADH_2$ enter the chain via CoQ, bypassing the NADH dehydrogenase step. For each mole of $FADH_2$ oxidized, six moles of protons are extruded across the inner mitochondrial membrane.

E. The ATP-ADP antiport. ATP produced within mitochondria is transferred to the cytosol in exchange for ADP by a transport protein in the inner mitochondrial membrane known as the ATP-ADP antiporter (adenine nucleotide translocase [ANT]) (Figure 5-8).

F. Inhibitors of the electron transport chain (summarized in Table 5-1).

t a b l e **5-1**	Inhibitors of the Electron Transport Chain	
Component of the Electron Transport Chain	**Substance**	**Effect**
Complex I	**Rotenone**, a fish poison and pesticide	Inhibits **NADH dehydrogenase** causing NADH to accumulate. It **does not block the transfer of electrons from $FADH_2$.**
Complex I	**Amytal**, a barbiturate sedative.	Blocks complex I
Complex III	**Antimycin**, a fungal antibiotic	Blocks the passage of electrons through the **cytochrome b-c_1 complex.**
Complex IV	**Cyanide** and **carbon monoxide (CO)**	Combine with **cytochrome oxidase** and **block the transfer of electrons to O_2**
	2-4-Dinitrophenol	An **ionophore** that allows protons from the cytosol to reenter the matrix without going through the pore in the ATP synthase complex. It is an **uncoupler, increasing** the rate of O_2 consumption (respiration), **electron transport**, the tricarboxylic acid cycle, and CO_2 production, while **generating heat, rather than energy.**
ATP Synthase	**Oligomycin**	**Binds to the stalk of the ATP synthase**, preventing proton reentry into the mitochondrial matrix. **Also acts as an uncoupler**
ATP-ADP antiport	**Atractyloside**, a plant toxin	Results in the depletion of mitochondrial ADP and the eventual depletion termination of ATP synthesis

III. REACTIVE OXYGEN SPECIES

A. **Oxygen radicals** (Figure 5-13)
1. Molecules with **extra electrons on the oxygen** are **free radicals**.
2. They are often a **byproduct** of normal metabolic pathways of **oxidative metabolism**.

B. **Sources of reactive oxygen species (ROS)**
1. **CoQ of the ETC**
   a. CoQ occasionally loses an electron in the transfer of reducing equivalents though the electron chain.
   b. This **electron is transferred** to dissolved O_2 for the production of **superoxide**.
   c. CoQ is the major source of superoxide within the cell.
2. **Production of ROS in the peroxisome**
   a. **Fatty oxidation** occurs within these organelles with the transfer of **2 electrons from FADH$_2$ to O$_2$**.
   b. **H$_2$O$_2$, hydrogen peroxide**, is formed within the peroxisome.
3. **Cytochrome P-450 mono-oxygenases**
   a. This group of enzymes is involved in the **detoxification of various drugs** that enter the body.
   b. The enzyme catalyses the transfer of electrons from **NADPH** (the reduced form of nicotinamide adenine dinucleotide phosphate) to O_2 and the various substrates to be detoxified.

> **CLINICAL CORRELATES** Consumption of alcohol and certain drugs induces expression of various cytochrome mono-oxidases. Patients who abuse such substances are more prone to the **deleterious effects of ROS** formed by these **P-450** enzymes.

   c. Free radical intermediates in these conversions are often created by "**leakage**" of electrons as the reactions take place.
4. **NADPH oxidase** (Figure 5-14)
   a. This enzyme is embedded in the membrane of the **phagolysosome within immune cells**.

> **CLINICAL CORRELATES** Chronic granulomatous disease (CGD) results from a deficiency of **NADPH oxidase** and the inability to effectively kill engulfed microbes, especially bacteria. Patients with CGD present with **serious recurrent bacterial infections**.

   b. Electrons are transferred from **NADPH to O$_2$** to form **superoxide**.
   c. The superoxide is used to **kill engulfed microbes** within the cell.
5. **Myeloperoxidase (MPO)** (Figure 5-14)
   a. This enzyme, too, is an important enzyme in immune cells, particularly **neutrophils**.

> **CLINICAL CORRELATES** The H$_2$O$_2$-MPO-halide system is one of the **most effective mechanisms for killing bacteria** within neutrophils. However, patients with defects in this system have **near-normal immune function** because bacteria are killed, albeit slower, by **superoxide** produced by the action of **NADPH oxidase**.

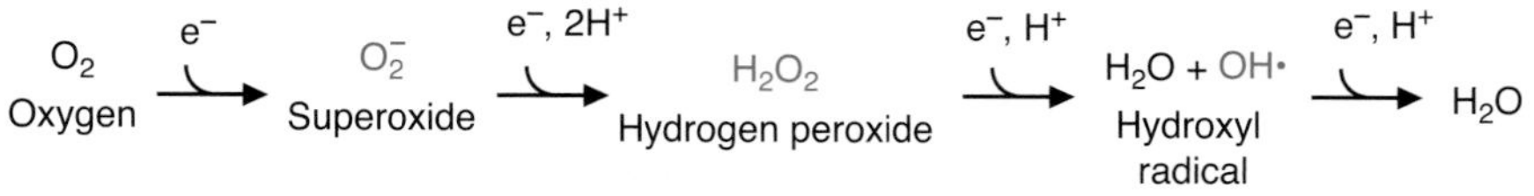

$$O_2 \xrightarrow{e^-} O_2^- \xrightarrow{e^-, 2H^+} H_2O_2 \xrightarrow{e^-, H^+} H_2O + OH\cdot \xrightarrow{e^-, H^+} H_2O$$

Oxygen · Superoxide · Hydrogen peroxide · Hydroxyl radical

FIGURE 5-13 The reduction of oxygen by four 1-electron steps with the creation of reactive oxygen species along the pathway.

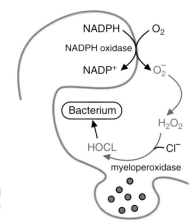

FIGURE 5-14 The generation of superoxide (O_2^-) and hypochlorous acid (HOCl) by NADPH oxidase and myeloperoxidase, respectively, within a neutrophil.

     b. It catalyzes the formation of hypochlorous acid (HOCl) from H_2O_2 in the presence of a halide ion, such as **chloride**.

  6. Ionizing radiation
     a. High-energy cosmic rays and human-made x-rays can deliver enough energy to split water into hydroxyl and hydrogen radicals.
     b. These radicals go on to damage tissue in mechanisms described later.

C. Deleterious effects of ROS (Figure 5-15)
  1. ROS chemically modify various biomolecules within the cell, causing deleterious effects and even cell death.
  2. Damage to lipids
     a. Free radicals can cause peroxidation of lipids.

CLINICAL CORRELATES The organic solvent **carbon tetrachloride** (CCl_4) is used in the **dry cleaning industry**. The P-450 cytochrome system converts CCL_4 to the free radical species $CCl_3\bullet$. This highly reactive species causes a chain reaction of **lipid peroxidation**, particularly in the liver, that leads to **hepatocellular necrosis**.

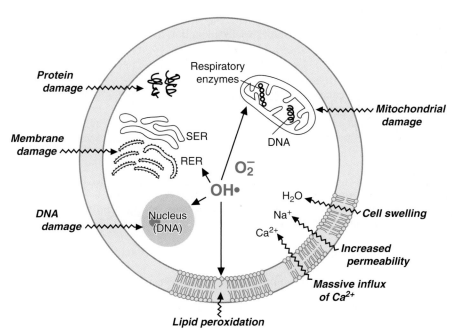

FIGURE 5-15 Free radical–induced cellular injury. O^-_2, superoxide; OH·, hydrogen radical.

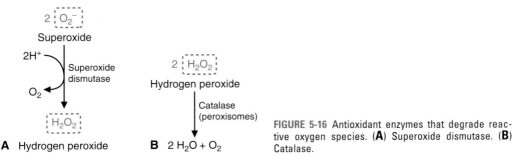

FIGURE 5-16 Antioxidant enzymes that degrade reactive oxygen species. (**A**) Superoxide dismutase. (**B**) Catalase.

    b. Lipid membranes become damaged, leading to increased cell permeability, influx of calcium (an important cofactor for proteolytic enzymes), and cell swelling.

  3. Peptide and protein damage

    a. ROS species react with iron and sulfur moieties of proteins, including sulfhydryl groups, methionine, ferredoxin, and heme.

    b. Oxidative decarboxylation, deamination of proteins, and cleavage of peptide bonds can occur.

  4. Damage to DNA

    a. ROS cause alteration in the nucleotide bases of the DNA molecule.

    b. ROS cause **breaks in the deoxyribose backbone**.

    c. DNA damage, if not repaired, often results in programmed cell death.

D. Antioxidants, the cell's defense against ROS

  1. The cell has developed enzymes and other molecules to help protect itself from the deleterious effects of ROS.

  2. Superoxide dismutase (SOD) (Figure 5-16A)

> **CLINICAL CORRELATES** Some patients with familial forms of **amyotrophic lateral sclerosis (ALS**, or **Lou Gehrig's disease)** have mutations in the intracellular forms of **SOD**. This disease is characterized by **progressive ascending paralysis**, with eventual death from **respiratory failure**.

    a. Isozymes of this enzyme are found in the mitochondria, cytosol, and even extracellularly.

    b. SOD catalyzes the conversion of superoxide anion to H_2O_2 **and** O_2.

  3. Catalase (Figure 5-16B)

> **CLINICAL CORRELATES** Many **bacterial pathogens**, such as *Staphylococcus*, produce **catalase**. These pathogens are of particular concern in patients **who lack NADPH oxidase**, as in those individuals hydrogen peroxide is the major agent that kills phagocytosed bacteria. Thus, infections involving catalase-positive organisms can be very deleterious in these patients, as the hydrogen peroxide will be degraded.

    a. This enzyme promotes the conversion of H_2O_2 to H_2O and O_2.

    b. This enzyme is mainly found within **peroxisomes**, where it protects the cell from the **endogenous production of hydrogen peroxide**.

  4. Glutathione

    a. Glutathione is a **tripeptide** that is oxidized to **donate reducing equivalents** to regenerate **oxidized cellular molecules**.

    b. Glutathione is generated as part of the γ-glutamyl cycle. It is most concentrated in the liver.

Review Test

Directions: Each of the numbered questions or incomplete statements in this section is followed by answers or by completions of the statement. Select the **one** lettered answer or completion that is **best** in each case.

1. A biochemistry graduate student isolates all the enzymes of the TCA cycle and adds OAA and acetyl CoA, including the appropriate energy precursors, cofactors, and water. Which of the following will not be a direct product of his experiment?

(A) ATP
(B) GTP
(C) NADH
(D) CO_2
(E) $FADH_2$

2. A 24-year-old woman presents with diarrhea, dysphagia, jaundice, and white transverse lines on the fingernails (Mee lines). The patient is diagnosed with arsenic poisoning, which inhibits which one of the following enzymes?

(A) Citrate synthase
(B) Isocitrate dehydrogenase
(C) Pyruvate dehydrogenase
(D) Malate dehydrogenase
(E) Succinate dehydrogenase

3. A 3-year-old boy presents to the pediatric clinic with the symptoms of hypotonia, lactic acidosis, and seizures. After an extensive workup, he is diagnosed with PDHC deficiency, an X-linked recessive disorder. Which one of the following cofactors is *not* required by this enzyme to convert pyruvate to acetyl CoA?

(A) Thiamine
(B) Lipoic acid
(C) Pantothenate
(D) Niacin
(E) Ascorbic acid

4. A medicinal chemist working for a pharmaceutical company is synthesizing the barbiturate, barbital, for a clinical trial. In the following pathway for the synthesis of the barbital, which substrate is most likely to inhibit the only membrane-bound enzyme of the Krebs cycle?

(A)   **(B)**   **(C)**   **(D)**   **(E)**

5. A 3-year-old boy presents to the emergency room after having a generalized tonic-clonic seizure. The child has a history of epilepsy, ataxia, and lactic acidosis. When questioned, the parents state that their child was born with a rare metabolic disease, pyruvate carboxylase deficiency. Which one of the following metabolites is this child unable to produce effectively?

(A) Pyruvate
(B) Alanine
(C) Acetyl CoA
(D) Oxaloacetate
(E) Acetoacetate

6. MELAS is a mitochondrial disorder characterized by mitochondrial encephalopathy, lactic acidosis, and strokelike episodes. If a cell were to contain 100% nonfunctional mitochondria, what would be the net ATP yield that would be produced from 1 mole of glucose?

(A) 1 mole
(B) 2 moles
(C) 4 moles
(D) 8 moles
(E) 0 moles

7. A scientist is studying oxidative phosphorylation in intact, carefully isolated mitochondria. Upon adding an oxidizable substrate, such as pyruvate, a constant rate of oxygen utilization is noted. The scientist then adds a compound that greatly enhances the rate of oxygen consumption. This compound is most likely which one of the following?

(A) Rotenone
(B) Carbon monoxide
(C) Antimycin

(D) Cyanide
(E) Dinitrophenol

8. A 53-year-old, previously successful man recently lost his job and is under investigation for racketeering. His wife returns home to find him slumped over the steering wheel of his idling car in the closed garage. He is unresponsive and has a cherry color to his lips and cheeks. Which of the following is inhibited by the carbon monoxide in the car's exhaust fumes?

(A) Complex I of the ETC
(B) Cytochrome oxidase
(C) The ATP-ADP antiporter
(D) The F_0 component of the F_0-F_1 ATPase
(E) The F_1 component of the F_0-F_1 ATPase

9. An 8-year-old boy is seen by an ophthalmologist for vision difficulties, and the physician notices a slowing of the boy's eye movements. The ophthalmologist finds ophthalmoplegia and pigmentary retinopathy and suspects the child has Kearns-Sayre syndrome. Assuming that the defect in this disorder is due to a mutation in complex II of the ETC, electron transfer from which substrate would be impaired?

(A) Malate
(B) α-Ketoglutarate
(C) Isocitrate
(D) Succinate
(E) Pyruvate

10. A 6-year-old child has been suffering from muscle weakness that has progressively worsened over the past 6 months. Measurement of oxygen consumption with mitochondria isolated from a muscle biopsy revealed normal rates of succinate oxidation but very poor rates of pyruvate oxidation. Assays conducted on extracts of the mitochondria revealed normal malate dehydrogenase and PDH activities. The patient may have a mutation in a mitochondrial gene encoding a subunit of which of the following?

(A) Complex I
(B) Complex II
(C) Complex III
(D) Complex IV
(E) ATP synthase

11. A 58-year-old man develops progressive lower extremity weakness, slurring of his words, and weakness of his hands. A neurologist performs a thorough workup, confirming the diagnosis of ALS. The patient recalls that his father had similar symptoms and eventually died of respiratory failure. Some patients with the familial form of ALS have a defect in the enzyme that normally catalyzes which of the following reactions?

(A) The conversion of peroxide to water and oxygen
(B) The conversion of superoxide to hydrogen peroxide and water
(C) The conversion of carbon tetrachloride to the $CCL_3·$ radical
(D) The regeneration of oxidized hemoglobin (methemoglobin)
(E) The conversion of carbonic acid to carbon dioxide and water

Answers and Explanations

1. **The answer is A.** The Krebs cycle does not directly produce ATP. The one substrate level phosphorylation reaction in the cycle generates GTP (the step catalyzed by succinate thiokinase). NADH is generated at three steps (catalyzed by isocitrate dehydrogenase, α-ketoglutarate dehydrogenase, and malate dehydrogenase) and $FADH_2$ at one step (catalyzed by succinate dehydrogenase). CO_2 is a product of the isocitrate and α-ketoglutarate dehydrogenase reactions.

2. **The answer is C.** Arsenic binds the sulfhydryl groups of lipoic acid, creating an inactive 6-membered ring. Because lipoic acid is one of the three cofactors of PDH, this inactivates the enzyme's ability to synthesize acetyl CoA from pyruvate. Because α-ketoglutarate dehydrogenase also utilizes lipoic acid, its activity would also be inhibited by arsenic. Citrate synthase is not inhibited by arsenic. The other dehydrogenases listed as answer choices—isocitrate dehydrogenase, malate dehydrogenase, and succinate dehydrogenase—do not require lipoic acid and are not directly inhibited by arsenic.

3. **The answer is E.** Ascorbic acid is a required cofactor for the hydroxylation reactions that occur in collagen formation. It has no role in TCA cycle reactions. The PDHC utilizes the other cofactors listed as answers. The conversion of pyruvate to acetyl CoA begins with the decarboxylation of pyruvate, which is bound to the cofactor thiamine pyrophosphate (TPP). The next reaction of the complex is the transfer of the 2-carbon acetyl group from acetyl TPP to lipoic acid, the covalently bound coenzyme of lipoyl transacetylase. The enzyme dihydrolipoyl dehydrogenase, with FAD as a cofactor, catalyzes the oxidation of the two sulfhydryl groups of lipoic acid. The final activity of the PDHC is the transfer of reducing equivalents from the $FADH_2$ of dihydrolipoyl dehydrogenase to NAD^+, forming FAD and NADH.

4. **The answer is A.** Succinate dehydrogenase is the only membrane-bound enzyme of the Krebs cycle. Malonate (choice A) resembles succinate (it is lacking a methylene group as compared to succinate) and binds to the active site of succinate dehydrogenase, yet it is not oxidized owing to the absence of an ethyl group between the carboxyl groups. Ethyl oxide and ethyl iodine (choice B) act as nucleophiles but have no inhibitory effects on the Krebs cycle. Diethyl ethyl malonate (choice C), urea (choice D), and barbital (choice E) differ greatly from the endogenous substrate succinate and, therefore, would likely not inhibit the enzyme.

5. **The answer is D.** Pyruvate carboxylase is a biotin-dependent mitochondrial enzyme that converts pyruvate to OAA. In the absence of pyruvate carboxylase activity, OAA can only be produced from the transamination of aspartate, so OAA levels cannot be replenished effectively. Pyruvate production is normal, and as pyruvate accumulates, lactate is formed. Alanine is also formed from pyruvate via a transamination reaction. The PDHC will convert pyruvate to acetyl CoA. Acetoacetate is a ketone body, which is made from acetyl CoA.

6. **The answer is B.** Mitochondria contain both the TCA cycle and the ETC. Therefore, diseases that compromise and fully reduce mitochondrial activity will result in energy production solely through glycolysis. This net energy production per mole of glucose is 2 moles of ATP and 2 moles of NADH, which are unable to undergo further oxidation via mitochondrial oxidative phosphorylation. The NADH will reduce pyruvate to form lactate such that glycolysis can continue. The ''L'' in MELAS stands for lactic acidosis.

7. **The answer is E.** An uncoupler was added to the mitochondria to greatly increase the rate of oxygen consumption. Dinitrophenol will allow free proton diffusion across the inner mitochondrial membrane, thereby dissipating the proton gradient and preventing ATP synthesis. Without an existing proton gradient to ''push'' against, electron flow through the electron transport chain is accelerated, resulting in enhanced oxygen consumption. Rotenone inhibits electron transfer from complex I to coenzyme Q. Carbon monoxide and cyanide block complex IV from

accepting electrons. Antimycin blocks electron flow from complex III. Since electron flow is blocked using rotenone, carbon monoxide, cyanide, or antimycin, oxygen uptake will cease.

8. **The answer is B.** In addition to binding the iron in hemoglobin and impairing oxygen transport, carbon monoxide also terminates cellular respiration by inhibiting cytochrome oxidase, which contains a heme iron. Amytal, a barbiturate, inhibits complex I of the ETC. There are no iron-containing cytochromes in complex I because complex I contains proteins with iron-sulfur centers. The ATP-ADP antiporter is inhibited by the plant toxin atractyloside. The F_0 component of the F_0-F_1 ATPase is inhibited by the drug oligomycin. There is no inhibitor for the F_1 component of the proton-translocating ATPase.

9. **The answer is D.** Succinate feeds electrons into complex II, which, in this case, would be impaired. The other substrates listed, malate, α-ketoglutarate, isocitrate, and pyruvate, all feed their electrons via NADH through complex I. Malate dehydrogenase, α-ketoglutarate dehydrogenase, isocitrate dehydrogenase, and PDH all generate NADH during the course of the reactions that they catalyze.

10. **The answer is A.** PDH activity was normal, which produces NADH, but oxidation of pyruvate was impaired, which suggests a defect in the sequence of electron flow from complex I, to coenzyme Q, to complex III, then IV, then to oxygen. Because succinate oxidation was normal, a defect in complex I is strongly suspected. Succinate oxidation transfers electrons from complex II to coenzyme Q, then to complex III, on to complex IV, and finally on to molecular oxygen, generating water. Because succinate oxidation is normal, electron flow through complexes II, III, and IV is normal. This localizes the defect to electron flow within complex I. If the ATP synthase were defective, neither pyruvate or succinate oxidation would be normal because oxidation and phosphorylation are coupled. The mitochondrial genome encodes subunits of complexes I, III, and IV and the ATP synthase, but not complex II.

11. **The answer is B.** Some patients with the familial form of ALS have mutations in the enzyme SOD, which normally catalyzes the conversion of superoxide to hydrogen peroxide and water. Catalase, in turn, converts the hydrogen peroxide to water and oxygen. Carbon tetrachloride (CCl_4), used in the dry cleaning business, is converted to the hepatotoxic free radical CCL_3· by the cytochrome P-450 system. Carbonic anhydrase stimulates the conversion of carbonic acid to carbon dioxide and water. Methemoglobin reductase, which utilizes NADPH, can reduce oxidized hemoglobin (methemoglobin, in which the iron is in the +3 state) to its normal state (in which iron is in the +2 state). Glutathione can also be used to regenerate hemoglobin from methemoglobin.

chapter 6

Glycogen Metabolism

I. OVERVIEW OF GLYCOGEN STRUCTURE AND METABOLISM (FIGURE 6-1)

A. Glycogen, the major storage form of carbohydrate in animals, consists of chains of α-1,4–linked D-glucose residues with branches that are attached by α-1,6 linkages (Figure 6-2).

B. Glycogen is synthesized from glucose.

C. Glycogen degradation produces glucose 1-phosphate as the major product, but free glucose is also formed.

D. Liver glycogen is used to maintain blood glucose during fasting or exercise.

E. Muscle glycogen is used to generate adenosine triphosphate (ATP) for muscle contraction.

II. GLYCOGEN STRUCTURE (FIGURE 6-2)

A. The **linkages** between glucose residues are α-**1,4** except at branch points, where the linkage is α-**1,6**. Branching is more frequent in the interior of the molecule and less frequent at the periphery, the average being an α-1,6 branch every 8 to 10 residues.

B. One glucose unit, located at the reducing end of each glycogen molecule, is attached to the protein **glycogenin.**

C. The glycogen molecule branches like a tree and has **many nonreducing ends** at which addition and release of glucose residues occur during synthesis and degradation, respectively.

III. GLYCOGEN SYNTHESIS

A. Synthesis of uridine diphosphate (UDP)-glucose (Figure 6-3)
   1. UDP-glucose is the precursor to glycogen synthesis.
   2. Glucose enters cells and is phosphorylated to glucose 6-phosphate by the enzyme **hexokinase** (or by **glucokinase** in the liver). ATP provides the phosphate group.
   3. **Phosphoglucomutase** converts glucose 6-phosphate to glucose 1-phosphate.

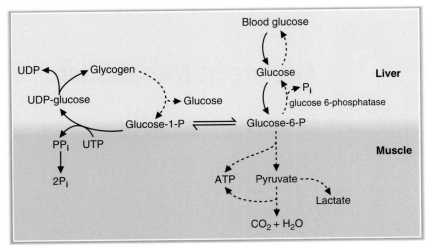

FIGURE 6-1 Overview of glycogen synthesis and degradation. *Solid arrows*, glycogen synthesis; *broken arrows*, glycogen degradation, glucose release in the liver, and glucose 6-phosphate utilization in the muscle; ATP, adenosine triphosphate; P, phosphate; P_i, inorganic phosphate; PP_i, inorganic pyrophosphate; UDP, uridine diphosphate; UTP, uridine triphosphate.

   4. Glucose 1-phosphate reacts with uridine triphosphate (UTP), forming **UDP-glucose** in a reaction catalyzed by **UDP-glucose pyrophosphorylase.** Inorganic pyrophosphate (PP_i) is released in this reaction.
   a. PP_i is cleaved by a pyrophosphatase to two inorganic phosphates (P_i).
   b. This removal of product helps to drive the process in the direction of glycogen synthesis.

B. Action of glycogen synthase (Figure 6-4A)
   1. Glycogen synthase is the key regulatory enzyme for glycogen synthesis. It transfers glucose residues from UDP-glucose to the nonreducing ends of a glycogen primer.
   2. UDP is released and reconverted to UTP by reaction with ATP.

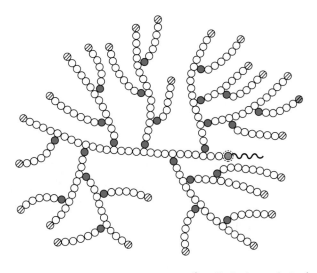

○ Glucose residue linked α-1,4   ⬤〰 Reducing end attached
                                          to glycogenin

⬤ Glucose residue linked α-1,6   ⊘ Nonreducing ends   **FIGURE 6-2** The structure of glycogen.

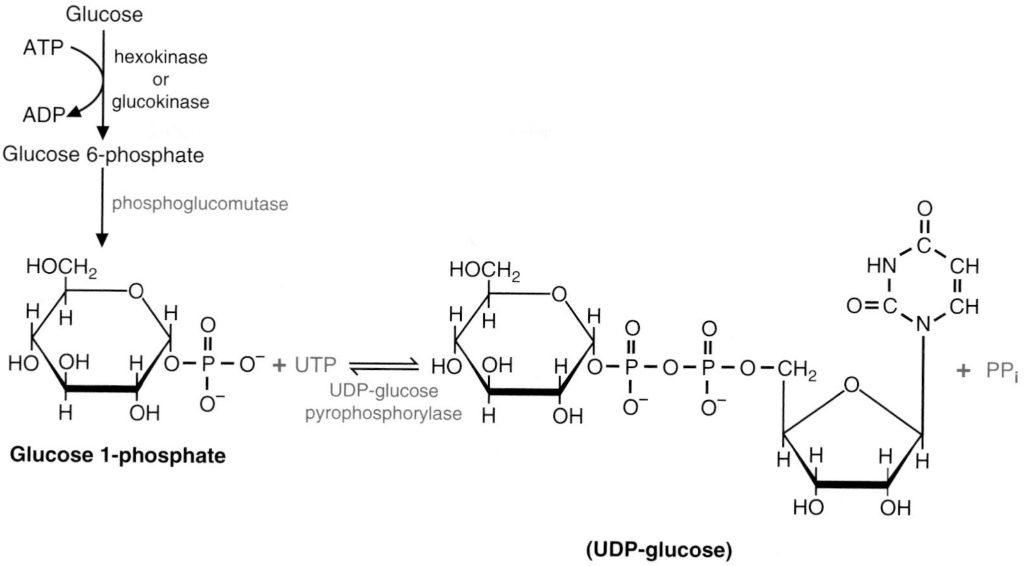

FIGURE 6-3 Formation of uridine diphosphate (UDP)-glucose from glucose. ADP, adenosine diphosphate; ATP, adenosine triphosphate; PP_i, inorganic pyrophosphate.

CLINICAL CORRELATES Genetic deficiency of **glycogen synthase** is also known as a **type 0** glycogen storage disease (GSD). This inborn error in metabolism results in **fasting hypoglycemia** with **occasional muscle cramping**. It can usually be managed with frequent meals and feeding of uncooked cornstarch to **prevent overnight hypoglycemia**.

---

3. The primers, which are attached to glycogenin, are glycogen molecules that were partially degraded in the liver during fasting or in muscle and liver during exercise.

C. **Formation of branches** (Figure 6-4A)
   1. When a chain contains 11 or more glucose residues, an **oligomer,** 6 to 8 residues in length, is removed from the nonreducing end of the chain. It is **reattached** via an α-**1,6 linkage** to a glucose residue within an α-1,4–linked chain.
   2. These branches are formed by the branching enzyme, a **glucosyl 4:6 transferase** that breaks an α-1,4 bond and forms an α-1,6 bond.
   3. The new branch points are at least 4 residues and an average of 7 to 11 residues from previously existing branch points.

CLINICAL CORRELATES **Andersen disease**, a **type IV** GSD, results from a genetic **deficiency of this branching enzyme**. Children **fail to thrive**. There is not an increased accumulation of glycogen, but rather, the **glycogen has very long outer branches**. This structural abnormality leads to a reduced solubility of the glycogen, causing progressive scarring of the liver (**cirrhosis**), which leads to death at about 5 years of age.

D. **Growth of glycogen chains**
   1. Glycogen synthase continues to add glucose residues to the **nonreducing ends** of newly formed branches as well as to the ends of the original chains.
   2. As the chains continue to grow, additional branches are produced by the branching enzyme.

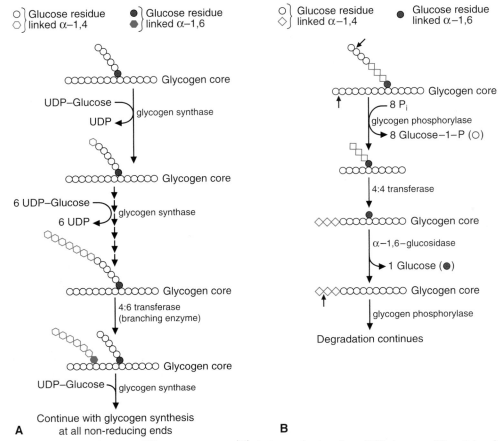

FIGURE 6-4 Glycogen synthesis **(A)** and degradation **(B)**. P_i, inorganic phosphate; UDP-glucose, uridine diphosphate glucose.

IV. GLYCOGEN DEGRADATION (FIGURE 6-4B)

A. Action of glycogen phosphorylase

1. **Glycogen phosphorylase**—the key regulatory enzyme for glycogen degradation—removes glucose residues, one at a time, from the nonreducing ends of glycogen molecules.

CLINICAL CORRELATES   A genetic deficiency of **liver phosphorylase** results in **Hers disease**, a type VI GSD. Because a complete deficiency of this enzyme would be fatal, patients typically have **partial deficiency of the protein**. As such, the disease can present with **extreme enlargement of the liver**, as a result of glycogen accumulation. However, some patients present with **only mild hypoglycemia** or no symptoms at all.

CLINICAL CORRELATES   **Muscle phosphorylase deficiency, McArdle disease**, is a type V GSD. The disorder presents with **exercise-induced cramps and pain secondary to rhabdomyolysis**. Most patients live normally, avoiding strenuous exercise; however, severe rhabdomyolysis leading to **myoglobinuria** can lead to life-threatening **renal failure**.

2. Phosphorylase uses P_i to cleave α-1,4 bonds, producing **glucose 1-phosphate**.

3. Phosphorylase can continue to hydrolyze α-1,4 linkages until it reaches a point four glucose units from an α-1,6 branch.

B. Removal of branches

1. The four units remaining at a branch are removed by the **debranching enzyme,** which has both glucosyl 4:4 transferase and α-1,6-glucosidase activity.

2. Three of the four glucose residues that remain at the branch point are removed as a trisaccharide and are attached to the nonreducing end of another chain by a **4:4 transferase,** which cleaves an α-1,4 bond and forms a new α-1,4 bond.

3. The last glucose unit at the branch point, which is linked α-1,6, is hydrolyzed by α-**1,6-glucosidase,** forming free glucose.

CLINICAL CORRELATES **Cori disease**, a type III GSD, results from a **deficiency of debranching enzyme**. Type IIIa is a deficiency of both liver and muscle enzymes and manifests with **hepatomegaly, hypoglycemia during fasting**, and **myopathy;** it is managed by **small meals** or continuous nasogastric feeding. The rarer type IIIb disease is a deficiency of the liver enzyme only, with no muscular involvement.

C. Degradation of glycogen chains

1. The **phosphorylase/debranching process is repeated**, generating glucose 1-phosphate and free glucose in about a 10:1 ratio that reflects the length of the chains in the outer region of the glycogen molecule.

D. Fate of glucosyl units released from glycogen (Figure 6-1)

1. In the **liver**, glycogen is degraded to **maintain blood glucose**.

    a. Glucose 1-phosphate is converted by **phosphoglucomutase** to glucose 6-phosphate.

    b. Inorganic phosphate is released from glucose 6-phosphate by **glucose 6-phosphatase**, and free glucose enters the blood. This enzyme also acts in gluconeogenesis.

2. In **muscle**, glycogen is degraded to provide **energy for contraction**.

    a. Phosphoglucomutase converts glucose 1-phosphate to glucose 6-phosphate, which enters the pathway of **glycolysis** and is converted either to lactate or to CO_2 and H_2O through the Krebs tricarboxylic acid cycle, leading to the generation of ATP via oxidative phosphorylation.

    b. Muscle does not contain glucose 6-phosphatase and, therefore, does not contribute to the maintenance of blood glucose.

V. LYSOSOMAL DEGRADATION OF GLYCOGEN

A. Glycogen is degraded by an α-**glucosidase** located in lysosomes.

B. Lysosomal degradation is not necessary for maintaining normal blood glucose levels.

CLINICAL CORRELATES **Pompe disease**, a type II GSD, is a **lysosomal storage disease. Accumulation of glycogen within the lysosome** results in the formation of large lysosomes, which ultimately compromises muscle cellular function. Type IIa is the infantile form that presents with muscle weakness (**floppiness**), **with death by 2 years** secondary to **heart muscle dysfunction**. The milder IIb (juvenile) and IIc (adult) forms have delayed and progressive onset and are dominated by skeletal muscle weakness.

VI. REGULATION OF GLYCOGEN DEGRADATION (FIGURE 6-5)

A. Glucagon, a peptide hormone, acts on liver cells, and **epinephrine** (adrenaline) acts on both liver and muscle cells to stimulate glycogen degradation.
  1. These hormones, via G proteins, activate **adenylate cyclase** in the cell membrane, which converts ATP to **3′,5′-cyclic adenosine monophosphate** (cAMP) (Figure 6-6).
  2. Adenylate cyclase is also called adenyl or adenylyl cyclase. (Step 1)

B. cAMP activates protein kinase A (Figure 6-5), which consists of two regulatory and two catalytic subunits. cAMP binds to the regulatory (inhibitory) subunits, releasing the catalytic subunits in an active form. (Step 2)

C. Protein kinase A phosphorylates **glycogen synthase,** causing it to be less active, thus decreasing glycogen synthesis. (Step 3)

D. Protein kinase A phosphorylates **phosphorylase kinase.** (Step 4)

E. Phosphorylase kinase phosphorylates **phosphorylase b,** converting it to its active form, phosphorylase a. (Step 5)

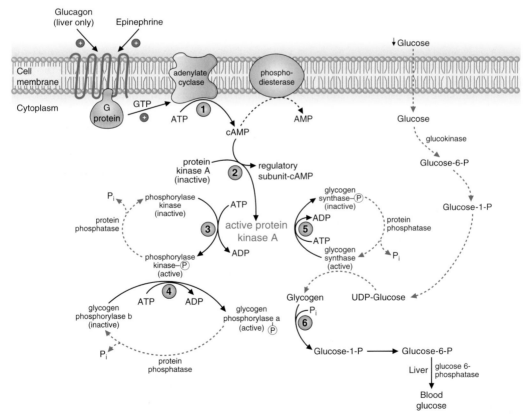

FIGURE 6-5 Hormonal regulation of glycogen synthesis and degradation. *Solid lines* indicate reactions that predominate when glucagon or epinephrine is elevated. Steps 1 through 6, indicated by *circled numbers,* correspond to section VI.A–F in the text. *Dashed lines* indicate reactions that predominate when insulin is elevated. Note that protein kinase A phosphorylates both phosphorylase kinase and glycogen synthase. ADP, adenosine diphosphate; ATP, adenosine triphosphate; cAMP, cyclic adenosine monophosphate; P_i, inorganic phosphate.

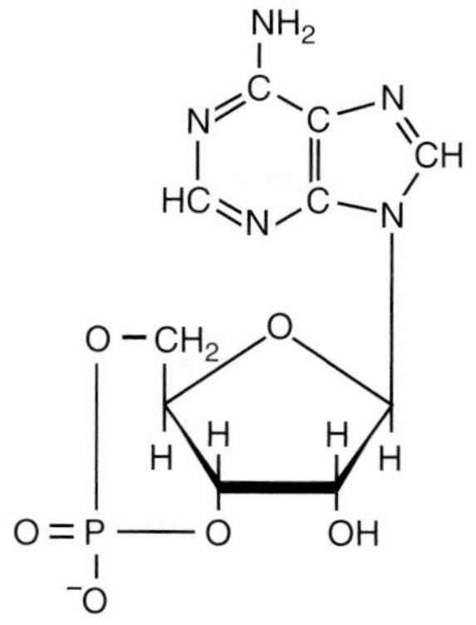

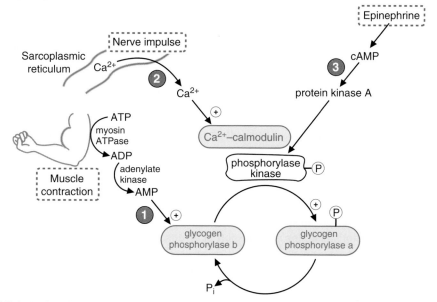

FIGURE 6-6 Cyclic adenosine monophosphate.

F. Phosphorylase a cleaves glucose residues from the nonreducing ends of glycogen chains, producing glucose 1-phosphate, which is oxidized or, in the liver, converted to blood glucose. (Step 6)

G. The cAMP cascade
1. The cAMP-activated process is a cascade in which the initial **hormonal signal is amplified** many times.
2. One hormone molecule, by activating the enzyme adenylate cyclase, produces many molecules of cAMP, which activate protein kinase A.
3. One active protein kinase A molecule phosphorylates many phosphorylase kinase molecules, which convert many molecules of phosphorylase b to phosphorylase a.
4. One molecule of phosphorylase a produces many molecules of glucose 1-phosphate from glycogen.
5. The net result is that one hormone molecule can generate tens of thousands of molecules of glucose 1-phosphate, which form glucose 6-phosphate. Oxidation of many thousands of molecules of glucose 6-phosphate can generate hundreds of thousands of molecules of ATP.

H. Additional **regulatory mechanisms in muscle** (Figure 6-7)
1. In addition to cAMP-mediated regulation, **adenosine monophosphate (AMP)** and **Ca^{2+}** stimulate glycogen breakdown in muscle.

FIGURE 6-7 Activation of muscle glycogen phosphorylase during exercise. ADP, adenosine diphosphate; AMP, adenosine monophosphate; ATP, adenosine triphosphate; cAMP, cyclic adenosine monophosphate.

2. **Phosphorylase b** is activated by the rise in **AMP**, which occurs during muscle contraction by the following reactions:

$$\text{contraction}$$
$$2\,\text{ATP} \rightarrow 2\,\text{ADP} + 2\,\text{P}_i$$
$$\text{adenylate kinase}$$
$$(\text{myokinase})$$
$$2\,\text{ADP} \rightarrow \text{AMP} + \text{ATP}$$
$$\text{Sum: ATP} \rightarrow \text{AMP} + 2\,\text{P}_i$$

3. **Phosphorylase kinase** is activated by Ca^{2+}, which is released from the sarcoplasmic reticulum during muscle contraction.
4. Ca^{2+} binds to **calmodulin,** which serves as a subunit of phosphorylase kinase.

CLINICAL CORRELATES Deficiency of **phosphorylase kinase** is a type IX GSD. It most commonly results in **hepatomegaly, growth retardation, delayed motor development,** and **increased blood lipids**. Phosphorylase kinase is a **complex enzyme,** consisting of multiple subunits that are encoded by different genes, located on separate chromosomes. Several different subtypes of this disease have been identified. The most common form is the **X-linked form**.

VII. REGULATION OF GLYCOGEN SYNTHESIS (FIGURE 6-5)

A. Factors that promote glycogen synthesis in the liver
   1. **Insulin**, a pancreatic peptide hormone, is elevated after a meal and stimulates the synthesis of glycogen in liver and muscle.
   2. In the **fed state**, glycogen degradation decreases because **glucagon** is **low**, and the cAMP cascade is not activated.
      a. cAMP is converted to AMP by a cell membrane **phosphodiesterase**.
      b. As **cAMP decreases,** the regulatory subunits rejoin the catalytic subunits of **protein kinase A,** and the enzyme is **inactivated**.
      c. **Dephosphorylation** of phosphorylase kinase and phosphorylase a causes these enzymes to be inactivated. **Insulin** causes activation of the **phosphatases** that dephosphorylate these enzymes.
   3. **Glycogen synthesis** is promoted by activation of **glycogen synthase** and by the increased concentration of glucose, which enters liver cells from the hepatic portal vein.
      a. The inactive, phosphorylated form of glycogen synthase is dephosphorylated, causing the enzyme to become active.
      b. **Insulin** causes activation of the **phosphatase** that catalyzes this reaction.

B. Factors that promote glycogen synthesis in muscle
   1. After a meal, muscle will have low levels of cAMP, AMP, and Ca^{2+} (if the muscle is not contracting), all agents that stimulate glycogen degradation. In addition, epinephrine, another agent that activates glycogenolysis, is low. Consequently, muscle glycogen degradation will not occur.
   2. **Insulin stimulates glycogen synthesis** by mechanisms similar to those in the liver.
   3. In addition, **insulin stimulates the transport of glucose** into muscle cells, providing increased substrate for glycogen synthesis.

Review Test

Directions: Each of the numbered questions or incomplete statements in this section is followed by answers or by completions of the statement. Select the **one** lettered answer or completion that is **best** in each case.

1. A newborn is found to have fasting hypoglycemia. The nursery staff begins overnight feeds by nasogastric tube because they find that the child has consistently low blood sugars. A liver biopsy and molecular studies demonstrate an absence of glycogen synthase. The normal function of this enzyme is to do which of the following?

(A) Remove glucose residues one at a time from glycogen in the liver
(B) Remove glucose residues one at a time from glycogen in muscles
(C) Transfer glucose from UDP-glucose to the nonreducing end of a glycogen primer
(D) Hydrolyze α-1,6 bonds of glycogen
(E) Function as a glucosyl 4:6 transferase

2. A newborn is experiencing failure to thrive. On physical examination, organomegaly is appreciated owing to accumulation of glycogen in the lysosomes of several organs, including the heart, muscle, and liver. You diagnose the condition as Pompe disease. Which one of the following biochemical deficits is seen in this disorder?

(A) A deficiency of glycogenin
(B) Loss of α-1,6-glucosidase activity
(C) Loss of glucose 6-phosphatase activity
(D) Loss of muscle glycogen phosphorylase activity
(E) Loss of a lysosomal glucosidase activity

3. A second-year medical student decides to do research in a nutrition laboratory that is studying the effects of caffeine on cellular metabolism. Caffeine inhibits cAMP phosphodiesterase. If caffeine were added to liver cells, in the presence of glucagon, which of the following enzymes would be phosphorylated and inactivated?

(A) Phosphorylase kinase
(B) Pyruvate kinase
(C) Phosphorylase
(D) Protein kinase A
(E) Calmodulin

4. A 28-year-old professional cyclist has been training for an opportunity to race in the Tour de France. His coach strongly suggests that he consume carbohydrates after each of his workouts to ensure that his muscle glycogen storage can endure the 28-day race. The activity of muscle glycogen synthase in resting muscles is increased by the action of which of the following?

(A) Epinephrine
(B) Glucagon
(C) Insulin
(D) Phosphorylation
(E) Fasting and starvation

5. A patient had large deposits of liver glycogen, which, after an overnight fast, contained shorter than normal branches. A defective form of which of the following could cause this abnormality?

(A) Glycogen phosphorylase
(B) Glucagon receptor
(C) Glycogenin
(D) Amylo-1,6-glucosidase (α-glucosidase)
(E) Amylo-4,6-transferase (4:6 transferase)

6. A sprinter is trying to optimize his performance. He has calculated that, even under anaerobic conditions, his glycogen stores will supply him with enough energy to last the race. What would the energy difference be between using glucose from a dietary source versus relying solely on glucose from glycogen stores as fuel for his race?

(A) Dietary would give 1 more mole of ATP/glucose
(B) Dietary would give 2 more moles of ATP/glucose
(C) Dietary would give the same ATP/glucose
(D) Dietary would give 1 less mole of ATP/glucose
(E) Dietary would give 2 less moles of ATP/glucose

7. A 32-year-old woman receives anesthesia in preparation for a laparoscopic cholecystectomy. The anesthesiologist notices a subtle twitch of the masseter muscle in the jaw, followed by sinus tachycardia and an increase of the end-expiratory CO_2. He immediately recognizes the early signs of malignant hyperthermia and administers dantrolene. Dantrolene is a muscle relaxant that acts specifically on skeletal muscle by interfering with the release of calcium from the sarcoplasmic reticulum. Which of the following enzymes would be affected by this action?

(A) Phosphoglucomutase
(B) Glucokinase
(C) Glycogen synthase
(D) Glycogen phosphorylase kinase
(E) Glucosyl 4:6 transferase

Answers and Explanations

1. **The answer is C.** Glycogen synthase is the first enzyme in the synthesis of glycogen. It transfers glucose from UDP-glucose to the nonreducing end of a glycogen primer and adds subsequent residues to the growing chain. The removal of glucose residues (answers A and B) during the catabolism of glycogen is mediated by glycogen phosphorylase, a deficiency of which results in Hers disease if in the liver and McArdle disease if in the muscle. Debranching enzyme hydrolyzes α-1,6 bonds of glycogen (answer D). Finally, deficiency of glucosyl 4:6 transferase (the branching enzyme) results in Andersen disease (answer E).

2. **The answer is E.** Pompe disease results from a deficiency of α-1,4-glucosidase (acid maltase), halting the release of glucose from glycogen found in lysosomes. McArdle syndrome is caused by a deficiency in muscle glycogen phosphorylase (answer D), which also cleaves the same α-1,4-glycosidic bond but, instead, presents with muscle symptoms, such as weakness and cramps. The difference between Pompe and McArdle symptoms is that Pompe disease results in a loss of lysosomal function, but not so McArdle disease. Glycogenin initiates glycogen synthesis, and therefore, a deficiency would result in a decrease in glycogen storage. An α-1,6-glucosidase deficiency results in the inability to liberate the 1,6 branch points of glycogen as seen in Cori disease, but does not have lysosomal involvement. Glucose 6-phosphatase deficiency, or von Gierke disease, results in hypoglycemia, hepatomegaly, hyperlipidemia, hyperuricemia, gouty arthritis, nephrolithiasis, and chronic renal failure, without lysosomal involvement.

3. **The answer is B.** Under the conditions of the experiment, cAMP levels would be elevated by glucagon treatment and would remain elevated owing to the presence of caffeine. This leads to constant activation of protein kinase A (PKA). PKA will phosphorylate pyruvate kinase, leading to its inactivation. Phosphorylase kinase and phosphorylase are activated by phosphorylation. PKA is not regulated by phosphorylation but by dissociation of inhibitory subunits that bind to cAMP. Calmodulin is a calcium-binding protein that serves as a subunit of phosphorylase kinase, but is not phosphorylated by PKA.

4. **The answer is C.** Glycogen synthesis occurs at times of rest and when the energy needs of the cells are being met. Of the hormones influencing the storage of glucose, insulin promotes the synthesis of energy stores through the dephosphorylation and activation of glycogen synthase. In fact, a helpful generalization is that glucagon and epinephrine typically mobilize energy stores through the activation of enzymes via direct phosphorylation, whereas insulin accomplishes the opposite. Fasting and starvation will not result in an increase in muscle glycogen stores.

5. **The answer is D.** If, after fasting, the branches were shorter than normal, phosphorylase must be functional and capable of being activated by glucagon. The branching enzyme (the 4:6 transferase) must be normal because branches are present. The protein glycogenin must be present in order for large amounts of glycogen to be synthesized and deposited. The defect most likely is in the debranching enzyme (which contains an α-1,6-glucosidase). If the debrancher is defective, phosphorylase would break the glycogen down to within four glucose residues of the branch points, but complete degradation would not occur. Therefore, short branches would be present in the glycogen. If the short branches contain only one glucose unit, the defect is in the α-1,6-glucosidase activity of the debrancher. If they contain four glucose units, the defect is in the 4:4 transferase activity of the debrancher.

6. **The answer is D.** Dietary glucose would enter the blood as free glucose, be transported into the muscle cell, and then be metabolized through the glycolytic pathway, producing lactate. The net yield would be 2 moles of ATP per mole of glucose metabolized (there is a loss of 2 moles of ATP for the hexokinase and phosphofructokinase-1 steps, and a gain of 4 moles of ATP from the phosphoglycerate kinase and pyruvate kinase steps). Glucose derived from glycogen, however, is

primarily released as glucose 1-phosphate (not free glucose), so the utilization of ATP at the hexokinase step is bypassed, resulting in a net yield of 3 moles of ATP per 1 mole of glucose residues released from glycogen. This calculation ignores the 10% of glucose residues in glycogen that are released as free glucose by the action of the debranching enzyme.

7. **The answer is D.** Glycogen regulation in skeletal muscle versus the liver is matched well to the functions of the muscle and liver. Muscle glycogen functions as storage for mechanical energy needs, whereas liver glycogen functions to maintain blood glucose levels. With regard to regulation, when a motor neuron stimulates the release of calcium from the sarcoplasmic reticulum, the calcium binds to calmodulin and activates glycogen phosphorylase kinase, which in turn activates glycogen phosphorylase. Thus, a reduction in calcium release from the sarcoplasmic reticulum would lead to inactivation of glycogen phosphorylase kinase. None of the other enzymes listed contains a calmodulin subunit, and they would not be regulated by calcium. Glucokinase (in the liver) converts glucose to glucose 6-phosphate. Phosphoglucomutase converts glucose 6-phosphate to glucose 1-phosphate. Glycogen synthase is activated via phosphorylation. Finally, glucosyl 4:6 transferase is the enzyme that creates branches in glycogen.

Gluconeogenesis and the Maintenance of Blood Glucose Levels

chapter **7**

I. OVERVIEW (FIGURE 7-1)

A. Gluconeogenesis, which **occurs mainly in the liver** and to a small degree in the kidney, is the synthesis of glucose from compounds that are not carbohydrates.

B. The major precursors for gluconeogenesis are **lactate, amino acids** (which form pyruvate or tricarboxylic acid [TCA] cycle intermediates), and **glycerol** (which forms dihydroxyacetone phosphate [DHAP]). Even-chain fatty acids do not produce any net glucose.

C. Gluconeogenesis involves several enzymatic steps that do not occur in glycolysis; thus, glucose is **not generated by a simple reversal of glycolysis.**

D. The synthesis of 1 mole of glucose from 2 moles of pyruvate requires the energy equivalent of about 6 moles of adenosine triphosphate (ATP).

E. Blood glucose levels are maintained within a very narrow range, even though the nature of a person's diet may vary widely, and the normal person eats periodically during the day and fasts between meals and at night. Even under circumstances when a person does not eat for extended periods of time, blood glucose levels decrease only slowly.

F. The major hormones that regulate blood glucose are **insulin** and **glucagon.**

G. After a meal, blood glucose is supplied by dietary carbohydrate. However, during fasting, the liver maintains blood glucose levels by the processes of glycogenolysis and gluconeogenesis.

H. All cells use glucose for energy; however, the production of glucose during fasting is particularly important for tissues such as the brain and red blood cells.

I. During exercise, blood glucose is also maintained by liver glycogenolysis and gluconeogenesis.

II. REACTIONS OF GLUCONEOGENESIS

A. Conversion of pyruvate to phosphoenolpyruvate (Figure 7-2)
  1. In the liver, pyruvate is converted to phosphoenolpyruvate (PEP) in two steps.
  2. **Pyruvate** (produced from lactate, alanine, and other amino acids) (Step 1) is first converted to oxaloacetate (OAA) (Step 2) by **pyruvate carboxylase,** a mitochondrial enzyme that requires biotin and ATP.

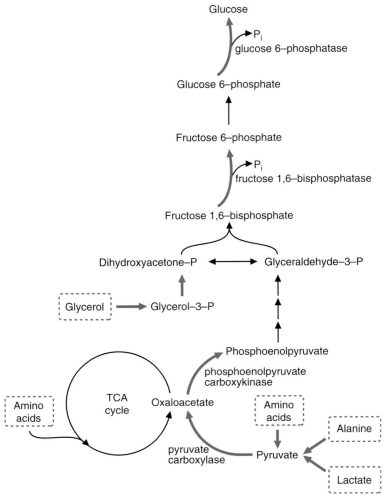

FIGURE 7-1 The key reactions of gluconeogenesis from the precursors alanine, lactate, and glycerol. *Heavy arrows* indicate steps that differ from those of glycolysis. P_i, inorganic phosphate; TCA, tricarboxylic acid cycle.

    a. OAA cannot directly cross the inner mitochondrial membrane.

    b. Therefore, it is converted to malate (Step 3) or to aspartate, which can cross the mitochondrial membrane and be reconverted to OAA in the cytosol.

  3. **OAA** is decarboxylated by **phosphoenolpyruvate carboxykinase (PEPCK)** to form PEP. (Step 4) This reaction requires guanosine triphosphate (GTP).

  4. **PEP** is converted to fructose 1,6-bisphosphate by reversal of the glycolytic reactions (see Figure 7-3).

B. **Conversion of fructose 1,6-bisphosphate to fructose 6-phosphate** (Figure 7-3)

  1. **Fructose 1,6-bisphosphate** is converted to fructose 6-phosphate in a reaction that releases inorganic phosphate and is catalyzed by **fructose-1,6-bisphosphatase (F-1,6-BP).**

  2. Fructose 6-phosphate is converted to glucose 6-phosphate by the same isomerase used in glycolysis.

C. **Conversion of glucose 6-phosphate to glucose**

  1. **Glucose 6-phosphate** releases inorganic phosphate (P_i), which produces free glucose that enters the blood. The enzyme is **glucose 6-phosphatase.**

  2. **Glucose 6-phosphatase** is involved in both **gluconeogenesis and glycogenolysis** (see Figure 6-5).

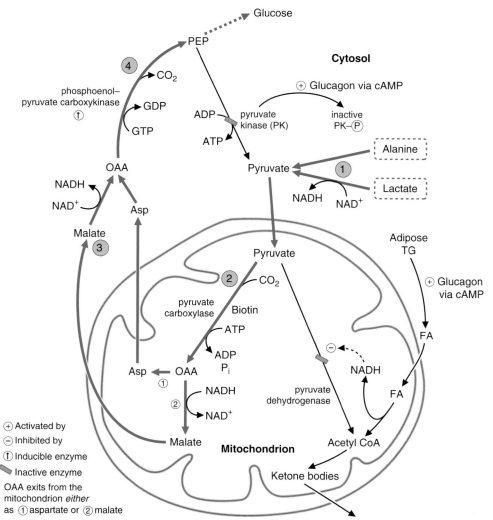

FIGURE 7-2 The conversion of pyruvate to phosphoenolpyruvate (PEP). Follow the diagram by starting with the precursors alanine and lactate (on the *right*). Asp, aspartate; ATP, adenosine triphosphate; cAMP, cyclic adenosine monophosphate; FA, fatty acid; GDP, guanosine diphosphate; GTP, guanosine triphosphate; OAA, oxaloacetate; P_i, inorganic phosphate; TG, triacylglycerol.

CLINICAL CORRELATES Deficiency of **glucose 6-phosphatase, von Gierke disease,** is a type I glycogen storage disease (GSD). Failure to convert glucose 6-phosphate to glucose results in intracellular accumulation of glucose 6-phosphate and **severe hypoglycemia** that can cause **lethargy, seizures,** and **brain damage.** Patients often have **hepatomegaly,** increased bleeding (due to platelet dysfunction), and **growth retardation. Frequent meals** and nighttime nasogastric feedings help control the disease.

D. Regulatory enzymes of gluconeogenesis

1. Under fasting conditions, **glucagon** is elevated and stimulates gluconeogenesis.
   a. Because of changes in the activity of certain enzymes, futile cycles are prevented, and the overall flow of carbon is from pyruvate to glucose (Figures 7-2 and 7-3).
   b. A futile cycle (also known as *substrate cycling*) is the continuous recycling of substrates and products with the net consumption of energy and no useful result.

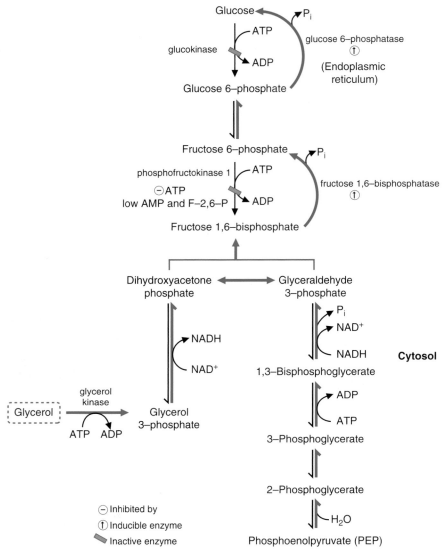

FIGURE 7-3 The conversion of phosphoenolpyruvate and glycerol to glucose. *Heavy arrows* indicate the pathway. F-2,6-P, fructose 2,6-bisphosphate; ADP, adenosine diphosphate; AMP, adenosine monophosphate; ATP, adenosine triphosphate; P_i, inorganic phosphate.

2. **Pyruvate dehydrogenase (PDH)** (Figure 7-2)
    a. Decreased insulin and increased glucagon stimulate the **release of fatty acids** from adipose tissue.
    b. **Fatty acids** travel to the liver and **are oxidized,** producing acetyl coenzyme A (CoA), NADH, and ATP, which cause inactivation of PDH.
    c. Because **PDH** is relatively **inactive,** pyruvate is converted to OAA, not to acetyl CoA.
3. **Pyruvate carboxylase**
    a. Pyruvate carboxylase, which converts pyruvate to OAA, is **activated by acetyl CoA.**
    b. Note that pyruvate carboxylase is active in both the fed and fasting states.
4. **PEPCK**
    a. PEPCK is an **inducible** enzyme.
    b. **Transcription** of the gene encoding PEPCK is stimulated by binding of proteins that are phosphorylated in response to cyclic adenosine monophosphate (cAMP) and by binding of glucocorticoid–protein complexes to regulatory elements in the gene.
    c. Increased production of PEPCK messenger RNA (mRNA) leads to increased translation, resulting in higher PEPCK levels in the cell.

5. **Pyruvate kinase (PK)**
   a. **Glucagon,** via cAMP and protein kinase A, causes PK to be phosphorylated and **inactivated.**
   b. Because PK is relatively inactive, PEP formed from OAA is not reconverted to pyruvate but, in a series of steps, forms fructose 1,6-bisphosphate, which is converted to fructose 6-phosphate.
6. **Phosphofructokinase-1** (Figure 7-3)
   a. Phosphofructokinase-1 is relatively **inactive** because the concentrations of its activators, adenosine monophosphate (AMP) and fructose 2,6-bisphosphate, are low and its inhibitor, ATP, is relatively high owing to the oxidation of fatty acids.
7. **F-1,6-Bisphosphatase**
   a. The level of **fructose 2,6-bisphosphate,** an inhibitor of F-1,6-bisphosphatase, is **low** during fasting. Therefore, F-1,6-bisphosphatase is **more active.**
   b. F-1,6-bisphosphatase is also **induced** in the fasting state.

8. **Glucokinase**
   a. **Glucokinase** is relatively **inactive** because it has a **high K_m** for glucose, and under conditions that favor gluconeogenesis, the glucose concentration is low. Therefore, free glucose is not reconverted to glucose 6-phosphate.

E. **Precursors for gluconeogenesis**
   1. Lactate, amino acids, and glycerol are the major precursors for gluconeogenesis in humans.
   2. **Lactate** is oxidized by NAD^+ in a reaction catalyzed by **lactate dehydrogenase** to form pyruvate, which can be converted to glucose (Figure 7-2). Sources of lactate include red blood cells and exercising muscle.

3. **Amino acids** for gluconeogenesis come from degradation of muscle protein.
   a. Amino acids are released directly into the blood from muscle, or carbons from amino acids are converted to alanine and glutamine and released.
      (1) **Alanine** is also formed by transamination of pyruvate that is derived by oxidation of glucose.
      (2) **Glutamine** is converted to alanine by tissues such as gut and kidney.
   b. Amino acids travel to the liver and provide carbon for gluconeogenesis. Quantitatively, **alanine is the major gluconeogenic amino acid.**
   c. Amino acid **nitrogen** is converted to **urea.**
4. **Glycerol,** which is derived from **adipose** triacylglycerols, reacts with ATP to form glycerol 3-phosphate, which is oxidized to DHAP and converted to glucose (Figure 7-3).

F. Role of fatty acids in gluconeogenesis
  1. **Even-chain fatty acids**
     a. Fatty acids are oxidized to acetyl CoA, which enters the TCA cycle.
     b. For every 2 carbons of acetyl CoA that enter the TCA cycle, 2 carbons are released as CO_2. Therefore, there is **no net synthesis of glucose from acetyl CoA.**
     c. The **PDH** reaction is irreversible; thus, acetyl CoA cannot be converted to pyruvate.
     d. Although even-chain fatty acids do not provide carbons for gluconeogenesis, β-oxidation of fatty acids provides **ATP** that drives gluconeogenesis.
  2. **Odd-chain fatty acids**
     a. The three carbons at the ω-end of an odd-chain fatty acid are converted to propionate.
     b. **Propionate** enters the TCA cycle as succinyl CoA, which forms **malate**, an intermediate in glucose formation (Figure 7-2).

G. Energy requirements for gluconeogenesis
  1. **From pyruvate** (Figures 7-2 and 7-3)
     a. Conversion of pyruvate to OAA by **pyruvate carboxylase** requires 1 mole of ATP.
     b. Conversion of OAA to PEP by phosphoenolpyruvate carboxykinase requires 1 mole of GTP (the equivalent of 1 mole of ATP).
     c. Conversion of 3-phosphoglycerate to 1,3-bisphosphoglycerate by **phosphoglycerate kinase** requires 1 mole of ATP.
     d. Because 2 moles of pyruvate are required to form 1 mole of glucose, **6 moles of high-energy phosphate are required for synthesis of 1 mole of glucose.**
  2. **From glycerol**
     a. Glycerol enters the gluconeogenic pathway at the DHAP level.
     b. Conversion of glycerol to glycerol 3-phosphate, which is oxidized to DHAP, requires 1 ATP.
     c. Because 2 moles of glycerol are required to form 1 mole of glucose, 2 moles of high-energy phosphate are required for synthesis of 1 mole of glucose.

III. MAINTENANCE OF BLOOD GLUCOSE LEVELS

A. Blood glucose levels in the fed state
  1. **Changes in insulin and glucagon levels** (Figure 7-4)
     a. **Blood insulin** levels increase as a meal is digested, following the rise in blood glucose.

CLINICAL CORRELATES   **Decreased production of insulin,** which is usually caused by autoimmune destruction of pancreatic β cells, results in **type 1** (formerly called insulin-dependent) diabetes mellitus. Type 1 diabetes is characterized by **hyperglycemia,** the result of decreased uptake of glucose by cells and increased output of glucose by the liver (due to low insulin and high glucagon levels in the blood). These patients are dependent on exogenous insulin to survive.

CLINICAL CORRELATES   **Decreased release of insulin** from the pancreas or **decreased sensitivity** of tissues to insulin (insulin resistance) results in **type 2** (formerly called non–insulin-dependent) **diabetes mellitus.** This condition also is characterized by **hyperglycemia.**

     (1) Glucose enters the **pancreatic β cells** via the insulin-independent glucose transporter, GLUT-2, which stimulates release of preformed insulin and promotes the synthesis of new insulin.
     (2) Additionally, amino acids (particularly **arginine** and **leucine**) cause the release of preformed insulin from β cells of the pancreas, although to a lesser extent than that released by glucose.

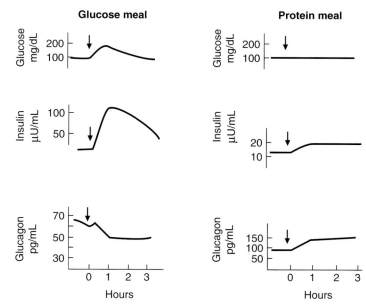

FIGURE 7-4 Changes in blood glucose, insulin, and glucagon levels in response to a glucose or protein meal.

---

    b. Blood glucagon levels change depending on the content of the meal.
      (1) A high-carbohydrate meal causes glucagon levels to decrease.
      (2) A high-protein meal causes glucagon to increase (Figure 7-4).
      (3) On a normal mixed diet, glucagon will remain relatively constant after a meal, while insulin increases.

---

  2. Fate of dietary glucose in the liver
    a. Glucose enters the hepatocyte via the insulin-independent **GLUT-2 transporter.**
    b. Glucose is **oxidized** for energy. Excess glucose is converted to **glycogen** and to the **triacylglycerols** of **very-low-density lipoprotein (VLDL).**
    c. The enzyme **glucokinase** has a **high K_m** for glucose (about 6 mM); thus, its velocity increases after a meal when glucose levels are elevated. On a high-carbohydrate diet, glucokinase is **induced.**
    d. Glycogen synthesis is promoted by insulin, which stimulates the phosphatase that dephosphorylates and activates glycogen synthase.
    e. Synthesis of triacylglycerols is also stimulated. The triacylglycerols are converted to VLDLs and released into the blood.
  3. Fate of dietary glucose in peripheral tissues
    a. All cells oxidize glucose for energy.
    b. Insulin stimulates the **transport** of glucose into **adipose** and **muscle** cells.

    c. In **muscle,** insulin stimulates the synthesis of **glycogen.**
    d. **Adipose** cells convert glucose to the **glycerol** moiety for synthesis of triacylglycerols.
4. **Return of blood glucose to fasting levels**
    a. The **uptake of dietary glucose** by tissues (particularly liver, adipose, and muscle) causes blood glucose to decrease.
    b. **By 2 hours after a meal,** blood glucose has returned to the fasting level of 5 mM or 80 to 100 mg/dL.

B. **Blood glucose levels in the fasting state** (Figure 7-5)
  1. **Changes in insulin and glucagon levels**
    a. During fasting, insulin levels decrease, and glucagon levels increase.
    b. These hormonal changes promote **glycogenolysis** and **gluconeogenesis** in the liver so that blood glucose levels are maintained.

  2. **Stimulation of glycogenolysis**
    a. Within a few hours after a meal, **glucagon** levels increase.
    b. As a result, **glycogenolysis** is stimulated and begins to supply glucose to the blood.
  3. **Stimulation of gluconeogenesis**
    a. **By 4 hours after a meal,** the liver is supplying glucose to the blood via gluconeogenesis and glycogenolysis (Figure 7-6).
    b. Regulatory mechanisms prevent futile cycles from occurring and promote the conversion of gluconeogenic precursors to glucose (Figures 7-2 and 7-3).
  4. **Stimulation of lipolysis** (Figure 7-5)
    a. During fasting, the **breakdown of adipose triacylglycerols** is stimulated, and fatty acids and glycerol are released into the blood.
    b. **Fatty acids** are **oxidized** by certain tissues and converted to **ketone bodies** by the liver. The ATP and NADH produced by β-oxidation of fatty acids promote gluconeogenesis in the liver.
    c. **Glycerol** is a source of carbon for gluconeogenesis in the liver.
  5. **Relative roles of glycogenolysis and gluconeogenesis in maintaining blood glucose** (Figure 7-6)
    a. **Glycogenolysis** is stimulated as blood glucose falls to the fasting level after a meal. It is the main source of blood glucose for the next 8 to 12 hours.
    b. **Gluconeogenesis** is stimulated within a few hours (up to 4 hours) after a meal and supplies an increasingly larger share of blood glucose as the fasting state persists.
    c. By 16 hours of fasting, **gluconeogenesis and glycogenolysis** are about **equal** as sources of blood glucose.

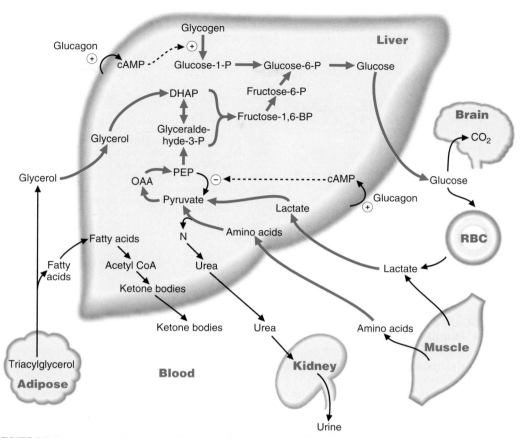

FIGURE 7-5 Tissue interrelationships in glucose production during fasting. Trace the precursors lactate, amino acids, and glycerol to blood glucose. cAMP, cyclic adenosine monophosphate; CoA, coenzyme A; DHAP, dihydroxyacetone phosphate; OAA, oxaloacetate; P, phosphate; PEP, phosphoenolpyruvate; RBC, red blood cell.

    d. As liver glycogen stores become depleted, **gluconeogenesis predominates.**
    e. By about 30 hours of fasting, liver glycogen is depleted, and thereafter, **gluconeogenesis** is the **only source** of blood glucose.

CLINICAL CORRELATES The class of drugs known as **biguanides,** of which **metformin** is an example, is important in the management of **type 2 diabetes mellitus.** Although the mechanism is fairly complex, these drugs work primarily by **inhibiting hepatic gluconeogenesis** because an "average" person with type 2 diabetes has three times the normal rate of gluconeogenesis. The effect of this drug is to **decrease circulating glucose concentrations** in the postabsorptive state.

C. Blood glucose levels during prolonged fasting (starvation)
    1. Even after 5 to 6 weeks of starvation, blood glucose levels are still in the range of 65 mg/dL.
    2. Changes in fuel utilization by various tissues prevent blood glucose levels from decreasing abruptly during prolonged fasting.
    3. The levels of ketone bodies rise in the blood, and the **brain uses ketone bodies** for energy, decreasing its utilization of blood glucose.
    4. The rate of **gluconeogenesis** and, therefore, of **urea** production by the liver **decreases.**
    5. Muscle protein is spared. Less muscle protein is used to provide amino acids for gluconeogenesis.

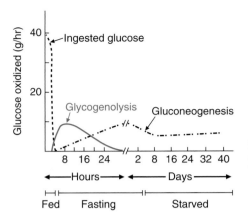

FIGURE 7-6 Sources of blood glucose in fed, fasting, and starved states. Note that the scale changes from hours to days.(Modified from Hanson RW Mehlman MA (eds.): *Gluconeogenesis: Its Regulation in Mammalian Species.* New York, John Wiley & Sons, 1976, p 518. Copyright © 1976 by John Wiley & Sons, Inc. Reprinted with permission from John Wiley & Sons, Inc.)

D. Blood glucose levels during exercise

  1. During exercise, blood glucose is maintained by essentially the same mechanisms that are used during fasting.

  2. Use of endogenous fuels

   a. As the exercising muscle contracts, **ATP** is used.

   b. ATP is regenerated initially from **creatine phosphate.**

   c. Muscle glycogen is oxidized to produce ATP. AMP activates phosphorylase b, and Ca^{2+}-calmodulin activates phosphorylase kinase. The hormone epinephrine causes the production of cAMP, which stimulates glycogen breakdown.

  3. Use of fuels from the blood

   a. As blood flow to the exercising muscle increases, blood glucose and fatty acids are taken up and oxidized by muscle.

   b. As blood glucose levels begin to decrease, the **liver,** by the processes of **glycogenolysis** and **gluconeogenesis,** acts to maintain blood glucose levels.

Review Test

Directions: Each of the numbered questions or incomplete statements in this section is followed by answers or by completions of the statement. Select the **one** lettered answer or completion that is **best** in each case.

Questions 1–4: Referring to the graph at the bottom of the page, match the appropriate types of insulin (questions 1-4) with their serum levels (indicated on the graph as A through D). There is one best answer per question.

1. Ultralente (Humulin U), glargine (Lantus), and detemir (Levemir) insulin

(A)
(B)
(C)
(D)

2. NPH (Humulin N) and Lente (Humulin L) insulin

(A)
(B)
(C)
(D)

3. Lispro (Humalog), aspart (NovoLog), and glulisine (Apidra) insulin

(A)
(B)
(C)
(D)

4. Regular insulin

(A)
(B)
(C)
(D)

5. Which one of the following occurs in an individual who is rested and has fasted for 12 hours?

(A) Gluconeogenesis is the major process by which blood glucose is maintained.
(B) Adenylate cyclase has been inactivated in liver.
(C) Liver glycogen stores have been depleted.
(D) Glycogen phosphorylase, pyruvate kinase, and glycogen synthase are phosphorylated in the liver.
(E) Glycogen synthase has been activated in liver.

6. A 32-year-old bodybuilder has decided to go on a diet consisting of only egg whites to ensure optimal protein for muscle growth. After a few weeks, he notices decreased energy and is found to be hypoglycemic. A nutritionist tells the patient that he most likely has a functional biotin deficiency. Which of the following enzymes is unable to catalyze a key step in synthesizing glucose from pyruvate?

(A) Pyruvate carboxylase
(B) Phosphoenolpyruvate carboxykinase
(C) Fructose 1,6-bisphosphatase
(D) Glucose 6-phosphatase
(E) Phosphoglycerate kinase

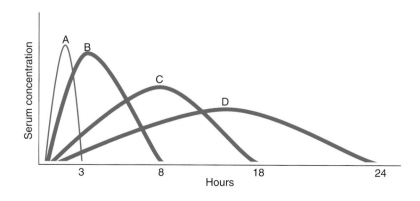

7. A 33-year-old, obese man with an impressive family history of type 2 diabetes is concerned he may develop the disease as well. During a health maintenance examination, his family physician orders several laboratory tests to evaluate the patient. Which of the following results would lead to a diagnosis of diabetes?

(A) A single random glucose level of 190 mg/dL

(B) The presence of a reducing sugar in his urine

(C) A single fasting blood glucose level of 160 mg/dL

(D) A 2-hour oral glucose tolerance test with a blood glucose level of 210 mg/dL

(E) A single fasting blood glucose level of 110 mg/dL

8. A 62-year-old, obese man complains of polydipsia (increased drinking), polyuria (increased urination), and fatigue. A glucose tolerance test confirms the diagnosis of diabetes. He is placed on metformin, which works by which of the following mechanisms?

(A) Inhibiting hepatic gluconeogenesis

(B) Increasing glucagon levels

(C) Increasing cellular responsiveness to circulating insulin

(D) Stimulating the release of preformed insulin

(E) Replacing the need for endogenous insulin

9. A 34-year-old woman presents with central obesity, relatively thin extremities, and purple stria on her abdomen. Further workup reveals an excessive serum cortisol level and a blood sugar level of 258 mg/dL. Which of the following is the most likely cause of her hyperglycemia?

(A) A pancreatic adenoma secreting adrenocorticotropic hormone (ACTH) and glucagon

(B) Glucocorticoid-enhanced transcription of PEPCK

(C) Increased substrates for gluconeogenesis due to excess fatty acid degradation

(D) Cortisol inhibition of insulin secretion

(E) Excess consumption of processed carbohydrates

Answers and Explanations

1. **The answer is D.** Ultralente, glargine (Lantus), and detemir (Levemir) insulin are slow-acting, but long-lived in the circulation, with peak levels occurring 12 to 16 hours after administration. Ultralente is prepared as a small crystal with zinc and a preservative agent, which slows its absorption from the injection site. Lantus is a recombinant insulin analog that differs from human insulin in that the asparagine at position A21 is replaced by glycine, and 2 molecules of arginine have been added to the carboxy terminal of the B-chain. This form of insulin has a solubility optimum of pH 4, so when injected, microprecipitates form, which slows insulin release into the blood. This slow release then leads to the long-acting insulin observed.

2. **The answer is C.** NPH and Lente insulin have a more rapid effect than Ultralente insulin, but they also have a more rapid turnover rate, so they are not as long lived. The crystalline structure of this insulin type is more easily absorbed than the Ultralente preparation.

3. **The answer is A.** Lispro (Humalog), aspart (NovoLog), and glulisine (Apidra) insulins are the most rapidly absorbed insulins, and are rapid acting, but they also exhibit a short half-life in circulation. Lispro is a chemically modified insulin in which amino acids at two positions of the B chain have been reversed; B28-B29 should be proline-lysine, but in lispro, they are lysine-proline. This agent is not crystallized with zinc and is rapidly absorbed from the injection site. Aspart has only a single amino acid different from human insulin; position B28 is aspartic acid instead of proline. This also leads to a more easily absorbed form of insulin.

4. **The answer is B.** Regular insulin peaks in concentration about 4 hours after injection and has a relatively short half-life, becoming absent from the circulation after about 8 hours.

5. **The answer is D.** After 12 hours of fasting, liver glycogen stores are still substantial (liver glycogen stores are not depleted until after about 30 hours of fasting). Glycogenolysis is stimulated by glucagon, which activates adenylate cyclase. The cAMP generated by adenylate cyclase activates protein kinase A, which phosphorylates glycogen phosphorylase kinase, pyruvate kinase (PK), and glycogen synthase. As a result, glycogen phosphorylase is activated, whereas glycogen synthase and PK are inactivated. Gluconeogenesis does not become the major process for maintaining blood glucose until fasting has occurred for 18 to 20 hours.

6. **The answer is A.** Pyruvate carboxylase requires the cofactor biotin to catalyze the irreversible carboxylation of pyruvate to OAA. Although the conversion of OAA to phosphoenolpyruvate is also irreversible and requires energy in the form of GTP, the enzyme catalyzing this step, PEPCK, does not require a cofactor. As with pyruvate carboxylase and PEPCK, F-1,6-bisphosphatase and glucose 6-phosphatase are used to bypass the irreversible steps of glycolysis. Neither of those enzymes requires biotin, which is used exclusively for carboxylation reactions. Phosphoglycerate kinase catalyzes a reversible reaction in which ATP is generated from 1,3-bisphosphoglycerate, or in which ATP is utilized to generate 1,3-bisphosphoglycerate during gluconeogenesis. Because no carboxylation reaction is involved in the phosphoglycerate reaction, biotin is not a required cofactor for that enzyme.

7. **The answer is D.** Of all the test values, the one that renders a diagnosis of diabetes in a single episode is a 2-hour oral glucose tolerance test yielding a blood glucose level of 200 mg/dL at the end of the test. A single random glucose level of more than 200 mg/dL (not 190 mg/dL) with symptoms of diabetes would confirm the diagnosis. Guidelines concerning fasting glucose levels indicate that to diagnose, diabetes fasting blood glucose levels of more than 126 mg/dL need to be observed on at least two occasions. Two fasting blood glucose levels between 100 and 125 mg/dL indicate impaired glucose tolerance, or what has been called prediabetes. The presence of a reducing sugar in the urine is not sufficient criteria for diabetes because patients with benign fructosuria would also be positive in such a test and not necessarily glucose intolerant (diabetic).

8. The answer is A. Metformin, a biguanide, is beneficial in the treatment of type 2 diabetes because it inhibits hepatic gluconeogenesis, which is often increased in patients with type 2 diabetes. No known agent to treat diabetes directly affects the secretion of glucagon. Thiazolidinediones are used in the treatment of diabetes because they increase cellular responsiveness to insulin. Sulfonylureas stimulate the release of preformed insulin. None of these agents completely replaces the need for exogenous insulin in patients with insulin-dependent diabetes.

9. The answer is B. Cushing syndrome results in increased circulating glucocorticoids, primarily cortisol. Glucocorticoids bind to cytosolic receptor proteins that traverse the nuclear envelope and bind to specific sequences in the *PEPCK* gene and cause an increase in *PEPCK* gene expression. PEPCK RNA is translated into PEPCK protein in the cytosol. The increased PEPCK protein levels then catalyze the formation of PEP from OAA, which is an initiating step of gluconeogenesis, resulting in hyperglycemia due to the inappropriate stimulation of gluconeogenesis. Tumors of the pancreas more commonly produce insulin or glucagon. There are documented cases of pancreatic tumors secreting ACTH, but this is much less likely than another form of Cushing syndrome, as described by the patient's signs and symptoms. Fatty acid degradation produces primarily acetyl CoA, which cannot be used to synthesize net glucose. Cortisol actually stimulates insulin secretion, although, paradoxically, it decreases the tissues' sensitivity to the hormone. Excess consumption of carbohydrates, on a short-term basis, does not lead to hyperglycemia because insulin release will lead to glucose uptake by the tissues and a return of blood glucose levels to a normal value.

8 Miscellaneous Carbohydrate Metabolism

I. FRUCTOSE AND GALACTOSE METABOLISM

A. Metabolism of fructose. The major dietary source of fructose is the disaccharide sucrose in table sugar and fruit, but it is also present as the monosaccharide in corn syrup, which is used as a sweetener.

   1. Conversion of fructose to glycolytic intermediates (Figure 8-1)

      a. Fructose is metabolized mainly in the **liver,** where it is converted to pyruvate or, under fasting conditions, to glucose.

         (1) Fructose is phosphorylated by adenosine triphosphate (ATP) to form fructose 1-phosphate. The enzyme is **fructokinase.**

> **CLINICAL CORRELATES** Deficiency of **fructokinase** is also known as **benign fructosuria.** It is an autosomal recessive disorder usually **diagnosed incidentally** because fructose accumulates in the urine and is **detected as a reducing sugar** that may give the indication of falsely high glucose readings.

         (2) Fructose 1-phosphate is cleaved by **aldolase B** to form dihydroxyacetone phosphate (DHAP) and glyceraldehyde, which is phosphorylated by ATP to form glyceraldehyde 3-phosphate. DHAP and glyceraldehyde 3-phosphate are intermediates of glycolysis. (Aldolase B is the same liver enzyme that cleaves fructose 1,6-bisphosphate in glycolysis.)

      b. In tissues other than liver, the major fate of fructose is phosphorylation by hexokinase to form fructose 6-phosphate, which enters glycolysis. Hexokinase has an affinity for fructose about 5% of that for glucose.

   2. Production of fructose from glucose

      a. Glucose is reduced to sorbitol by **aldose reductase,** which reduces the aldehyde group to an alcohol (Figure 8-2).

      b. Sorbitol is then reoxidized at carbon 2 by **sorbitol dehydrogenase** to form fructose.

B. Metabolism of galactose

> **CLINICAL CORRELATES** The disaccharide **lactose,** found in milk or milk products, is the major dietary source of galactose. It is also found in many artificial sweeteners and as "filler" in some medications.

   1. Conversion of galactose to intermediates of glucose pathways (Figure 8-3)

      a. Galactose is phosphorylated by ATP to galactose 1-phosphate. The enzyme is **galactokinase.**

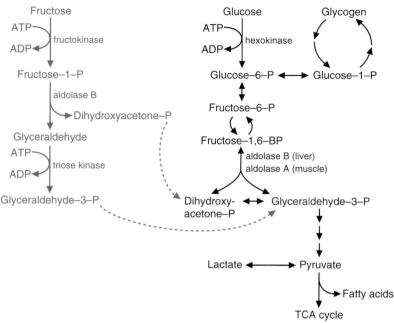

FIGURE 8-1 Conversion of fructose to intermediates of glycolysis. ADP, adenosine diphosphate; ATP, adenosine triphosphate; P, phosphate; TCA, tricarboxylic acid.

CLINICAL CORRELATES   **Galactokinase deficiency** results in increased levels of galactose in the blood (galactosemia) and urine (galactosuria). This results in the development of **cataracts** in infants without appropriate dietary restriction; however, these patients are **otherwise asymptomatic,** unlike the more severe classic galactosemia.

---

b. **Galactose 1-phosphate** reacts with uridine diphosphate (UDP)-glucose and forms glucose 1-phosphate and UDP-galactose. The enzyme is **galactose 1-phosphate uridylyltransferase.**

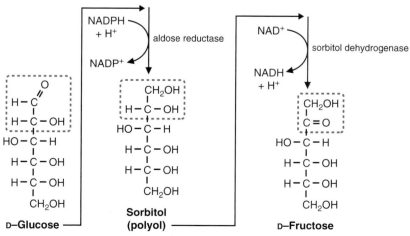

FIGURE 8-2 Reduced forms of sugars. Sorbitol is produced by reduction of glucose and can be reoxidized at carbon 2 to form fructose. Galactitol is produced by reduction of galactose.

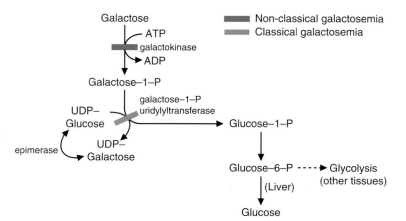

FIGURE 8-3 Conversion of galactose to intermediates of glucose metabolism. Galactose 1-phosphate uridylyltransferase is deficient in classic galactosemia. ADP, adenosine diphosphate; ATP, adenosine triphosphate; P, phosphate.

CLINICAL CORRELATES **Classic galactosemia** is a serious disorder that results from a deficiency of **galactose 1-phosphate uridylyltransferase.** The disorder typically presents with **hepatomegaly,** jaundice, **hypoglycemia, convulsions,** and **lethargy.** The infant may have difficulty feeding, poor weight gain, and the development of **cataracts.** Infants are at increased risk for **neonatal sepsis** due to *Escherichia coli.* **Neonatal screening** tests typically detect the disorder early, allowing for the elimination of all dietary galactose and preventing the development of more serious complications, including **mental retardation** and cirrhosis.

   c. **UDP-galactose** is epimerized to UDP-glucose in a reaction that is readily reversible. The enzyme is **UDP-glucose epimerase.**

CLINICAL CORRELATES **Deficiency of UDP-glucose epimerase** occurs in two distinct forms. The first is a benign condition, in which there is a deficiency in only leukocytes and erythrocytes. The second is more serious because it involves all tissues and has symptoms similar to classic galactosemia with the addition of hypotonia and nerve deafness. Again, the management requires the elimination of dietary galactose.

   d. Repetition of reactions described previously (in sections a–c) results in conversion of galactose to **UDP-glucose** and **glucose 1-phosphate.**
      (1) In the **liver,** these glucose derivatives are converted to blood glucose during fasting or to glycogen after a meal.
      (2) In various tissues, the glucose 1-phosphate forms glucose 6-phosphate and feeds into glycolysis.
2. **Other fates of UDP-galactose** (Figure 8-4)
   a. UDP-galactose can be produced either from galactose or from glucose via UDP-glucose and an epimerase.
   b. UDP-galactose supplies galactose moieties for the synthesis of **glycoproteins, glycolipids,** and **proteoglycans.** The enzyme that adds galactose units to growing polysaccharide chains is **galactosyl transferase.**
   c. UDP-galactose reacts with glucose in the **lactating mammary gland** to produce the milk sugar **lactose.** The modifier protein, α-**lactalbumin,** reacts with galactosyl transferase, lowering its K_m (Michaelis constant) for glucose so that glucose adds to galactose (from UDP-galactose), forming lactose.
3. **Conversion of galactose to galactitol.** Aldose reductase reduces the aldehyde of galactose to an alcohol, forming galactitol.

CLINICAL CORRELATES **Galactitol,** like **sorbitol,** accumulates in cells, increasing their osmotic pressure and **promoting cell swelling.** It is this swelling that ultimately leads to **damage of nerves, lens of the eye,** and **liver cells** in the defects in galactose metabolism described earlier.

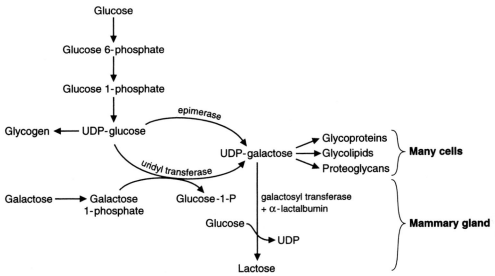

FIGURE 8-4 Metabolism of uridine diphosphate (UDP)-galactose. UDP-galactose can be produced from dietary glucose or galactose.

II. PENTOSE PHOSPHATE PATHWAY

A. Reactions of the pentose phosphate pathway (Figure 8-5)
  1. Oxidative reactions (Figure 8-6)
    a. Glucose 6-phosphate is converted, via the enzyme **glucose 6-phosphate dehydrogenase**, to 6-phosphogluconolactone, and $NADP^+$ is reduced to $NADPH + H^+$.

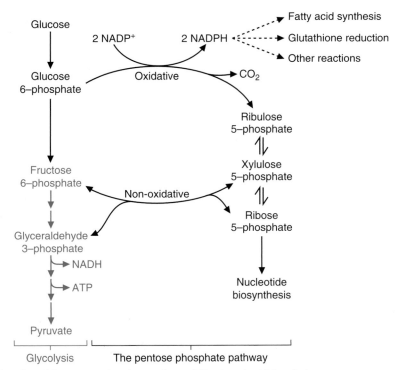

FIGURE 8-5 Overview of the pentose phosphate pathway. ATP, adenosine triphosphate.

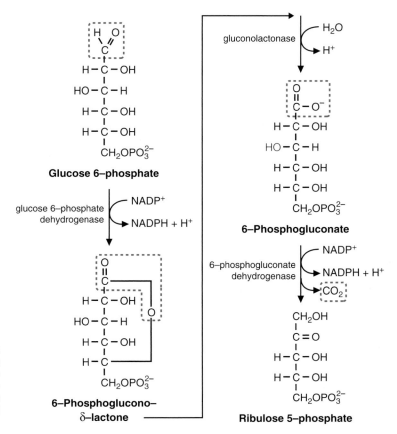

FIGURE 8-6 The oxidative reactions of the pentose phosphate pathway. These reactions are irreversible. Deficiency of glucose 6-phosphate dehydrogenase can result in hemolytic anemia.

---

    b. 6-Phosphogluconolactone is hydrolyzed to 6-phosphogluconate, with the help of the enzyme **gluconolactonase.**

    c. 6-Phosphogluconate is oxidatively decarboxylated. The enzyme involved is **6-phosphogluconate dehydrogenase.**

       (1) CO_2 is released, and a second NADPH + H$^+$ is generated from NADP$^+$.

       (2) The remaining carbons form ribulose 5-phosphate.

2. Nonoxidative reactions (Figure 8-5)

    a. Ribulose 5-phosphate is isomerized to ribose 5-phosphate or epimerized to xylulose 5-phosphate.

    b. Ribose 5-phosphate and **xylulose 5-phosphate** undergo reactions, catalyzed by **transketolase** and **transaldolase,** that transfer carbon units, ultimately forming fructose 6-phosphate and glyceraldehyde 3-phosphate.

       (1) Transketolase, which requires **thiamine pyrophosphate,** transfers two-carbon units (Figure 8-7).

       (2) Transaldolase transfers three-carbon units.

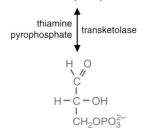

Xylulose 5–phosphate

+

H O
\ //
C
|
H − C − OH
|
H − C − OH
|
H − C − OH
|
$CH_2OPO_3^{2-}$

Ribose 5–phosphate

thiamine
pyrophosphate ┃ transketolase

H O
\ //
C
|
H − C − OH
|
$CH_2OPO_3^{2-}$

Glyceraldehyde 3–phosphate

+

CH₂OH
|
C = O
|
HO − C − OH
|
H − C − OH
|
H − C − OH
|
H − C − OH
|
$CH_2OPO_3^{2-}$

Sedoheptulose 7–phosphate

FIGURE 8-7 A two-carbon unit transferred by transketolase. Thiamine pyrophosphate is a cofactor for this enzyme.

3. **Overall reactions of the pentose phosphate pathway** (Figure 8-8)

$$3 \text{ glucose–6–P} + 6 \text{ NADP}^+ \rightarrow 3 \text{ ribulose–5–P} + 3 \text{ CO}_2 + 6 \text{ NADPH}$$

$$3 \text{ ribulose–5–P} \rightarrow 2 \text{ xylulose–5–P} + \text{ribose–5–P}$$

$$2 \text{ xylulose–5–P} + \text{ribose–5–P} \rightarrow 2 \text{ fructose–6–P} + \text{glyceraldehyde–3–P}$$

B. **Functions of NADPH** (Figure 8-5)
   1. The pentose phosphate pathway produces NADPH for **fatty acid synthesis.** Under these conditions, the fructose 6-phosphate and glyceraldehyde 3-phosphate generated in the pathway reenter glycolysis.

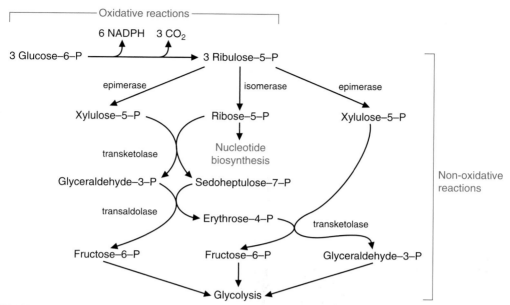

FIGURE 8-8 The reactions of the pentose phosphate pathway.

2. NADPH is also used to **reduce glutathione** (γ-glutamylcysteinylglycine).
   a. Glutathione helps to prevent oxidative damage to cells by reducing hydrogen peroxide (H_2O_2).
   b. Glutathione is also used to transport amino acids across the membranes of certain cells by the γ-glutamyl cycle.

C. **Generation of ribose 5-phosphate** (Figure 8-5)
   1. When **NADPH levels are low,** the oxidative reactions of the pathway can be used to generate ribose 5-phosphate for nucleotide biosynthesis.
   2. When **NADPH levels are high,** the reversible nonoxidative portion of the pathway can be used to generate ribose 5-phosphate for nucleotide biosynthesis from fructose 6-phosphate and glyceraldehyde 3-phosphate.

III. PROTEOGLYCANS, GLYCOPROTEINS, AND GLYCOLIPIDS

A. **Proteoglycans**
   1. **Synthesis of proteoglycans**
      a. The **protein** is synthesized on the endoplasmic reticulum (ER).
      b. **Glycosaminoglycans** are produced by the addition of sugars to serine or threonine residues of the protein. UDP sugars serve as the precursors.
      c. In the ER and the Golgi, the glycosaminoglycan chains grow by sequential addition of sugars to the nonreducing end.
         (1) **Sulfate groups,** donated by 3'-phosphoadenosine 5'-phosphosulfate (PAPS), are added after the hexosamine is incorporated into the chain.
         (2) Because of the uronic acid and sulfate groups, the glycosaminoglycans are **negatively charged,** causing the chains to be heavily hydrated.

CLINICAL CORRELATES   **Glycosaminoglycans** are important **components of the fluid in joints (synovial fluid)** and the vitreous humor of the eye. These solutions are mucous and **highly compressible** because water can be "squeezed out" from between the chains. Patients with **osteoarthritis** have a relative **deficiency** of these important "cushioning" molecules, resulting in damage to the joint.

  d. **Proteoglycans** are **secreted** from the cell.
  e. Proteoglycans can associate noncovalently with **hyaluronic acid** (a glycosaminoglycan), forming large aggregates, which act as molecular sieves that can be penetrated by small, but not by large, molecules.
  2. **Degradation of proteoglycans by lysosomal enzymes**
  a. Because proteoglycans are located outside the cell, they are taken up by **endocytosis**. The endocytic vesicles fuse with lysosomes.
  b. **Lysosomal enzymes** specific for each monosaccharide remove the sugars, one at a time, from the nonreducing end of the chain.
  c. **Sulfatases** remove the sulfate groups before the sugar residue is hydrolyzed.
  d. Several rare diseases, known as **mucopolysaccharidoses, result from deficiencies of these lysosomal enzymes,** with subsequent accumulation of substrate. Tissues become engorged with these "residual bodies," and their function is impaired (Table 8-1).

B. **Glycoproteins**
  1. **Synthesis of glycoproteins**
  a. The protein is synthesized on the ER. In the ER and the Golgi, the **carbohydrate chain** is produced by the sequential addition of monosaccharide units to the nonreducing end. UDP sugars, guanosine diphosphate (GDP)-mannose, GDP-L-fucose, and cytidine monophosphate-N-acetylneuraminic acid (CMP-NANA) act as precursors.
  b. For O-linked glycoproteins, the initial sugar is added to a **serine or threonine** residue in the protein, and the carbohydrate chain is then elongated.

t a b l e **8-1** Mucopolysaccharidoses			
Disease	**Enzyme Deficiency**	**Accumulated Products**	**Clinical Consequence**
Hurler syndrome (MPS I)	α-L-Iduronidase	Heparan sulfate, dermatan sulfate	**Deficiency** of this enzyme results in **mental retardation, micrognathia, coarsening of facial features** with **macroglossia** (enlarged tongue), retinal degeneration, **corneal clouding**, and **cardiomyopathy.**
Hunter syndrome (MPS II)	Iduronate sulfatase	Heparan sulfate, dermatan sulfate	This **X-linked deficiency** is generally milder than Hurler syndrome, **without corneal clouding.** However, it is associated with **variable mental retardation.**
Sanfilippo syndrome A **Sanfilippo syndrome B** **Sanfilippo syndrome C** (MPS IIIA to C)	Heparan sulfamidase *N*-acetylglucosaminidase *N*-acetylglucosamine 6-sulfatase	Heparan sulfate Heparan sulfate Heparan sulfate	This biochemically heterogenous syndrome results in **developmental delay, severe hyperactivity, spasticity, and progressive loss of motor skills,** with death by the second decade.
Morquio syndrome (MPS IV)	Galactose 6-sulfatase	Keratan sulfate, chondroitin 6-sulfate	Unlike other MPS syndromes, Morquio syndrome **is not associated with CNS involvement.** The disease is predominated by **severe skeletal dysplasia** and short stature. Motor involvement results from spinal cord impingement on motor neurons.
Sly syndrome (MPS VII)	β-Glucuronidase	Heparan sulfate, dermatan sulfate, chondroitin 4-,6-sulfate	This syndrome results in **hepatomegaly, skeletal deformity** with short stature, corneal clouding, and **developmental delay.** Although rare, much work has been accomplished in terms of **gene therapy** and **bone marrow transplantation** as a cure for this MPS.

CNS, central nervous system, MPS, mucopolysaccharidosis.

Blood group antigens are *O*-linked glycoproteins and lipid ceramides. Most individuals produce a **fructose linked to a galactose at the nonreducing end** of the blood group antigen, the so-called **H substance**. Individuals with **A blood group** produce an *N*-acetylgalactosamine transferase, which transfers an *N*-acetylgalactosamine moiety to the H substance. Individuals with **B blood group** produce a galactosyltransferase that adds **galactose to the H substance**. Individuals with **AB blood group produce both transferases,** whereas individuals with **O blood type produce neither** and, therefore, have only the H substance at the nonreducing end (Figure 8-9).

   c. **Dolichol phosphate** is involved in the synthesis of *N*-linked glycoproteins in which the carbohydrate moiety is attached to the amide N of asparagine.
     (1) Dolichol phosphate, a long-chain alcohol containing about 20 five-carbon isoprene units, can be synthesized from acetyl coenzyme A (CoA).
     (2) Sugars are added sequentially to dolichol phosphate, which is associated with the membrane of the ER.
     (3) The branched polysaccharide chain is transferred to an amide N of an asparagine residue in the protein.
     (4) In the ER and the Golgi, sugars are removed from the chain, and other sugars are added.
   d. **Glycoproteins** are **segregated** into lysosomes within the cell, **attached** to the cell membrane, or **secreted** by the cell.
     (1) **Lysosomal enzymes** are glycoproteins. A mannose phosphate residue targets these glycoproteins to lysosomes.

I-cell disease results from a defect in the addition of the **mannose 6-phosphate** tag on enzymes destined for the **lysosome**. As such, these **hydrolytic enzymes** end up being secreted from the cell. **Substrates within lysosomes accumulate, resulting in large inclusion bodies,** hence I-cells. Patients have **skeletal abnormalities, joint impairment, coarse facial features,** and **psychomotor impairment** culminating in death by the age of 8 years.

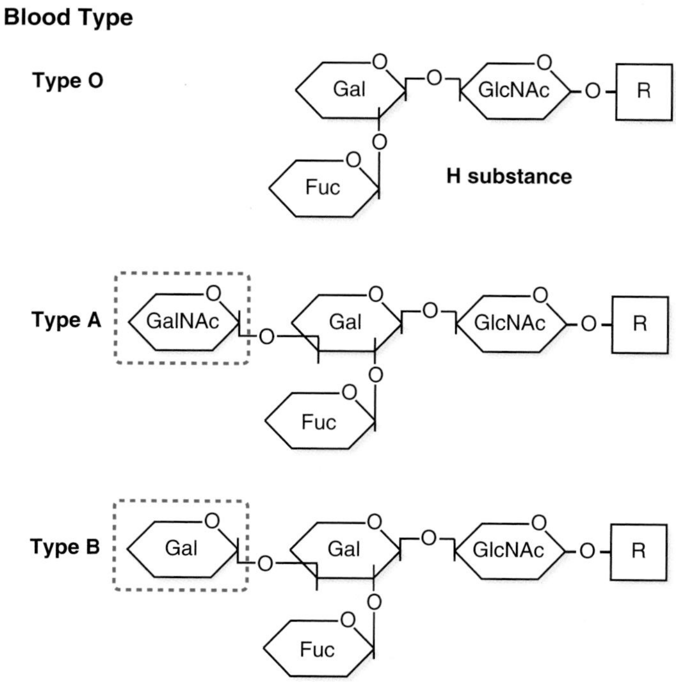

FIGURE 8-9 Structures of blood group substances. Note that these structures are the same except that type A has *N*-acetylgalactosamine (GalNAc) at the nonreducing end, type B has galactose (Gal), and type O has neither. R is either a protein or the lipid ceramide.

(2) When a glycoprotein is attached to the **cell membrane,** the carbohydrate portion extends into the extracellular space, and a hydrophobic segment of the protein is anchored in the membrane.

2. **Degradation of glycoproteins**
   - **Lysosomal enzymes** specific for each monosaccharide remove sugars sequentially from the nonreducing ends of the chains.

Review Test

Directions: Each of the numbered questions or incomplete statements in this section is followed by answers or by completions of the statement. Select the **one** lettered answer or completion that is **best** in each case.

1. A newborn undergoes a physical examination relevant for hepatomegaly, inguinal hernia, and deformed chest (pectus carinatum). A family history of mucopolysaccharidosis (MPS) leads you to check enzyme activities from a sample of fibroblasts. The findings were significant for decreased activity in β-glucuronidase, which is indicative of which of the following syndromes?

(A) Hurler syndrome (MPS type I)
(B) Morquio syndrome (MPS type IV)
(C) Hunter syndrome (MPS type II)
(D) Sanfilippo A syndrome (MPS type III)
(E) Sly syndrome (MPS type VII)

2. A 14-day-old breast-fed neonate fails to gain weight during infancy. Although concerned, the mother continues to breast-feed and wait. The infant subsequently develops cataracts, an enlarged liver, and mental retardation. Urinalysis is significant for high levels of galactose in the urine, as well as galactosemia. What food product in the baby's diet is leading to these symptoms?

(A) Fructose
(B) Lactose
(C) Phenylalanine
(D) Glucose
(E) Sorbitol

Questions 3–7: Using answers choices (A) through (E) below, match the clinical vignette with the appropriate defective or deficient enzyme.
(A) Glucose 6-phosphate dehydrogenase
(B) Galactose 1-phosphate uridylyltransferase
(C) *N*-acetylglucosamine 1-phosphate transferase
(D) Galactokinase
(E) Fructokinase

3. An immigrant 4-month-old child who did not receive prenatal or antenatal care appears ill. The child presents with hepatomegaly, jaundice, hypoglycemia, and convulsions. Blood work shows an elevated white blood cell count of 14,000, 16%

bands, and blood cultures that grow out *Escherichia coli*, signifying a bacterial infection.

(A)
(B)
(C)
(D)
(E)

4. A native of East Africa presents with jaundice and splenomegaly after eating fava beans. A blood smear reveals hemolysis.

(A)
(B)
(C)
(D)
(E)

5. A healthy, well-appearing child with no pertinent medical history has 3+ glucose on a urine dipstick.

(A)
(B)
(C)
(D)
(E)

6. A 15-month-old child has obvious signs of developmental delay. This includes an inability to roll over and poor head control. Gingival hypertrophy, coarse facial features, and an umbilical and aortic insufficiency are also noted in this child on physical examination.

(A)
(B)
(C)
(D)
(E)

7. A 12-month-old, otherwise healthy male has cataracts and galactosemia.

(A)
(B)

(C)
(D)
(E)

8. A 19-year-old, African American male military recruit is about to be sent to Iraq on his assignment. In preparation for his tour of duty, he is given a prophylactic dose of primaquine to prevent malaria. Several days after he begins taking the drug, he develops fatigue and hemolytic anemia. Which of the following proteins is likely deficient?

(A) Fructokinase
(B) Aldolase B
(C) Glucose 6-phosphate dehydrogenase
(D) Galactokinase
(E) Galactosyl transferase

9. A 3-year-old girl presents with developmental delay and growth failure. The physical examination is remarkable for coarse facial features, craniofacial abnormalities, gingival hyperplasia, prominent epicanthal fold, and macroglossia. The patient was diagnosed with I-cell diseases. Lysosomal proteins are mistargeted in this disorder. Rather than being targeted to the cell's lysosomes, lysosomal proteins in this disease are found in which of the following?

(A) In the endoplasmic reticulum (ER)
(B) In the Golgi apparatus
(C) In the mitochondria
(D) Exported from the cell
(E) In the cytoplasm

10. A 65-year-old man with a long history of uncontrolled diabetes presents to his physician after failing the driver's license renewal eye examination. Despite having abnormally high blood glucose levels and a hemoglobin A_{1C} of 10.4, the patient wants a more specific explanation. You begin by explaining that glucose enters the lens of the eye, where it is converted to sorbitol. Which of the following converts glucose to sorbitol?

(A) Hexokinase
(B) Aldose reductase
(C) Aldose mutase
(D) Sorbitol dehydrogenase
(E) Aldose oxidase

Answers and Explanations

1. **The answer is E.** Sly syndrome is one of the few lysosomal storage disorders with clinical manifestations in utero or at birth. The signs of coarse facial feature (gargoyle facies), mental developmental problems, and short stature can be seen in Sly syndrome as well as all the mucopolysaccharidoses. Hurler syndrome is due to a lack of α-L-iduronidase; Morquio syndrome to a lack of galactose 6-sulfatase; Hunter syndrome to a lack of iduronate sulfatase; and Sanfilippo A syndrome to a lack of heparan sulfamidase.

2. **The answer is B.** This patient has classic galactosemia, resulting from the inability to process galactose once the lactose in the breast milk is cleaved to its monomers, galactose and glucose. This disease results from an autosomal recessively inherited mutation in galactose 1-phosphate uridylyltransferase. Logically, treatment is removal of lactose and galactose from the diet. The enzyme defect does not allow galactose 1-phosphate to react with UDP-glucose, leading to the accumulation of both galactose 1-phosphate and galactose. The high galactose levels lead to galactitol accumulation and cataract formation. The high galactose 1-phosphate inhibits phosphoglucomutase, which leads to the hepatomegaly.

3. **The answer is B.** This child is exhibiting the signs of classic galactosemia, a lack of galactose 1-phosphate udriyltransferase. The lack of this enzyme leads to hypoglycemia due to galactose 1-phosphate inhibition of phosphoglucomutase, and jaundice due to the liver's inability to conjugate bilirubin. Sepsis is a common complication of untreated galactose 1-phosphate uridylyltransferase deficiency.

4. **The answer is A.** The patient has a defect in glucose 6-phosphate dehydrogenase (G6PDH). A lack of G6PDH leads to a reduced ability to generate NADPH, which is required to regenerate the protective form (the reduced form) of glutathione. This is particularly evident in red blood cells (RBCs) because they lack mitochondria and can only generate NADPH through G6PDH. In the presence of strong oxidizing agents (which are present in fava beans), the RBC cannot regenerate reduced glutathione, which protects the membrane from oxidative damage. This results in RBC membrane damage and cell lysis results. The jaundice results from the excess heme (from hemoglobin) released from the RBCs being converted to bilirubin and overwhelming the conjugation system of the liver.

5. **The answer is E.** The child has a fructokinase deficiency. A deficiency in fructokinase will not allow fructose to be metabolized (fructose cannot be converted to fructose 1-phosphate), resulting in elevated serum fructose after eating a meal containing sucrose or fructose. The elevated fructose leads to no metabolic problems, but does enter the urine for excretion. Because fructose is a reducing sugar (as is glucose), it will react positively in a glucose dipstick test. A more specific glucose oxidase test would need to be run to demonstrate that the positive result on the dipstick test was or was not due to elevated glucose.

6. **The answer is C.** The child has the symptoms of I-cell disease, which is a defect in N-acetylglucosamine 1-phosphate transferase. This results in an inability to appropriately tag lysosomal enzymes so that they can be routed to the lysosomes. Instead, they are secreted from the cell. This results in a loss of lysosomal function and a severe lysosomal storage disease.

7. **The answer is D.** The child has a galactokinase deficiency. Galactose cannot be converted to galactose 1-phosphate, so galactose accumulates whenever lactose is present in the diet. The elevated galactose is converted to the sugar alcohol galactitol in the lens of the eye by aldose reductase, which leads to cataract formation. This is a less severe disorder than galactose 1-phosphate uridylyltransferase deficiency because the toxic metabolite galactose 1-phosphate does not accumulate. Galactokinase deficiency is considered the nonclassic form of galactosemia.

8. **The answer is C.** Drugs that cause oxidative stress, like primaquine and sulfa-containing drugs, result in hemolytic disease in patients with G6PDH deficiency. In the presence of strong oxidizing agents, patients lacking G6PDH cannot adequately regenerate reduced glutathione in the red blood cells, which ultimately leads to membrane damage and lysis of the cells. Deficiency of fructokinase is a benign disorder. Deficiency of aldolase B leads to hereditary fructose intolerance. Galactokinase deficiency leads to galactosemia, a slightly milder form than is seen with galactose 1-phosphate uridylyltransferase deficiency. Galactosyl transferase is important in the glycosylation of proteins as well as in the metabolism of substances like bilirubin.

9. **The answer is D.** If lysosomal proteins are not appropriately tagged with mannose 6-phosphate in the ER and Golgi apparatus, the proteins will be exported from the cell. The lysosomal proteins do not contain the appropriate targeting signals to be sent to the ER, Golgi apparatus, or mitochondria. Because these enzymes are synthesized on membrane-bound ribosomes (the rough ER), they will not be found in the cytoplasm (cytoplasmic proteins are synthesized on cytoplasmic ribosomes). Although the child's physical abnormalities are similar to other storage diseases, gingival hyperplasia is a unique clinical feature to I-cell disease.

10. **The answer is B.** Glucose enters tissues such as nerves, kidney, and the lens of the eye by an insulin-independent mechanism. In these tissues, glucose is reduced to sorbitol by aldose reductase. The damage to these tissues is believed to be due to an osmotic effect because the sorbitol is unable to escape these tissues readily. Sorbitol dehydrogenase converts sorbitol to fructose. Hexokinase phosphorylates glucose to glucose 6-phosphate. There are no enzymes named aldose oxidase and aldose mutase.

9 Fatty Acid Metabolism

I. FATTY ACID AND TRIACYLGLYCEROL SYNTHESIS

A. Conversion of glucose to acetyl CoA for fatty acid synthesis (Figure 9-1)
1. **Glucose** enters liver cells and is converted via glycolysis to pyruvate, which enters mitochondria.
2. **Pyruvate** is converted to acetyl coenzyme A (CoA) by pyruvate dehydrogenase and to **oxalo-acetate** (OAA) by pyruvate carboxylase.
3. Because acetyl CoA cannot directly cross the mitochondrial membrane and enter the cytosol to be used for the process of fatty acid synthesis, acetyl CoA and OAA condense to form **citrate,** which can cross the mitochondrial membrane.
4. In the cytosol, **citrate is cleaved** to OAA and acetyl CoA by citrate lyase, an enzyme that requires adenosine triphosphate (ATP) and is induced by insulin.
   a. **OAA** from the citrate lyase reaction is reduced in the cytosol by NADH, producing NAD^+ and **malate.** The enzyme is cytosolic malate dehydrogenase.
   b. In a subsequent reaction, **malate** is converted to pyruvate, NADPH is produced, and CO_2 is released. The enzyme is **malic enzyme** (or $NADP^+$-dependent malate dehydrogenase).
      (1) **Pyruvate** reenters the mitochondrion and is reutilized.
      (2) **NADPH** supplies reducing equivalents for reactions on the fatty acid synthase complex.
      (3) **NADPH** is produced by **malic enzyme** and the **pentose phosphate pathway.**
5. **Acetyl CoA** (from the citrate lyase reaction or from other sources) supplies carbons for fatty acid synthesis in the cytosol.

B. Synthesis of fatty acids by the fatty acid synthase complex (Figure 9-2)
1. **Fatty acid synthase** is a multienzyme complex located in the cytosol. It has two large identical subunits with seven catalytic activities.
   a. This enzyme contains a **phosphopantetheine residue,** derived from the vitamin pantothenic acid, and a **cysteine residue;** both contain sulfhydryl groups that can form thioesters with acyl groups.
   b. The growing fatty acyl chain moves during the synthesis of two carbon units from one to the other of these sulfhydryl residues as it is elongated.
2. **Addition of two-carbon units**
   a. Initially, **acetyl CoA** reacts with the phosphopantetheinyl residue, and then the acetyl group is transferred to the cysteinyl residue.
   b. A malonyl group from **malonyl CoA** forms a **thioester** with the phosphopantetheinyl sulf-hydryl group.
      (1) **Malonyl CoA** (two carbons) is formed from acetyl CoA by a carboxylation reaction that requires **biotin** and ATP. The enzyme catalyzing this reaction is acetyl CoA carboxylase.
      (2) **Acetyl CoA carboxylase** is inhibited by phosphorylation, activated by dephosphoryl-ation and by citrate, and induced by insulin.
   c. The **acetyl group** on the fatty acid synthase complex condenses with the malonyl group; the CO_2 that was added to the malonyl group by acetyl CoA carboxylase is released; and a β-**ketoacyl group,** now containing four carbons, is produced.

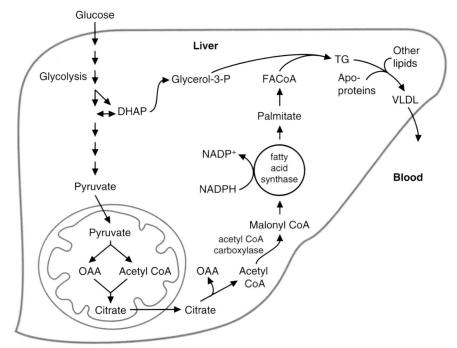

FIGURE 9-1 Lipogenesis, the synthesis of fatty acids (FA) and triacylglycerols (TG) from glucose, occurs mainly in the liver. CoA, coenzyme A; DHAP, dihydroxyacetone phosphate; OAA, oxaloacetate; VLDL, very-low-density lipoprotein.

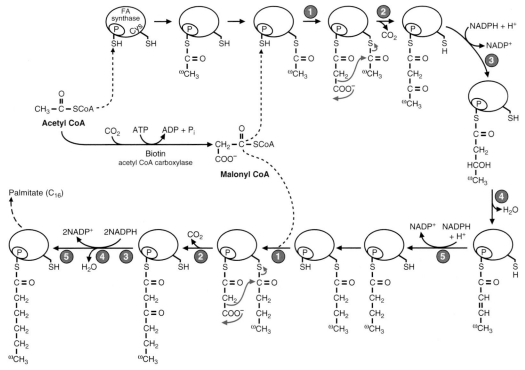

FIGURE 9-2 Fatty acid (FA) synthesis (palmitate). Malonyl coenzyme A (CoA) provides the two-carbon units that are added to the growing fatty acyl chain. The addition and reduction steps (1 to 5) are repeated until palmitic acid is produced. ADP, adenosine diphosphate; ATP, adenosine triphosphate; Cys-SH, a cysteinyl residue; P, a phosphopantetheinyl group attached to the FA synthase complex; P_i, inorganic phosphate.

3. **Reduction of the β-ketoacyl group**
   a. The β-keto group is **reduced** by NADPH to a β-hydroxy group.
   b. Then **dehydration** occurs, producing a double bond between carbons 2 and 3.
   c. Finally, the double bond is reduced by NADPH, and a **four-carbon acyl group** is formed.
   d. **NADPH** is produced by the **pentose phosphate pathway** and **malic enzyme.**
4. **Elongation of the growing fatty acyl chain**
   a. The acyl group is transferred to the cysteinyl sulfhydryl group, and **malonyl CoA** reacts with the phosphopantetheinyl group. Condensation of the acyl and malonyl groups releases CO_2, followed by three reactions reducing the β-keto group. The chain grows by two carbons.
   b. This sequence of reactions repeats until the growing chain is 16 carbons in length.
   c. **Palmitate,** a 16-carbon saturated fatty acid, is the final product released by hydrolysis from the fatty acid synthase complex.

C. **Elongation and desaturation of fatty acids**
   1. **Palmitate** can be elongated and desaturated to form **long-chain saturated and unsaturated fatty acids**.
   2. **Elongation of long-chain fatty acids** occurs on the endoplasmic reticulum by reactions similar to those that occur on the fatty acid synthase complex.
      a. **Malonyl CoA** provides two-carbon units adding to palmitoyl CoA.
      b. Malonyl CoA condenses with the carbonyl group of the fatty acyl residue, and CO_2 is released.
      c. The β-keto group is reduced by NADPH to a β-hydroxy group; dehydration occurs; and a double bond is formed, which is reduced by NADPH.
   3. **Desaturation of fatty acids** requires O_2, NADPH, and cytochrome b_5.
      a. In humans, desaturases may add double bonds at the 9 to 10 position of a fatty acyl CoA and between carbon 9 and the carboxyl group.
      b. Plants introduce double bonds between carbon 9 and the ω-carbon; animals cannot. These unsaturated fatty acids from plants are essential in the human diet.
      c. **Linoleate** (18:2, $\Delta^{9,12}$) and **α-linolenate** (18:3, $\Delta^{9,12,15}$) are the major sources of the essential fatty acids, required for synthesis of **arachidonic acid** and other polyunsaturated fatty acids of the eicosanoid (e.g., prostaglandins) family.

CLINICAL CORRELATES   Total parenteral nutrition (TPN) is an **intravenous** form of nutrition containing **essential fatty acids** required in the diet. TPN is used in chronic illness, infection, trauma, burn injuries, postsurgery recovery, starvation, and kidney or liver failure. TPN avoids **using the gastrointestinal tract.**

D. **Synthesis of triacylglycerols** (Figure 9-3)
   1. **In intestinal epithelial** cells, triacylglycerol synthesis occurs by a different pathway than in other tissues. This triacylglycerol becomes a component of chylomicrons. Ultimately, the fatty acyl groups are stored in adipose triacylglycerols.
   2. **In liver and adipose tissue,** glycerol 3-phosphate provides the glycerol moiety that reacts with two fatty acyl CoA molecules to form **phosphatidic acid.** The phosphate group is cleaved to form a diacylglycerol, which reacts with another fatty acyl CoA to form a triacylglycerol.

CLINICAL CORRELATES   Elevated **triglyceride (triacylglycerol) > 1000 mg/dL** can cause **pancreatitis,** an inflammation of the pancreas that causes severe abdominal pain.

      a. **The liver** can use glycerol to produce glycerol 3-phosphate by a reaction that requires ATP and is catalyzed by glycerol kinase.

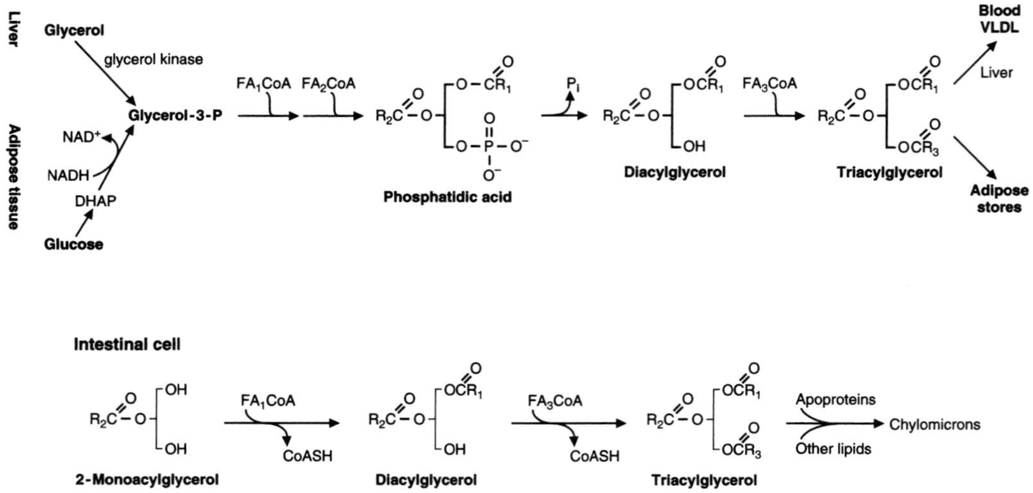

FIGURE 9-3 Synthesis of triacylglycerols in liver, adipose tissue, and intestinal cells. DHAP, dihydroxyacetone phosphate; glycerol-3-P, glycerol 3-phosphate; R, aliphatic chain of a fatty acid; P_i, inorganic phosphate; VLDL, very-low-density lipoprotein.

    b. **Adipose tissue,** which **lacks glycerol kinase,** *cannot* generate glycerol 3-phosphate from glycerol.

    c. **Both liver and adipose tissue** can convert glucose, through glycolysis, to **dihydroxyacetone phosphate (DHAP),** which is reduced by NADH to glycerol 3-phosphate.

    d. **Triacylglycerol** is **stored in adipose tissue.**

    e. In the **liver,** triacylglycerol is incorporated into **very-low-density lipoprotein (VLDL),** entering blood. Ultimately, fatty acyl groups are stored in adipose triacylglycerols.

CLINICAL CORRELATES   Chylous ascites is the **extravasation of milky chyle** (lymph) with a triglyceride (triacylglycerol) level of more than 200 mg/dL **into the peritoneal cavity of the abdomen.** (Fluid collection in the peritoneum is ascites.) Chylous ascites occurs in **abdominal surgery, abdominal trauma,** and **cancers** such as lymphomas, in which the lymphatic system is obstructed.

E. **Regulation of triacylglycerol synthesis from carbohydrate**
  1. Synthesis of triacylglycerols from carbohydrate occurs in the liver in the **fed state.**
  2. **Key regulatory enzymes** are activated and induced by carbohydrate.
    a. The glycolytic enzymes **glucokinase, phosphofructokinase 1,** and **pyruvate kinase** are active.
    b. **Pyruvate dehydrogenase** is dephosphorylated and active.
    c. **Pyruvate carboxylase** is activated by acetyl CoA.
    d. **Citrate lyase** is inducible.
    e. **Acetyl CoA carboxylase** is induced, activated by citrate, and converted to its active, dephosphorylated state by a phosphatase that is stimulated by insulin.
    f. The **fatty acid synthase complex** is inducible.
  3. **NADPH,** the reductant for fatty acid synthesis, is produced by the inducible **malic enzyme** and the pentose phosphate pathway enzymes: **glucose 6-phosphate dehydrogenase** and **6-phosphogluconate dehydrogenase.**
  4. **Malonyl CoA,** the product of the acetyl CoA carboxylase reaction, **inhibits carnitine acyltransferase I** (carnitine palmitoyl transferase I), thereby preventing newly synthesized fatty acids from entering mitochondria and undergoing β-oxidation. (Figure 9-4)

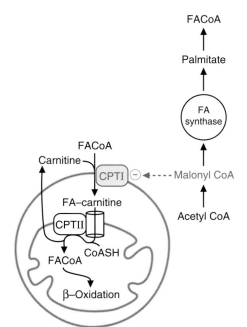

FIGURE 9-4 Inhibition of carnitine acyltransferase I (carnitine palmitoyl transferase I [CPTI]) by malonyl coenzyme A (CoA). This mechanism prevents newly synthesized fatty acids (in the cytoplasm) from being immediately oxidized by being transported into the mitochondria. CoASH, unreacted coenzyme A; FA, fatty acyl group.

II. FORMATION OF TRIACYLGLYCEROL STORES IN ADIPOSE TISSUE

A. **Hydrolysis of triacylglycerols of chylomicrons and VLDL** (Figure 9-5)
   1. The triacylglycerols of chylomicrons and VLDL are hydrolyzed to **fatty acids** and **glycerol** by lipoprotein lipase in the capillary walls of adipose tissue.
   2. **Lipoprotein lipase** is synthesized in adipose cells and secreted from the cell in response to insulin. This results in elevated lipoprotein lipase levels after consuming a meal. **Apoprotein C-II,** which is transferred from high-density lipoprotein (HDL) to chylomicrons and VLDL once those particles enter the circulation, activates lipoprotein lipase.

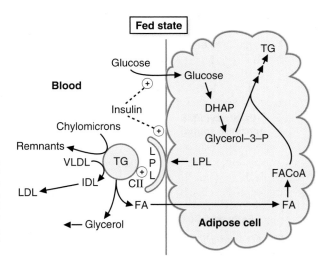

FIGURE 9-5 Formation of triacylglycerol (TG) stores in adipose tissue in the fed state. CII, apoprotein C-II; CoA, coenzyme A; DHAP, dihydroxyacetone phosphate; FA, fatty acid; IDL, intermediate-density lipoprotein; LPL, lipoprotein lipase; +, stimulated by; circled TG, triacylglycerol of chylomicrons; VLDL, very-low-density lipoprotein.

B. **Synthesis of triacylglycerols in adipose tissue**
   1. **Fatty acids** released from chylomicrons and VLDL by lipoprotein lipase are taken up by adipose cells and converted to triacylglycerols, but glycerol is not used because adipose tissue lacks glycerol kinase (Figure 9-3).
      a. **Transport of glucose** into adipose cells is **stimulated by insulin.**
      b. Glucose is converted to **DHAP** and reduced by NADH to form **glycerol 3-phosphate,** which produces the glycerol moiety of the triacylglycerol.
   2. The triacylglycerols are stored in large fat globules in adipose cells.

III. FATTY ACID OXIDATION

A. **Activation of fatty acids**
   1. In the cytosol, long-chain fatty acids are activated by **ATP** and **CoA,** forming **fatty acyl CoA** (Figure 9-6). Short-chain fatty acids are activated in mitochondria.
   2. **ATP** is converted to **adenosine monophosphate (AMP) and pyrophosphate (PP_i)** when a fatty acid is activated. The PPi produced during the reaction is cleaved by pyrophosphatase to two inorganic phosphates (P_i). Thus, two high-energy bonds are required for fatty acid activation.

B. **Transport of fatty acyl CoA from the cytosol into mitochondria** (Figure 9-7)
   1. **Cytosolic fatty acyl CoA** reacts with **carnitine** in the outer mitochondrial membrane, forming fatty acyl carnitine via **carnitine acyl transferase I (CAT I),** also called carnitine palmitoyl transferase I (CPT I). **Fatty acyl carnitine** passes to the inner membrane, where it reacts with carnitine acyl transferase II (CAT II) to **reform fatty acyl CoA,** which enters the mitochondrial matrix.

CLINICAL CORRELATES   **Primary carnitine deficiency** is a deficiency of the plasma membrane carnitine transporter, leading to **urinary wasting of carnitine.** Subsequent depletion of intracellular carnitine impairs transport of long-chain fatty acids into mitochondria, limiting fatty acid availability for oxidation and energy production.

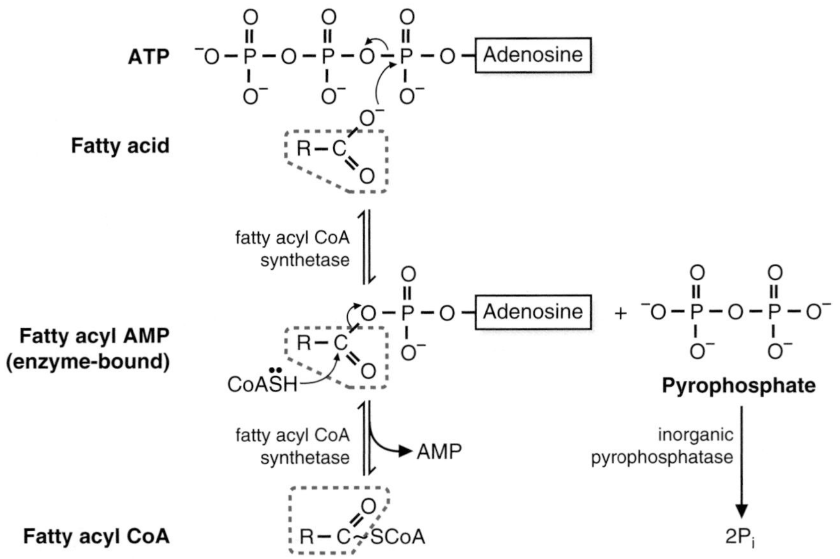

FIGURE 9-6 Activation of a fatty acid by fatty acyl coenzyme A (CoA) synthetase. AMP, adenosine monophosphate; ATP, adenosine triphosphate; P_i, inorganic phosphate.

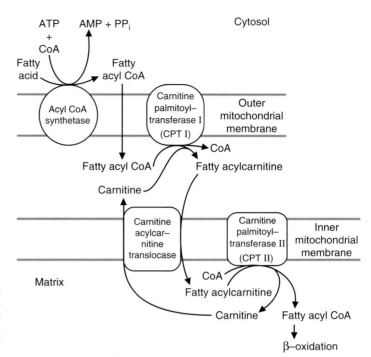

FIGURE 9-7 Transport of long-chain fatty acids into the mitochondria. AMP, adenosine diphosphate; ATP, adenosine triphosphate; CoA, coenzyme A; PPᵢ, inorganic pyrophosphate.

2. **CAT I,** which catalyzes the transfer of acyl groups from coenzyme A to carnitine, is **inhibited by malonyl CoA,** an intermediate in fatty acid synthesis. Therefore, when fatty acids are synthesized in the cytosol, malonyl CoA inhibits their transport into mitochondria, preventing a futile cycle (synthesis followed by immediate degradation).

CLINICAL CORRELATES CAT I deficiency results in intermittent **ataxia, oculomotor palsy** (cranial nerve [CN] III), hypotonia, **mental confusion,** and disturbance of consciousness.

3. Inside the mitochondrion, fatty acyl CoA undergoes β-**oxidation.**

C. β-**Oxidation of even-chain fatty acids**
   1. β-**Oxidation** (oxidizing the β-carbon of a fatty acyl CoA) is a four-step spiral.
      a. The first three steps are similar to the tricarboxylic acid (TCA) cycle reactions that convert succinate to OAA.
      b. These steps are repeated until all carbons of even-chain fatty acyl CoA are converted to acetyl CoA (Figure 9-8). (Step 1)
   2. **Flavin adenine dinucleotide (FAD) accepts hydrogens** and electrons from fatty acyl CoA in step 1.
      a. A double bond is produced between the α- and β-carbons, and an enoyl CoA is formed.
      b. $FADH_2$ produced interacts with the electron transport chain, generating ATP.
      c. The enzyme mediating this reaction is **acyl CoA dehydrogenase.**
   3. **H₂O adds across the double bond,** via **enoyl CoA hydratase,** and a β-hydroxyacyl CoA is formed. (Step 2)

CLINICAL CORRELATES Medium-chain acyl CoA dehydrogenase (MCAD) deficiency is a **deficiency of one of the acyl CoA dehydrogenases,** which oxidizes fatty acids between 6 and 10 carbons long. The defect is manifested when serum glucose levels are low (**hypoglycemia**) because of fasting, infection, or increased amount of time between feedings. **Fatty acids cannot be fully oxidized** as an alternate form of energy in individuals with this disorder.

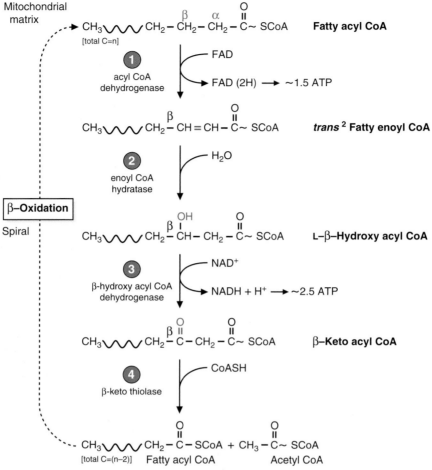

FIGURE 9-8 Steps of β-oxidation. The four steps are repeated until the even-chain fatty acid is completely converted to acetyl coenzyme A (CoA). ATP, adenosine triphosphate.

4. **β-Hydroxyacyl CoA is oxidized** by NAD^+ to a β-ketoacyl CoA.
    a. NADH produced interacts with the electron transport chain, generating ATP.
    b. The enzyme is L-3-hydroxyacyl CoA dehydrogenase (specific for the L-isomer). (Step 3)
5. The **bond between the α- and β-carbons** of the β-ketoacyl CoA is cleaved by a **thiolase** that requires coenzyme A.
    a. Acetyl CoA is produced from the two carbons at the carboxyl end of the fatty acyl CoA, with remaining carbons forming a fatty acyl CoA that is two carbons shorter than the starting fatty acid.
    b. The enzyme is β-**keto thiolase.** (Step 4)
6. The shortened **fatty acyl CoA repeats** these four steps. The spiral continues until all the carbons of the original fatty acyl CoA are converted to acetyl CoA.
    a. The complete oxidation of the 16-carbon palmitoyl CoA undergoes seven repetitions of the oxidation spiral.
    b. In the last repetition, a four-carbon fatty acyl CoA (butyryl CoA) is cleaved to 2 molecules of acetyl CoA.
7. **Energy is generated** from the products of β-oxidation.
    a. When 1 mole of palmitoyl CoA is oxidized, 7 moles of $FADH_2$, 7 moles of NADH, and 8 moles of acetyl CoA are formed.
        (1) Each of the 7 moles of $FADH_2$ generates about 1.5 moles of ATP, for a total of about 10.5 moles of ATP.
        (2) Each of the 7 moles of NADH generates about 2.5 moles of ATP, for a total of about 17.5 moles of ATP.

(3) Each of the 8 moles of acetyl CoA can enter the TCA cycle, each producing about 10 moles of ATP, for a total of about 80 moles of ATP.

(4) With oxidation of one mole of palmitoyl CoA to CO_2 and H_2O, a total of about 108 moles of ATP are produced.

   b. The **net ATP** produced from one mole of palmitate is about 106 moles because palmitate undergoes activation (requiring two high-energy bonds pre mole) before oxidation (108 ATP – 2 ATP [to represent the two high-energy bonds] = 106 ATP).

   c. **Oxidation of other fatty acids** will yield different amounts of ATP.

D. Oxidation of odd-chain and unsaturated fatty acids

1. **Odd-chain fatty acids** produce acetyl CoA and propionyl CoA.

   a. These fatty acids repeat the four steps of the β-oxidation spiral, producing **acetyl CoA** until the last cleavage when the three remaining carbons are released as propionyl CoA.

   b. **Propionyl CoA,** but not acetyl CoA, is converted to glucose.

2. **Unsaturated fatty acids** comprise about half the fatty acids in human lipids. Their oxidation requires new enzymes in addition to the four enzymes that catalyze the steps of the β-oxidation spiral. The pathways differ depending on the position in which the double bond is located.

   a. For fatty acids that contain a double bond at an odd carbon number (e.g., between carbons 9 and 10), β-**oxidation** occurs until the double bond of the unsaturated fatty acid reaches position 3 of the acyl CoA. At this point, an isomerase will convert the cis Δ3 double bond to a *trans* Δ2 double bond. The normal steps of β-oxidation can then proceed.

   b. For fatty acids that contain a double bond at an even carbon position (e.g., between carbons 12 and 13), β-oxidation occurs until the double bond of the unsaturated acid reaches position 4 of the acyl CoA. After the acyl CoA dehydrogenase creates the *trans* double bond between carbons 2 and 3, the enzyme 2,4-dienoyl CoA reductase reduces the two double bonds into one, generating a *trans* Δ3 double bond. The *trans* Δ3 double bond is then isomerized to *trans* Δ2, so that the normal steps of β-oxidation can then proceed.

E. ω-Oxidation of fatty acids (Figure 9-9)

1. The **(omega)-carbon** (the terminal methyl carbon) of fatty acids is oxidized to a carboxyl group in the smooth endoplasmic reticulum.

2. β-Oxidation then occurs in mitochondria at this end as well as from the original carboxyl end, assuming that β-oxidation is functional. **Dicarboxylic acids** are produced.

F. Oxidation of very-long-chain fatty acids in peroxisomes (Figure 9-10)

1. The process differs from β-oxidation in that **molecular O_2** is used in the first oxidation step, which forms **hydrogen peroxide** (H_2O_2), without the generation of $FADH_2$. NADH is generated in the second oxidation step of peroxisomal fatty acid oxidation.

2. Shorter-chain fatty acids travel to mitochondria, where β-oxidation occurs, generating ATP.

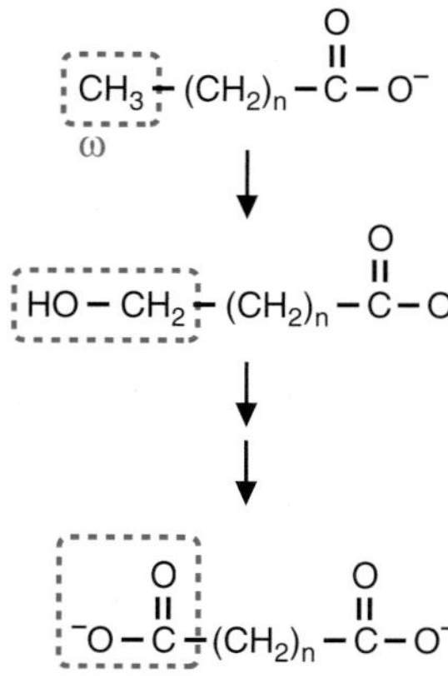

FIGURE 9-9 ω-Oxidation of fatty acids converts them to dicarboxylic acids.

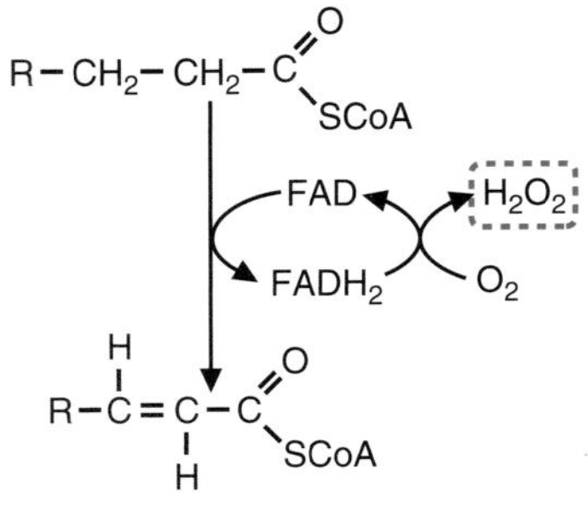

FIGURE 9-10 The first step of β-oxidation of fatty acids in peroxisomes. This step is catalyzed by a flavin adenine dinucleotide (FAD)–containing oxidase, which donates its electrons to oxygen to form hydrogen peroxide.

CLINICAL CORRELATES **Zellweger syndrome** is a peroxisomal disorder resulting in **accumulation of very-long-chain fatty acids** because the **peroxisome is not properly formed.** Clinical manifestations include congenital craniofacial dysmorphism, psychomotor retardation, and seizures. Death results in the first year of life.

CLINICAL CORRELATES **Adrenoleukodystrophy** is a rare metabolic disorder. **Very-long-chain fatty acids accumulate** in the brain (causing demyelination) and in the adrenal cortex (causing degeneration) because of an **inability to transport very-long-chain fatty acids into peroxisomes.** Clinical manifestations include psychomotor retardation and seizures.

G. α-Oxidation of fatty acids

1. **Branched-chain fatty acids** are oxidized at the α-carbon (in brain and nervous tissue), and the carboxyl carbon is released as CO_2.
2. Once the carboxyl carbon is released, in most cases, normal β-oxidation can degrade the rest of the branched-chain fatty acid.

IV. HIGH YIELD COMPARISON FROM FATTY ACID SYNTHESIS AND OXIDATION (TABLE 9-1)

table 9-1	High-Yield Comparison of Fatty Acid Synthesis and Oxidation	
Issue	**Fatty Acid Synthesis**	**Fatty Acid (β)-Oxidation**
Intracellular location	Cytoplasm	Mitochondria
Electron transfer coenzymes	NADPH	FAD, NAD+
Carrier	Acyl carrier protein	CoA
Activation by citrate?	Yes	No
Inhibited by palmitate?	Yes	No
Process favored by?	High ATP	High ADP
Acyl/acetyl group carrier	Citrate (mito to cyto)	Carnitine (cyto to mito)
Product	Palmitate	Acetyl CoA
Highest activity	Carbohydrate, fed state	Fasting and starvation
Hormonal state (insulin/glucagon)	High	Low
Repetitive process	Condensation Reduction Dehydration Reduction	Oxidation Hydration Oxidation Thiolysis

ADP, adenosine monophosphate; ATP, adenosine triphosphate; CoA, coenzyme A; FAD, flavin adenine dinucleotide.

Review Test

Directions: Each of the numbered questions or incomplete statements in this section is followed by answers or by completions of the statement. Select the **one** lettered answer or completion that is **best** in each case.

1. A 41-year-old woman presents with severe, sharp epigastric abdominal pain that radiates to her back and with nausea and vomiting. Laboratory results indicate a serum triglyceride level of 5000 mg/dL. She is diagnosed with pancreatitis, in part owing to her elevated serum triacylglycerol levels. To form triacylglycerol from diacylglycerol, which of the following compounds is also required?

(A) Glycerol
(B) Glycerol 3-phosphate
(C) Fatty acyl CoA
(D) Acetyl CoA
(E) Malonyl CoA

2. An 18-year-old woman presents with xanthomas on her eyelids and is found to have a rare genetic deficiency of lipoprotein lipase. She is diagnosed with type I hyperlipidemia. In this disorder, chylomicrons are abnormally elevated in the serum. In which cell or tissue does triacylglycerol packaging into chylomicrons occur?

(A) Intestinal epithelial cell
(B) Liver cell
(C) Muscle cell
(D) Heart cell
(E) Adipose cell

3. A 2-week-old child underwent complex congenital heart malformation repair. The cardiothoracic surgeon accompanies the patient back from the operating room and tells the pediatric intensive care unit staff that the ASD (atrial septal defect) and VSD (ventricular septal defect) were successfully repaired. However, the thoracic duct was accidentally cut, and daily echocardiograms will be needed to evaluate for cor pulmonale (alterations in the right ventricle of the heart). Which one of the following statements is true concerning fat metabolism in this patient?

(A) The thoracic duct carries a substantial volume of lymph and triglycerides from the enteric circulation to the venous system.

(B) Triacylglycerol is primarily stored in the liver.
(C) In the intestinal cell, glucose is converted to triacylglycerol by phosphatidic acid.
(D) In adipose cells, triacylglycerol is converted to VLDL.
(E) Somatostatin has no role in the treatment of chylothorax in children.

4. An 18-year-old obese woman maintains a sedentary lifestyle and eats a high-fat, high-carbohydrate diet. Maintenance of this diet and lifestyle has led to lipogenesis and obesity. Which of the following statements correctly describes an aspect of lipogenesis?

(A) The primary source of carbons for fatty acid synthesis is glycerol.
(B) Fatty acids are synthesized from acetyl CoA in the mitochondria.
(C) Fatty acid synthesis and esterification to glycerol to form triacylglycerols occurs primarily in muscle cells.
(D) The fatty acyl chain on the fatty acid synthase complex is elongated two carbons at a time.
(E) $NADP^+$, which is important for fatty acid synthesis, is produced by the pentose phosphate pathway.

5. A 45-year-old man presents with multiple gunshot wounds to the abdomen requiring an emergent laparotomy, jejunectomy, and colectomy. After surgery, he is placed on intravenous nutrition (i.e., TPN). Which of the following compounds should be a component of TPN?

(A) Palmitate
(B) Linoleate
(C) Phosphatidic acid
(D) Glycerol
(E) Glucose

6. A 16-year-old girl presents with extreme slenderness. Her body weight is 35% below expected. She feels as though she is obese and severely restricts her food intake. She is diagnosed with anorexia nervosa. In this patient, breakdown of fatty acids is required to provide energy. Before being oxidized, fatty acids are activated in the cytosol to form which of the following?

(A) ATP
(B) CoA
(C) Fatty acyl CoA
(D) Carnitine
(E) Malonyl CoA

7. After surgical resection of part of her small intestine, a 40-year-old woman presents with chronic foul-smelling diarrhea and weight loss. She is diagnosed with short bowel syndrome. In this syndrome, fat cannot be properly absorbed, so long-chain fatty acids are mobilized from adipose tissue to generate energy for cell survival. The initiating substrate for fatty acid oxidation is which of the following?

(A) Long-chain fatty acid
(B) Fatty acyl carnitine
(C) Fatty acyl CoA
(D) β-Hydroxyacyl CoA
(E) Acetyl CoA

8. An infant is born with a high forehead, abnormal eye folds, and deformed ear lobes and shows little muscle tone and movement. After multiple tests, he is diagnosed with Zellweger syndrome, a disorder caused by peroxisome malformation. What type of fatty acid would you expect to accumulate in patients with Zellweger syndrome?

(A) Short-chain fatty acids
(B) Acetyl CoA
(C) Dicarboxylic acids
(D) Long-chain fatty acids
(E) Very-long-chain fatty acids

9. A 4-month-old infant presents with a seizure. His mother reports that her infant has been irritable and lethargic over the past several days. The infant is found to be profoundly hypoglycemic and have low ketones. Short-chain dicarboxylic acids are found to be elevated in the serum. The most likely enzyme deficiency is which of the following?

(A) Medium-chain acyl CoA dehydrogenase (MCAD)
(B) Carnitine acyltransferase I
(C) Hormone-sensitive lipase
(D) Pyruvate carboxylase
(E) Fatty acyl CoA synthetase

10. A 12-year-old Jamaican boy presents with intractable vomiting, abdominal pain, and lethargy and is profoundly hypoglycemic. His symptoms are caused by Jamaican vomiting syndrome, a sickness caused by ingestion of hypoglycin, which is present in unripe ackee fruit. Hypoglycin is metabolized to a form of nonmetabolizable carnitine, which interferes with normal fatty acid oxidation. What is the primary role of carnitine?

(A) Activates long-chain fatty acids in the cytosol
(B) Transport of acyl groups across the inner mitochondrial membrane
(C) Is converted to enoyl CoA
(D) Is converted to β-hydroxyacyl CoA
(E) Is involved in breakdown of even-chain, but not odd-chain, fatty acids

Answers and Explanations

1. **The answer is C.** Triacylglycerol is formed when a diacylglycerol reacts with a fatty acyl CoA. Glycerol and glycerol 3-phosphate form the backbone of the triacylglycerol. Acetyl CoA and malonyl CoA are involved in fatty acid synthesis, and not directly in triacylglycerol synthesis.

2. **The answer is A.** Intestinal epithelial cells are the site of chylomicron formation. Dietary triacylglycerols are bound to apoproteins and other lipids to form the chylomicrons. In the liver, triacylglycerols are incorporated into VLDLs, which enter the blood. Triacylglycerols are stored in adipose tissue. The muscle, heart, and adipose cells do not package triacylglycerol into particles for export into the circulation.

3. **The answer is A.** The thoracic duct carries lymph and triglyceride from the enteric circulation to the venous system. Chylothorax is the accumulation of chylous fluid from a compromised thoracic duct. Nontraumatic causes (e.g., malignant erosion) or traumatic causes (e.g., blunt trauma, cardiothoracic surgery) result in the slow accumulation of a milky fluid rich in triglycerides in the chest cavity. Treatment is medical (somatostatin in children) and surgical (percutaneous drainage or thoracostomy tube drainage). Triglyceride is primarily stored in the adipose cells. Intestinal cells do not produce triglyceride from glucose; these cells pass glucose directly into the circulation. VLDL is produced by the liver, not adipose tissue.

4. **The answer is D.** The primary source of carbons for fatty acid synthesis is dietary carbohydrate. Fatty acids are synthesized from acetyl CoA in the hepatocyte cytosol, and esterification to glycerol to form triacylglycerols also occurs primarily in the liver. The fatty acyl chain on the fatty acid synthase complex is elongated two carbons at a time. With each two-carbon addition to the elongating chain, the β-keto group is reduced in a reaction that requires NADPH. NADPH is a reducing equivalent produced by the pentose phosphate pathway and the malic enzyme. $NADP^+$ is a product of fatty acid biosynthesis, not a substrate.

5. **The answer is B.** Linoleate and α-linolenate are the essential fatty acids required in the human diet. Palmitate (C16:0) is synthesized by the fatty acid synthase complex. Phosphatidic acid is an intermediate in triacylglycerol synthesis, which is formed using glycerol as a precursor in the liver and using glucose as a precursor in adipose tissue. It can be synthesized without the need for an essential fatty acid.

6. **The answer is C.** Long-chain fatty acids are activated, in a reaction requiring ATP and CoA, to a fatty acyl CoA. Carnitine reacts with fatty acyl CoA, forming fatty acyl carnitine, in order to transport the fatty acid across the mitochondrial membrane. Malonyl CoA is an intermediate in fatty acid synthesis.

7. **The answer is C.** Fatty acyl CoA undergoes β-oxidation in a spiral involving four steps. Long-chain fatty acids are released from adipose cells and must be activated and transported into mitochondria for oxidation. Fatty acyl CoA reacts with carnitine, forming fatty acyl carnitine, which crosses the inner mitochondrial membrane. The acyl group is then transferred back to CoA, forming fatty acyl CoA in the mitochondrial matrix. Subsequent reactions convert the fatty acyl CoA to $trans^2$ fatty enoyl CoA, β-hydroxy acyl CoA, and keto acyl CoA. The end product of fatty acid oxidation is acetyl CoA, which is oxidized via the TCA cycle and oxidative phosphorylation to produce carbon dioxide, water, and ATP.

8. **The answer is E.** Very-long-chain fatty acids are initially oxidized in peroxisomes, generating hydrogen peroxide, NADH, and acetyl CoA. Once the fatty acids have been shortened to about 8 to 10 carbons in length, they are transferred to the mitochondria to finish their oxidation via traditional β-oxidation. Thus, very-long-chain fatty acids will accumulate with this peroxisomal disorder. Short-chain and long-chain fatty acids are oxidized within the mitochondria via β-oxidation. Acetyl CoA will not accumulate with a peroxisomal disorder because it will also be

oxidized in the mitochondria. Dicarboxylic acids accumulate when there is a defect in mito-chondrial β-oxidation, and ω-oxidation begins to play a larger role in generating energy.

9. **The answer is A.** The infant has MCAD deficiency. The child can only partially oxidize fatty acids (to the 6- to 10-carbon stage), leading to reduced energy generation and low acetyl CoA levels. The low acetyl CoA reduces gluconeogenesis because pyruvate carboxylase cannot be fully activated. The reduced energy also contributes to the reduced levels of gluconeogenesis because that pathway requires energy to proceed. The dicarboxylic acids result from ω-oxidation of the medium-chain acyl CoAs, to try and generate more energy. Defects in CAT I or hormone-sensitive lipase would result in a complete lack of fatty acid oxidation, and the dicarboxylic acids would not be observed. A defect in pyruvate carboxylase, although negatively affecting gluco-neogenesis, would not affect fatty acid oxidation.

10. **The answer is B.** In the outer mitochondrial membrane, carnitine reacts with fatty acyl CoA to form fatty acyl carnitine, which can then pass to the inner mitochondrial membrane. Therefore, carnitine is important for the transport of fatty acyl CoA from the cytosol to the mitochondria and allow for β-oxidation to occur. Carnitine is not involved in activation of fatty acids or β-oxidation itself (which eliminates answer choices A, C, D, and E). As a note of interest, hypo-glycin leads to inhibition of gluconeogenesis (due to a lack of fatty acid oxidation, leading to low ATP and acetyl CoA levels). Profound hypoglycemia results, which is how hypoglycin was named.

10 Cholesterol Metabolism and Blood Lipoproteins

I. CHOLESTEROL AND BILE SALT METABOLISM

A. Cholesterol is synthesized from **cytosolic acetyl coenzyme A (CoA)** by a sequence of reactions. (Figure 10-1)

1. **Glucose** is a major source of carbon for acetyl CoA. Acetyl CoA is produced from glucose by the same sequence of reactions used to produce cytosolic acetyl CoA for fatty acid biosynthesis (Figure 10-2).

2. **Cytosolic acetyl CoA** forms acetoacetyl CoA, which condenses with another acetyl CoA to form hydroxymethylglutaryl CoA (HMG-CoA) (Figure 10-1). Acetyl CoA undergoes similar reactions in the mitochondrion, where HMG-CoA is used for ketone body synthesis.

3. **Cytosolic HMG-CoA,** a key intermediate in cholesterol biosynthesis, is reduced in the endoplasmic reticulum to mevalonic acid by the regulatory enzyme HMG-CoA reductase.

   a. **HMG-CoA reductase** is inhibited by cholesterol.

   b. HMG-CoA reductase is also inhibited by phosphorylation by the adenosine monophosphate (AMP)-activated protein kinase.

   c. In the liver, HMG-CoA reductase is also inhibited by bile salts and is induced when blood insulin levels are elevated.

CLINICAL CORRELATES   **Statins** are medications that function as **competitive inhibitors of HMG-CoA reductase,** thus **reducing the serum level of cholesterol.** Statins have been effective in regulating circulating cholesterol levels in patients with hypercholesterolemia.

---

4. **Mevalonic acid** is phosphorylated and decarboxylated to form the five-carbon (C-5) isoprenoid, isopentenyl pyrophosphate (Figure 10-1).

5. Two **isopentenyl pyrophosphate** units condense, forming a C-10 compound, geranyl pyrophosphate, which reacts with another C-5 unit to form a C-15 compound, farnesyl pyrophosphate (Figure 10-1).

6. **Squalene** is formed from two C-15 units and then oxidized and cyclized, forming lanosterol (Figure 10-1).

7. **Lanosterol** is converted to **cholesterol** in a series of steps (Figure 10-1).

8. The **ring structure** of cholesterol **cannot be degraded** in the body. The bile salts in the feces are the major form in which the steroid nucleus is excreted.

CLINICAL CORRELATES   **Gallstones** can be made of cholesterol. **Ursodeoxycholate** is a medication used to inhibit the formation of cholesterol gallstones. This medication is a hydrophilic bile salt that **decreases the content of cholesterol in bile.**

B. Bile salts are synthesized in the liver from cholesterol (Figure 10-3)

1. An α-**hydroxyl group** is added to carbon 7 of cholesterol. A **7α-hydroxylase,** which is inhibited by bile salts, catalyzes this rate-limiting step.

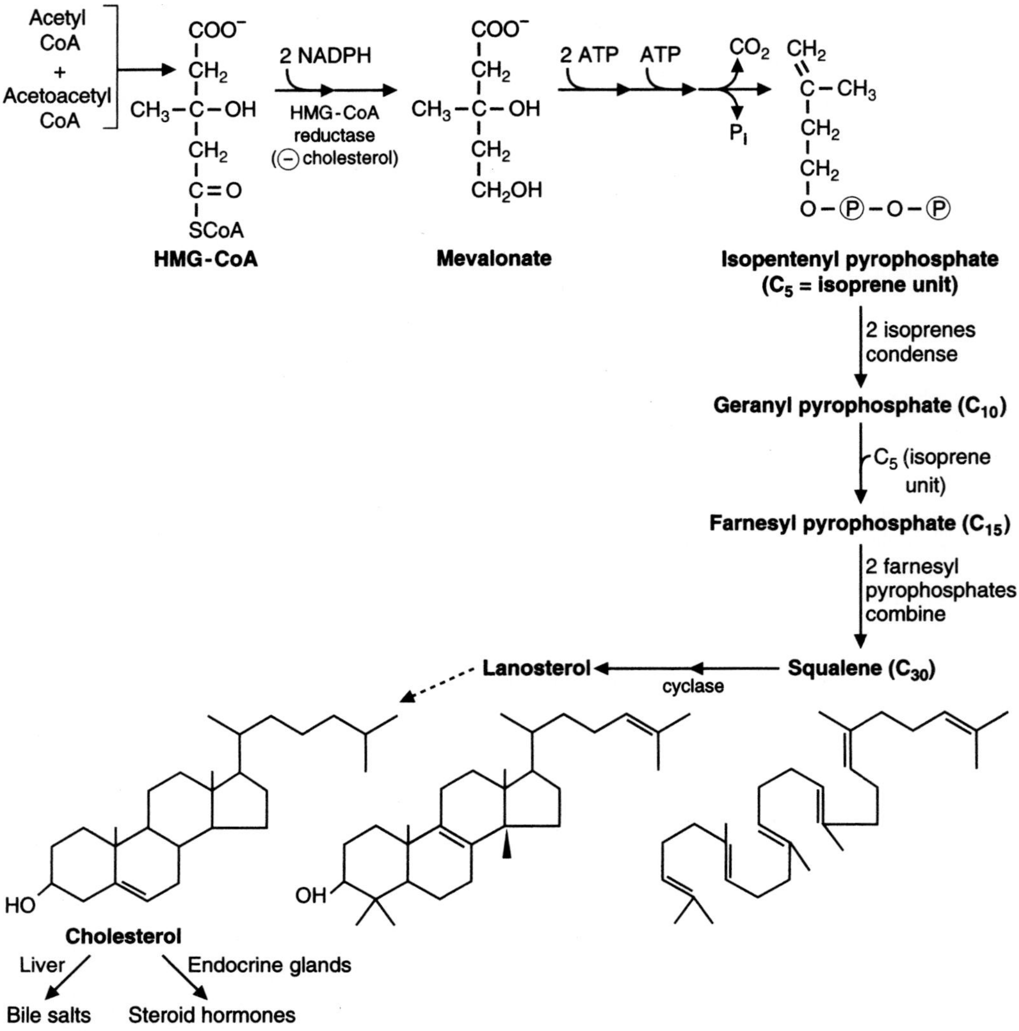

FIGURE 10-1 Cholesterol biosynthesis. HMG-CoA, hydroxymethylglutaryl coenzyme A; $\ominus$, inhibited by; $\textcircled{P}$ phosphate.

CLINICAL CORRELATES   **Atherosclerosis** is the **buildup of lipid-rich plaques** in the intima layer of **arteries.** Blood clots can form on these lipid-rich plaques, or part of the plaque may suddenly break loose, occluding a coronary or cerebral artery. **Occlusion of a coronary artery** can cause a **myocardial infarct** (heart attack), and **occlusion of a cerebral artery** can cause an ischemic cerebrovascular accident (**stroke**).

---

2. The **double bond** of cholesterol is **reduced,** and **further hydroxylations** occur, resulting in two compounds. One has α-hydroxyl groups at positions 3 and 7; and the other has α-hydroxyl groups at positions 3, 7, and 12.
3. The **side chain is oxidized** and converted to a branched, five-carbon chain, containing a carboxylic acid at the end.
   a. The bile acid with hydroxyl groups at positions 3 and 7 is **chenocholic acid.** The bile acid with hydroxyl groups at positions 3, 7, and 12 is **cholic acid.**
   b. These bile acids each have a **pK** of about **6.**
      (1) Above pH 6, the molecules are salts (i.e., they ionize and carry a negative charge).

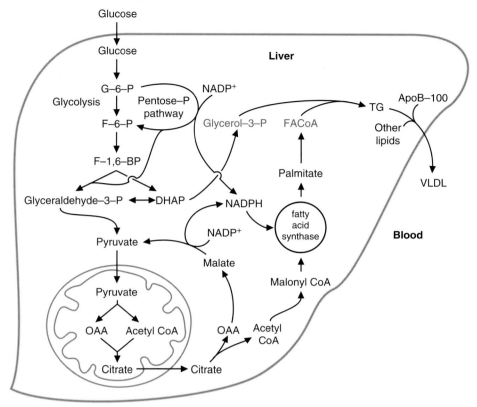

FIGURE 10-2 Synthesis of fatty acids and triaglycerols from glucose. DHAP, dihydroxyacetone phosphate; F-6-P, fructose 6-phosphate; F-1,6-BP, fructose 1,6-biphosphate; G-6-P, glucose 6-phosphate; OAA, oxaloacetate; VLDL, very-low-density lipoprotein.

(2) At pH 6 (the pH in the intestinal lumen), half of the molecules are ionized and carry a negative charge.

(3) Below pH 6, the molecules become protonated, and their charge decreases as the pH is lowered.

4. *Conjugation of the bile salts* (Figure 10-3, *middle*)

  a. The bile salts are activated by adenosine triphosphate (ATP) and coenzyme A, forming their CoA derivatives, which can form conjugates with either **glycine** or **taurine.**

  b. Glycine, an amino acid, forms an amide with the carboxyl group of a bile salt, forming **glycocholic acid or glycochenocholic acid.**

   (1) These bile salts each have a **pK** of about **4.**

   (2) This pK is lower than the unconjugated bile salts, so the conjugated bile salts are more completely ionized at pH 6 in the gut lumen and serve as better detergents.

  c. Taurine, which is derived from the amino acid cysteine, forms an amide with the carboxyl group of a bile salt.

   (1) Because of the sulfite group on the taurine moiety, the **taurocholic** and **taurochenocholic acids** have a **pK** of about **2.**

   (2) They ionize very readily in the gut and are the best detergents among the bile salts.

5. *Fate of the bile salts* (Figure 10-3, *bottom*)

  a. Cholic acid, chenocholic acid, and their conjugates are known as the **primary bile salts.** They are made in the liver and secreted via the **bile** through the **gallbladder** into the **intestine,** where, because they are amphipathic (contain both hydrophobic and hydrophilic regions), they aid in **lipid digestion.**

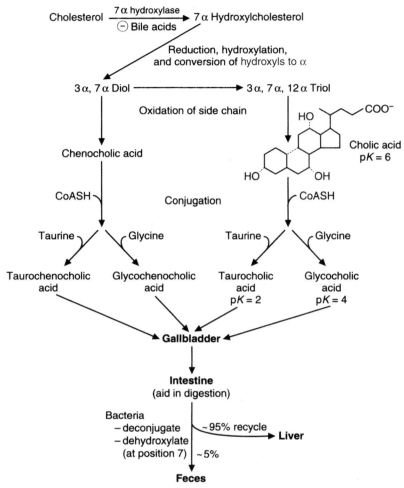

FIGURE 10-3 Synthesis and fate of bile salts. CoASH, nonreacted coenzyme A.

  b. In the intestine, bile salts can be **deconjugated** and **dehydroxylated** (at position 7) **by intestinal bacteria.**

  c. Bile salts are **resorbed** in the ileum and return to the liver, where they can be reconjugated with glycine or taurine. However, they are not rehydroxylated. Those that lack the 7α-hydroxyl group are called **secondary bile salts.**

  d. The **liver recycles** about 95% of the bile salts each day; 5% are lost in the feces.

CLINICAL CORRELATES **Bile acid sequestrants,** such as cholestyramine, **bind with bile acids in the intestinal lumen.** The insoluble complex of bile acid sequestrant and bile acid is eliminated in the stool. This **causes fecal loss of cholesterol.** As the body loses dietary cholesterol, the cells take up low-density lipoprotein (LDL) from circulation, which results in a lowering of circulating cholesterol.

C. Steroid hormones are synthesized from cholesterol, and 1,25-dihydroxycholecalciferol (active **vitamin D$_3$**) is synthesized from a precursor of cholesterol.

II. BLOOD LIPOPROTEINS

A. Composition of the blood lipoproteins (Table 10-1)

1. The major components of lipoproteins are triacylglycerols, cholesterol, cholesterol esters, phospholipids, and proteins. The protein components (called *apoproteins*) are designated A, B, C, and E.

2. **Chylomicrons** are the least dense of the blood lipoproteins because they have the most triacylglycerol and the least protein.

3. **Very-low-density lipoprotein (VLDL)** is more dense than chylomicrons but still has a high content of triacylglycerol.

4. **Intermediate-density lipoprotein (IDL),** which is derived from VLDL, is denser than VLDL and has less than half the amount of triacylglycerol of VLDL.

5. **LDL** has less triacylglycerol than IDL and more protein and, therefore, is denser than the IDL from which it is derived. LDL has the highest content of cholesterol and its esters.

6. **High-density lipoprotein (HDL)** is the densest lipoprotein. It has the lowest triacylglycerol content and the highest protein content of all the lipoprotein particles.

B. Metabolism of chylomicrons (Figure 10-4)

1. Chylomicrons are **synthesized in intestinal epithelial cells.** Their triacylglycerols are derived from dietary lipid, and their major apoprotein (apo) is apo B-48.

2. Chylomicrons travel through the lymph into the blood. (Step 1) **Apo C-II,** the activator of lipoprotein lipase, and **apo E** are transferred to nascent chylomicrons **from HDL,** and mature chylomicrons are formed. (Step 2)

3. In peripheral tissues, particularly adipose and muscle, the triacylglycerols are **digested by lipoprotein lipase.** As the chylomicron loses triacylglycerol, a chylomicron remnant is formed.

4. The chylomicron remnants interact with receptors on liver cells and are taken up by **endocytosis.** The contents are degraded by **lysosomal enzymes,** and the products (amino acids, fatty acids, glycerol, cholesterol, and phosphate) are released into the cytosol and reused.

C. Metabolism of VLDL (Figure 10-4)

1. **VLDL** is synthesized in the **liver,** particularly after a high-carbohydrate meal. It is formed from triacylglycerols that are packaged with cholesterol, apoproteins (particularly apo B-100), and phospholipids, and it is released into the blood. (Step 3)

2. In **peripheral tissues,** particularly adipose and muscle, VLDL triacylglycerols are **digested by lipoprotein lipase,** and VLDL is converted to IDL.

CLINICAL CORRELATES The agent **gemfibrozil,** a member of the **fibrate** class of lipid-lowering agents, activates the transcription of lipoprotein lipase by activating the PPAR (peroxisome proliferator-activated receptors) family of receptors. Therefore, the drug **decreases the level of VLDLs** and other triglyceride-rich lipoproteins.

t a b l e 10-1 Composition of the Blood Lipoproteins

Component	Chylomicrons	VLDL	IDL	LDL	HDL
Triacylglycerol	85%	55%	26%	10%	8%
Protein	2%	9%	11%	20%	45%
Apolipoprotein type	B, C, E	B, C, E	B, E	B	A, C, E
Cholesterol	1%	7%	8%	10%	5%
Cholesterol ester	2%	10%	30%	35%	15%
Phospholipid	8%	20%	23%	20%	25%

HDL, high-density lipoprotein; IDL, intermediate-density lipoprotein; LDL, low-density lipoprotein; VLDL, very-low-density lipoprotein.

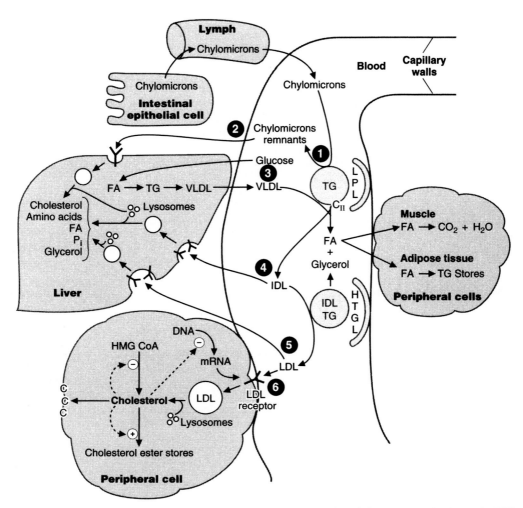

FIGURE 10-4 Metabolism of chylomicrons and very-low-density lipoprotein (VLDL). C, cholesterol; FA, fatty acid; HTGL, hepatic triglyceride lipase; LPL, lipoprotein lipase; TG, triacylglycerol; (TG), triacylglycerol of chylomicrons and VLDL; ⊖, inhibits; ⊕, stimulates; ❶ to ❸, fate of chylomicrons; ❸ to ❻, fate of VLDL.

3. **IDL** returns to the liver, is taken up by endocytosis, and is degraded by **lysosomal enzymes.** (Step 4) IDL can also be further degraded, forming LDL. (Step 5)

4. **LDL** reacts with receptors on various cells, is taken up by endocytosis, and is digested by **lysosomal enzymes.** (Step 6)
   a. **Cholesterol,** released from cholesterol esters by a lysosomal esterase, can be used for the synthesis of cell **membranes** or for the synthesis of bile salts in the liver or **steroid hormones** in endocrine tissue.
   b. Cholesterol **inhibits HMG-CoA reductase** (a key enzyme in cholesterol biosynthesis) and, thus, decreases the rate of cholesterol synthesis by the cell.
   c. Cholesterol **inhibits synthesis of LDL receptors** (downregulation) and, thus, reduces the amount of cholesterol taken up by cells.
   d. Cholesterol **activates acyl:cholesterol acyltransferase (ACAT),** which converts cholesterol to cholesterol esters for storage in cells.

D. **Familial hypercholesterolemia (types I, IIa, IIb, III, IV, V)** (Table10-2)

E. **Metabolism of HDL** (Figure 10-5)
   1. **HDL** is synthesized by the **liver** and released into the blood as small, disk-shaped particles. The major **protein** of HDL is **apo A.**

table 10-2 Hyperlipidemias

Disease	Description	Etiology of Lipid Disorder	Biochemical Finding
Type I	Hyperlipoproteinemia (rare genetic disorders)	Lipoprotein lipase deficiency or apo C-II deficiency	Chylomicrons high
Type IIa	Familial hypercholesterolemia (common autosomal dominant inheritance)	LDL receptor deficiency	Elevated LDL only
Type IIb	Familial combined hyperlipoproteinemia (common autosomal dominant inheritance)	Decreased LDL receptor and increased Apo B	LDL and VLDL high and triglycerides < 1000 mg/dL
Type III	Familial dysbetalipoproteinemia (rare)	Apo E defect	Increased IDL (a VLDL remnant)
Type IV	Familial hyperlipemia (common)	VLDL overproduction along with decreased clearance	Increased VLDLs
Type V	Hypertriglyceridemia with chylomicronemia (uncommon)	Increased VLDL production and decreased lipoprotein lipase production	Chylomicrons and VLDL elevated

HDL, high-density lipoprotein; IDL = intermediate-density lipoprotein; LDL, low-density lipoprotein; VLDL, very-low-density lipoprotein.

CLINICAL CORRELATES   **Tangier disease** is a disease of **cholesterol transport.** The first case was identified in a patient who lived on the island of Tangier and who had characteristic **orange-colored tonsils,** a **very low HDL** level, and an **enlarged liver and spleen.** Because of a mutation in a transport protein, **cholesterol cannot properly exit the cell to bind to apo A** (forming HDL). This results in a very low HDL level.

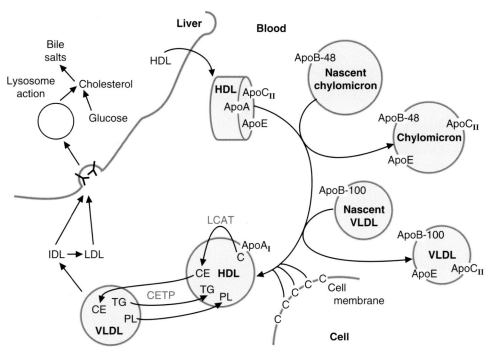

FIGURE 10-5 High-density lipoprotein (HDL) function and metabolism. Apo, apoprotein; C, cholesterol; CE, cholesterol ester; CETP, cholesterol ester transfer protein; IDL, intermediate-density lipoprotein; LCAT, lecithin:cholesterol acyltransferase; LDL, low-density lipoprotein; PL, phospholipid; TG, triacylglycerol; VLDL, very-low-density lipoprotein.

2. **Apo C-II,** which is transferred by HDL to chylomicrons and VLDL, serves as an **activator of lipoprotein lipase.**
   a. **Apo E** is also transferred and serves as a **recognition factor** for **cell surface receptors.**
   b. Apo C-II and apo E are transferred back to HDL after digestion of triacylglycerols of chylomicrons and VLDL.
3. **Cholesterol,** obtained by HDL from cell membranes or from other lipoproteins, is converted to **cholesterol esters** within the HDL particle by the **lecithin:cholesterol acyltransferase (LCAT) reaction,** which is activated by apo A-I.
   a. A fatty acid from position 2 of lecithin (phosphatidylcholine), a component of HDL, forms an ester with the 3-hydroxyl group of cholesterol, producing lysolecithin and a cholesterol ester.
   b. As cholesterol esters accumulate in the core of the lipoprotein, HDL particles become spheroids.

CLINICAL CORRELATES   **LCAT deficiency** results in an **inability to convert cholesterol associated with HDL to cholesterol esters.** Ordinarily, these **cholesterol esters would be transferred to other lipoproteins,** which would then be **taken up by receptors in the liver.** Therefore, by inducing esterification of cholesterol, LCAT is important for the **continued removal of cholesterol from the periphery.** Clinical manifestations include defects in the kidneys, red blood cells, and the cornea of the eyes.

---

4. **HDL transfers cholesterol esters** to other lipoproteins in exchange for various lipids. Cholesterol ester transfer protein (CETP) mediates this exchange. VLDL and other lipoproteins carry the cholesterol esters back to the liver.
5. **HDL particles** and other lipoproteins are taken up by the liver by endocytosis and **hydrolyzed by lysosomal enzymes.**
6. Cholesterol, released from cholesterol esters, can be packaged by the liver in VLDL and released into the blood or converted to bile salts and secreted into the bile.

Review Test

Directions: Each of the numbered questions or incomplete statements in this section is followed by answers or by completions of the statement. Select the **one** lettered answer or completion that is **best** in each case.

1. Which of the following apoproteins is an activator of lipoprotein lipase?

(A) Apo A
(B) Apo B
(C) Apo C-II
(D) Apo D
(E) Apo E

2. The major carriers of triacylglycerols are which of the following?

(A) Chylomicrons and VLDL
(B) IDL and LDL
(C) VLDL and LDL
(D) HDL and LDL
(E) Chylomicrons and LDL

3. A 40-year-old Hispanic woman with a body mass index of 34 presents with acute right upper quadrant pain, nausea, and vomiting after eating a meal rich in lipids. She is diagnosed with having cholelithiasis and is placed on a bile salt analog that is used to inhibit the formation of cholesterol gallstones. Which of the following is an example of a bile salt?

(A) HMG-CoA
(B) Mevalonate
(C) Squalene
(D) Lanosterol
(E) Chenocholic acid

4. An 8-year-old boy presents with orange-colored tonsils, a very low HDL level, and an enlarged liver and spleen and is diagnosed with Tangier disease. Which of the following statements best describes HDL?

(A) It is produced in skeletal muscle.
(B) It scavenges cholesterol from cell membranes.
(C) Its major protein is apo E.
(D) It is formed when VLDL is digested by lipoprotein lipase.
(E) It activates ACAT.

5. A 40-year-old man presents with chest pain that radiates to his left jaw and shoulder. He is diagnosed with a myocardial infarction and is prescribed a statin medication. Statins are competitive inhibitors of HMG-CoA reductase, which converts HMG-CoA to which of the following?

(A) Mevalonate
(B) Isopentenyl pyrophosphate
(C) Geranyl pyrophosphate
(D) Farnesyl pyrophosphate
(E) Cholesterol

6. A 45-year-old woman presents with oily, foul-smelling stool, which appears to be due to an obstruction of the bile duct. Which of the following statements correctly describes bile salts?

(A) They can act as detergents, aiding in lipid digestion.
(B) They are stored in the intestines.
(C) Ninety-five percent of bile salts are excreted in the feces, and 5% are recycled back to the liver.
(D) Bile salts are synthesized in the intestines.
(E) Squalene and lanosterol are examples of bile salts.

7. A 55-year-old woman presents with crushing substernal chest pain and shortness of breath. A coronary artery is occluded owing to an atherosclerotic plaque, and a high myocardial infarct is diagnosed. High serum HDL levels are protective against the development of atherosclerosis because HDL does which of the following?

(A) Inhibits cholesterol production by the liver
(B) Inhibits HMG-CoA reductase
(C) Increases VLDL production
(D) Increases LDL production
(E) Brings cholesterol esters back to the liver

8. A 30-year-old man presents with weakness in his right upper and lower extremities. He is diagnosed with an acute middle cerebral artery stroke secondary to atherosclerosis. Genetic studies show that he has familial hypercholes-terolemia, type II, a disorder caused by a defi-ciency of LDL receptors. Which of the following statements best describes patients with type II familial hypercholesterolemia?

(A) After LDL binds to the LDL receptor, the LDL is degraded extracellularly.
(B) The number of LDL receptors on the sur-face of hepatocytes increases.
(C) Cholesterol synthesis by hepatocytes increases.
(D) Excessive cholesterol is released by LDL.
(E) The cholesterol level in the serum decreases.

9. A 40-year-old woman presents with an LDL serum level of 400 (recommended level is <130), and a triglyceride level of 170 (recom-mended level is <150). She is diagnosed with type II familial hypercholesterolemia. In this disorder, a mutated LDL receptor is formed, such that it cannot bind to LDL. Which of the following would result?

(A) Cellular HMG-CoA reductase activity is not inhibited.
(B) The triglycerides in chylomicrons cannot be degraded.
(C) The VLDL level in the serum increases.
(D) The HDL level in the serum increases.
(E) The VLDL cannot be converted to IDL.

10. A 25-year-old woman presents with a low red blood cell count, corneal opacities, and kid-ney insufficiency. She is diagnosed with LCAT deficiency. LCAT is involved in which of the following processes?

(A) Converting cholesterol to cholesterol esters
(B) The transfer of cholesterol esters from HDL to other lipoproteins
(C) Endocytosis of HDL particles into hepatocytes
(D) Hydrolysis of HDL
(E) Decreased uptake of cholesterol by hepatocytes

Answers and Explanations

1. **The answer is C.** Apo C-II is an activator of lipoprotein lipase, Apo A is the major apolipoprotein of HDL, Apo B100 is the major apolipoprotein of LDL and VLDL (and apo B48 is the major apolipoprotein of chylomicrons), and Apo E is transferred by HDL to nascent chylomicrons and nascent VLDL to form mature forms of those particles. Apo D is unlike all the other apolipoproteins, and its role in metabolism has yet to be clearly defined.

2. **The answer is A.** The major carriers of triacylglycerols are chylomicrons (synthesized in the intestine from dietary fat) and VLDL (synthesized in the liver). The triacylglycerols are digested in capillaries by lipoprotein lipase. The fatty acids that are produced are used for energy by cells or are converted back to triacylglycerols and stored. IDL and LDL are digestion products of VLDL, which have reduced amounts of triglyceride compared with VLDL. HDL has the least amount of triglyceride of any lipoprotein particle.

3. **The answer is E.** Chenocholic acid is an example of a bile salt. HMG-CoA, mevalonate, squalene, and lanosterol are intermediates in cholesterol synthesis. Bile salts are synthesized from cholesterol in the liver, are stored in the gallbladder, and are released to facilitate lipid digestion in the intestines.

4. **The answer is B.** HDL scavenges cholesterol from cell membranes and lipoproteins. HDL is produced in the liver (not muscle), and its major apoprotein is apo A. IDL is formed when VLDL is digested by lipoprotein lipase. Cholesterol activates ACAT, which converts cholesterol to cholesterol esters for storage in cells.

5. **The answer is A.** HMG-CoA reductase converts HMG-CoA to mevalonate, using two NADPH molecules. Isopentenyl pyrophosphate, geranyl pyrophosphate, and farnesyl pyrophosphate are intermediates in cholesterol synthesis. Mevalonate is required to synthesize isopentenyl pyrophosphate, which leads to geranyl and farnesyl pyrophosphate production.

6. **The answer is A.** Bile salts, synthesized in the liver and stored in the gallbladder, act as detergents, aiding in lipid digestion. The bile salts are secreted into the intestine in response to cholecystokinin. An inadequate concentration of bile salts in the intestines can lead to oily, foul-smelling stool with a high fat content, a condition known as *steatorrhea*. Ninety-five percent of bile salts are recycled back to the liver, and 5% are excreted in the feces. Squalene and lanosterol are intermediary compounds in cholesterol synthesis, not bile acid synthesis.

7. **The answer is E.** HDL is known as the "good" lipoprotein particle because HDL scavenges cholesterol from the periphery (from cell membranes and from other lipoproteins) and brings cholesterol esters back to the liver, where they can be converted to and excreted as bile salts. This is known as *reverse cholesterol transport*. HDL does not inhibit cholesterol production by the liver. Statin medications inhibit HMG-CoA reductase activity, not HDL production. Increasing VLDL or LDL will facilitate the development of atherosclerosis, not protect against its development.

8. **The answer is C.** Familial hypercholesterolemia, type II, is due to a mutation in the LDL receptor, which, in a variety of mechanisms, prevents endocytosis of the receptor with bound LDL. Cholesterol synthesis by hepatocytes increases in patients with this disorder because HMG-CoA reductase is not properly inhibited. Normally, after LDL binds to the LDL receptor, the receptor–LDL complex is internalized, the LDL is degraded intracellularly, and the cholesterol released from the LDL migrates to the cytosol. The increase in intracellular cholesterol inhibits HMG-CoA reductase, resulting in decreased cholesterol synthesis by hepatocytes. Because the LDL receptor is deficient in patients with this disease, LDL cannot be taken up by hepatocytes (to release cholesterol), and an extremely high serum cholesterol level results, both from increased cellular synthesis and release of VLDL, and high levels of LDL particles in the circulation.

9. **The answer is A.** Normally, LDL, after binding to its receptor and internalization into the cell, is digested by lysosomal enzymes to release cholesterol. High levels of intracellular cholesterol inhibit HMG-CoA reductase, and cholesterol synthesis decreases in hepatocytes. In familial hypercholesterolemia type II, LDL cannot be taken up into hepatocytes. Because HMG-CoA reductase is not properly inhibited, excessive cholesterol levels result. Triglyceride digestion in chylomicrons, the level of VLDL, the level of HDL, and conversion of VLDL to IDL are not affected in type II hypercholesterolemia.

10. **The answer is A.** LCAT converts cholesterol to cholesterol esters, which accumulate in the core of HDL. This is an important part of reverse cholesterol transport. These cholesterol esters are transferred from HDL to VLDL and LDL (via the cholesterol ester transfer protein reaction), which are then taken up by receptors in the liver. Therefore, LCAT is important for removing cholesterol from peripheral cells by inducing esterification of cholesterol, thus allowing eventual cholesterol uptake by the liver. LCAT is not involved in endocytosis of HDL into hepatocytes, in the transfer of cholesterol esters from HDL to other lipoproteins, or in hydrolysis of HDL.

chapter 11

Ketones and Other Lipid Derivatives

I. KETONE BODY SYNTHESIS AND UTILIZATION (FIGURE 11-1)

A. **Synthesis of ketone bodies** (Figure 11-1, *top*) occurs in **liver mitochondria** when fatty acids are in high concentration in the blood (during fasting, starvation, or as a result of a high-fat diet).

1. **β-Oxidation** produces NADH and adenosine triphosphate (ATP) and results in the accumulation of acetyl coenzyme A (CoA), owing to allosteric inhibition of tricarboxylic acid (TCA) cycle enzymes. The liver is also producing glucose using oxaloacetate (OAA), so there is decreased condensation of acetyl CoA with OAA to form citrate.

2. **Two molecules of acetyl CoA** condense to produce acetoacetyl CoA. This reaction is catalyzed by thiolase or an isoenzyme of **thiolase.**

3. Acetoacetyl CoA and acetyl CoA form hydroxymethylglutaryl CoA (HMG-CoA) in a reaction catalyzed by HMG-CoA synthase.

4. **HMG-CoA** is cleaved by HMG-CoA lyase to form acetyl CoA and acetoacetate.

5. **Acetoacetate** can be reduced by an NAD-requiring dehydrogenase (3-hydroxybutyrate dehydrogenase) to **3-hydroxybutyrate (also known as β-hydroxybutyrate).** This is a reversible reaction.

6. Acetoacetate is also spontaneously **decarboxylated** in a nonenzymatic reaction, forming **acetone** (the source of the odor on the breath of ketotic diabetic patients).

CLINICAL CORRELATES   **Type 1 diabetes mellitus** is due to a **deficiency of insulin,** which is caused by autoimmune destruction of insulin-producing cells in the pancreas. Insulin is required for glucose to be used by cells. Deficiency of insulin leads to a state known as **diabetic ketoacidosis,** which manifests as a **severely elevated serum glucose level, increased ketone body synthesis,** and formation of **acetone** due to decarboxylation of acetoacetate.

---

7. The **liver** lacks the enzyme needed to metabolize ketone bodies (succinyl CoA-acetoacetate-CoA transferase, a thiotransferase), so it **cannot use the ketone bodies it produces.** Therefore, acetoacetate and 3-hydroxybutyrate are released into the blood by the liver.

B. **Utilization of ketone bodies** (Figure 11-1, *bottom*)

1. When ketone bodies are released from the liver into the blood, they are taken up by peripheral tissues such as **muscle and kidney,** where they are oxidized for energy. During **starvation,** ketone bodies in the blood increase to a level that permits entry into **brain** cells, where they are oxidized.

2. **Acetoacetate** can enter cells directly, or it can be produced from the oxidation of 3-hydroxybutyrate by 3-hydroxybutyrate dehydrogenase. NADH is produced by this reaction and can generate adenosine triphosphate (ATP).

3. Acetoacetate is activated by reacting with succinyl CoA to form **acetoacetyl CoA** and succinate. The enzyme is succinyl CoA-acetoacetate-CoA transferase (a thiotransferase).

4. Acetoacetyl CoA is cleaved by **thiolase** to form two molecules of acetyl CoA, which enter the TCA cycle and are oxidized to molecules of CO_2.

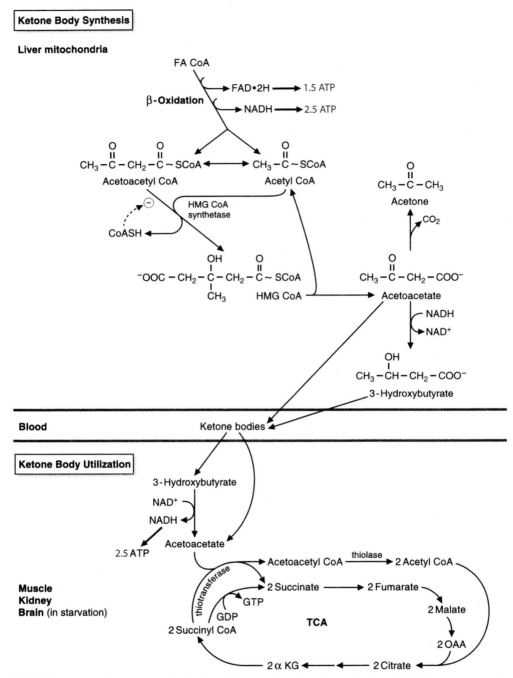

FIGURE 11-1 Ketone body synthesis and utilization. ATP, adenosine triphosphate; FA, fatty acid; FAD, flavin adenine dinu-cleotide; αK, α-ketoglutarate; HMG-CoA, hydroxymethylglutaryl coenzyme A; OAA, oxaloacetate; TCA, tricarboxylic acid. The thiotransferase is succinyl CoA–acetoacetate-CoA transferase.

5. **Energy is produced** from the oxidation of ketone bodies.
   a. One acetoacetate produces two acetyl CoA, each of which can generate about 10 ATP, or a total of about 20 ATP via the TCA cycle.
   b. However, activation of acetoacetate results in the generation of one less ATP because guanosine triphosphate (GTP), the equivalent of ATP, is not produced when succinyl CoA is used to activate acetoacetate. (In the TCA cycle, when succinyl CoA forms

succinate, GTP is generated.) Therefore, the oxidation of acetoacetate produces a net yield of only 19 ATP.

c. When **3-hydroxybutyrate** is oxidized, 2.5 additional ATP are formed because the oxidation of 3-hydroxybutyrate to acetoacetate produces NADH.

II. PHOSPHOLIPID AND SPHINGOLIPID METABOLISM

A. Synthesis and degradation of phosphoglycerides

1. The phosphoglycerides are synthesized by a process similar in its initial steps to triacylglycerol synthesis (glycerol 3-phosphate combines with two fatty acyl CoA to form **phosphatidic acid**).

2. **Synthesis of phosphatidylinositol**

   a. **Phosphatidic acid** reacts with cytidine triphosphate (CTP) to form cytidine diphosphate (CDP)-diacylglycerol, which reacts with inositol to form phosphatidylinositol.

   b. **Phosphatidylinositol** can be further phosphorylated to form phosphatidylinositol 4,5-bisphosphate, which is cleaved in response to various stimuli to form the compounds inositol 1,4,5-trisphosphate (IP_3) and diacylglycerol (DAG), which serve as second messengers.

3. **Synthesis of phosphatidylethanolamine, phosphatidylcholine, and phosphatidylserine** (Figure 11-2)

   a. **Phosphatidic acid** releases inorganic phosphate, and diacylglycerol is produced. **DAG** reacts with compounds containing cytidine nucleotides to form **phosphatidylethanolamine** and **phosphatidylcholine**.

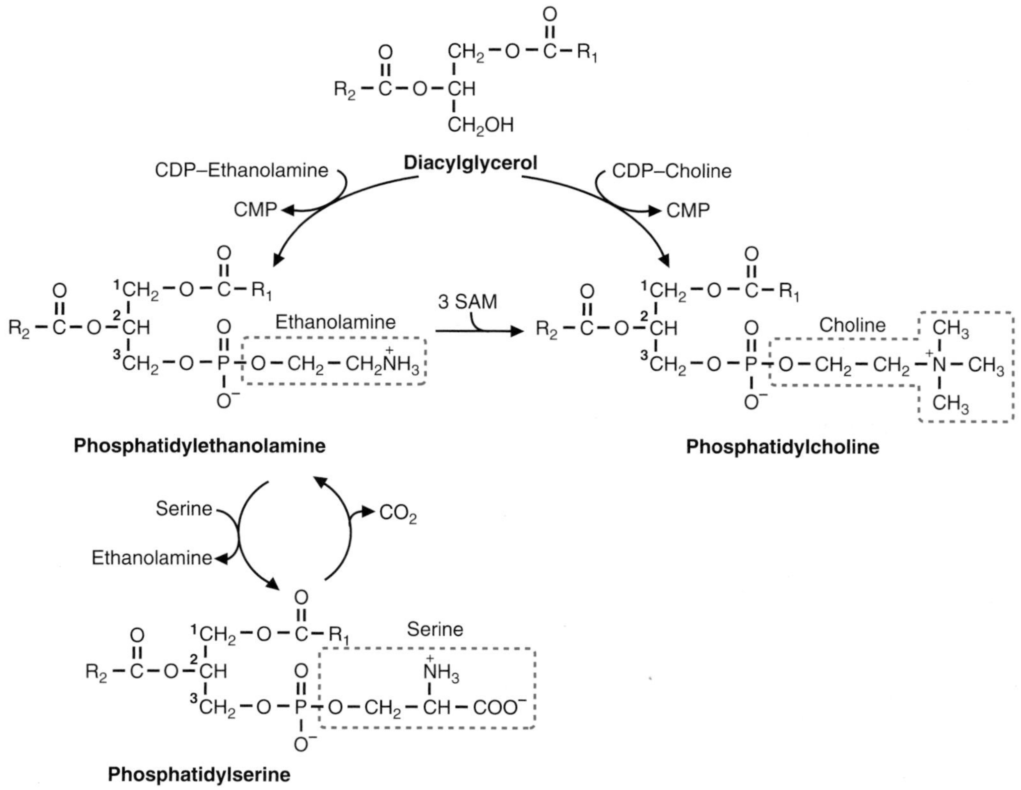

FIGURE 11-2 Synthesis of phospholipids. CDP, cytidine diphosphate; CMP, cytidine monophosphate, SAM, *S*-adenosylmethionine.

b. Phosphatidylethanolamine
(1) DAG reacts with CDP-ethanolamine to form phosphatidylethanolamine.
(2) Phosphatidylethanolamine can also be formed by decarboxylation of phosphatidylserine.

c. Phosphatidylcholine
(1) DAG reacts with CDP-choline to form **phosphatidylcholine (lecithin)**.
(2) Phosphatidylcholine can also be formed by methylation of phosphatidylethanolamine. S-Adenosylmethionine (SAM) provides the methyl groups.
(3) In addition to being an important component of cell membranes and the blood lipoproteins, phosphatidylcholine provides the fatty acid for the synthesis of cholesterol esters in high-density lipoprotein (HDL) by the **lecithin:cholesterol acyltransferase (LCAT) reaction** and, as the dipalmitoyl derivative, serves as a component of **lung surfactant.** If choline is deficient in the diet, phosphatidylcholine can be synthesized de novo from glucose (Figure 11-2).

> **CLINICAL CORRELATES** **Respiratory distress syndrome** (RDS) of the newborn occurs in **premature infants** due to a **deficiency of surfactant in the lungs,** which leads to a decrease in lung compliance. **Dipalmitoyl phosphatidylcholine** (DPPC, also called *lecithin*), is the **primary phospholipid in surfactant,** which lowers surface tension at the alveolar air–fluid interface. Surfactant is normally produced at gestational week 30.

d. Phosphatidylserine
(1) Phosphatidylserine is formed when phosphatidylethanolamine reacts with serine.
(2) Serine replaces the ethanolamine moiety (Figure 11-2).

4. Degradation of phosphoglycerides
a. Phosphoglycerides are hydrolyzed by phospholipases.
b. Phospholipase A_1 releases the fatty acid at position 1 of the glycerol moiety; phospholipase A_2 releases the fatty acid at position 2; phospholipase C releases the phosphorylated head group (e.g., choline) at position 3; and phospholipase D releases the free head group.

B. Synthesis and degradation of sphingolipids (Figure 11-3)
1. Sphingolipids are derived from **serine** rather than glycerol.
2. **Serine** condenses with **palmitoyl CoA** in a reaction in which the serine is decarboxylated by a pyridoxal phosphate–requiring enzyme.
3. The product of the condensation reaction is a derivative of **sphingosine.** Subsequent reactions convert this product to sphingosine.
4. A fatty acyl CoA forms an amide with the nitrogen of sphingosine, and the resulting compound is **ceramide.**
5. The hydroxymethyl moiety of ceramide combines with various compounds to form **sphingolipids and sphingoglycolipids.**
   a. **Phosphatidylcholine** reacts with ceramide to form **sphingomyelin.**
   b. Uridine diphosphate (UDP)-sugars react with ceramide to form galactocerebrosides or glucocerebrosides.
   c. A series of sugars can add to ceramide, with UDP sugars serving as precursors. **CMP-NANA** (N-acetylneuraminic acid, a sialic acid) can form branches from the carbohydrate chain. These ceramide-oligosaccharide compounds are **gangliosides.**
6. Sphingolipids are degraded by **lysosomal enzymes.** Genetic deficiencies of enzymes involved in the degradation of sphingolipids are well characterized (Table 11-1).

III. METABOLISM OF THE EICOSANOIDS

A. Prostaglandins, prostacyclins, and thromboxanes (Figure 11-4)
1. **Polyunsaturated fatty acids** containing 20 carbons, and three to five double bonds (e.g., arachidonic acid) are usually esterified to position 2 of the glycerol moiety of phospholipids in cell membranes. These fatty acids require **essential fatty acids,** such as dietary linoleic acid ($18:2, \Delta^{9,12}$), for their synthesis.

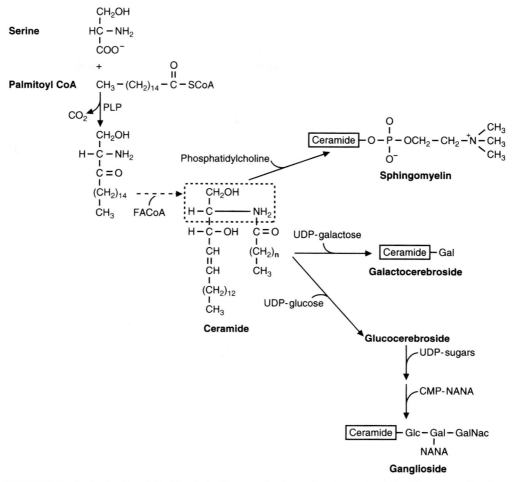

FIGURE 11-3 Synthesis of sphingolipids. The *dashed box* contains the portion of ceramide derived from serine. The *dotted arrow* indicates that some intermediate steps have been skipped going from the initial condensation of palmitoyl coenzyme A and serine to ceramide production. FA, fatty acyl groups; Gal, galactose; GalNAc, *N*-acetylgalactosamine; Glc, glucose; NANA, *N*-acetylneuraminic acid; PLP, pyridoxal phosphate.

2. The polyunsaturated fatty acid is cleaved from the membrane phospholipid by **phospholipase A₂**, which is inhibited by the steroidal anti-inflammatory agents (steroids).

CLINICAL CORRELATES   **Steroids,** such as cortisone and prednisone, are often prescribed for **inflammatory or autoimmune diseases,** such as rheumatoid arthritis, a debilitating inflammatory joint disease.

---

3. Oxygen is added, and a five-carbon ring is formed by the enzyme **cyclooxygenase,** which produces the initial prostaglandin. The initial prostaglandin is converted to other classes of **prostaglandins** and to the **thromboxanes.**
   a. **Aspirin, acetaminophen,** and other nonsteroidal anti-inflammatory agents **inhibit** this isozyme of cyclo-oxygenase.
   b. The **prostaglandins** have a multitude of effects that differ from one tissue to another and include inflammation, pain, fever, and aspects of reproduction. These compounds are known as **autocoids** because they exert their effects primarily in the tissue in which they are produced.
   c. Certain **prostacyclins** (PGI₂), produced by vascular endothelial cells, **inhibit platelet aggregation,** whereas certain **thromboxanes** (TXA₂) **promote platelet aggregation.**

t a b l e **11-1**	Sphingolipidoses		
Disease	Enzyme Deficiency	Accumulated Products	Clinical Consequence
Niemann-Pick disease	Sphingomyelinase	Sphingomyelin in the brain and blood cells	**Mental retardation, spasticity, seizures,** and **ataxia.** Death usually results by age 2-3 years. Inheritance is **autosomal recessive.**
Fabry disease	α-Galactosidase A	Glycolipids in brain, heart, and kidney, resulting in ischemia of affected organs	Severe pain in the extremities (**acroparesthesia),** skin lesions (**angiokeratomas),** **hypohidrosis,** and ischemic infarction of the kidney, heart, and brain
Krabbe disease	β-Galactosidase	Glycolipids causing destruction of myelin-producing oligodendrocytes	Clinical consequences of demyelination include **spasticity** and rapid neurodegeneration leading to death. Clinical signs include **hypertonia and hyperreflexia,** leading to **decerebrate posturing,** blindness, and deafness. Inheritance is autosomal recessive.
Gaucher disease	Glucocerebrosidase	Glucocerebrosides in blood cells, liver, and spleen	Enlarged liver and spleen (**hepatosplenomegaly),** anemia, low platelet count (**thrombocytopenia),** bone pain, and Erlenmeyer flask deformity of the distal femur. This **autosomal recessive** deficiency is prevalent in Ashkenazi Jews.
Tay-Sachs disease	Hexosaminidase A	GM₂ gangliosides in neurons	Progressive **neurodegeneration, developmental delay,** and early death. This **autosomal recessive** deficiency is prevalent in Ashkenazi Jews.
Metachromatic leukodystrophy	Arylsulfatase A	Sulfated glycolipid (sulfatide) compounds accumulate in neural tissue, causing demyelination of central nervous system and peripheral nerves.	Clinical consequences of demyelination include loss of cognitive and motor functions, intellectual decline in school performance, **ataxia, hyporeflexia,** and seizures.

CLINICAL CORRELATES   **Aspirin** has been shown to be **cardioprotective** in myocardial infarction. Although PGI₂ is also inhibited, the cardioprotective effect is mediated by **inhibiting TXA₂.**

4. Inactivation of the prostaglandins occurs when the molecule is oxidized from the carboxyl and ω-methyl ends to form **dicarboxylic acids** that are excreted in the urine.

B. Leukotrienes
1. **Arachidonic acid,** derived from membrane phospholipids, is the major precursor for synthesis of the leukotrienes.
2. In the first step, oxygen is added by lipoxygenases, and a family of linear molecules, hydroperoxyeicosatetraenoic acids (**HPETEs**), is formed.
3. A series of compounds, comprising the family of leukotrienes, is produced from these HPETEs. The leukotrienes are involved in **allergic reactions.**

CLINICAL CORRELATES   **Asthma** causes severe breathing difficulty due to **hyperreactivity and narrowing of the airways.** Because leukotrienes cause bronchoconstriction, **leukotriene receptor antagonists** can be prescribed as a treatment.

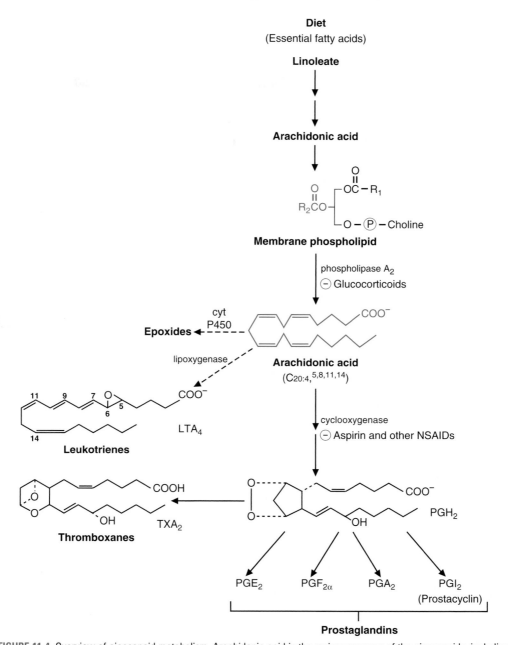

FIGURE 11-4 Overview of eicosanoid metabolism. Arachidonic acid is the major precursor of the eicosanoids, including leukotriene (LT), prostaglandin (PG), and thromboxane (TX). NSAIDs, nonsteroidal anti-inflammatory drugs; ⊖, inhibits.

IV. SYNTHESIS OF THE STEROID HORMONES

A. Steroid hormones are derived from **cholesterol** (Figure 11-5), which forms **pregnenolone** by cleavage of its side chain.

B. **Progesterone** is produced by oxidation of the A ring of **pregnenolone**.

C. **Testosterone** is produced from **progesterone** by removal of the side chain of the D ring. Testosterone is also produced from **pregnenolone** via dehydroepiandrosterone (DHEA).

D. **17β-Estradiol** (E₂) is produced from **testosterone** by aromatization of the A ring.

E. **Cortisol and aldosterone,** the adrenal steroids, are produced from **progesterone**.

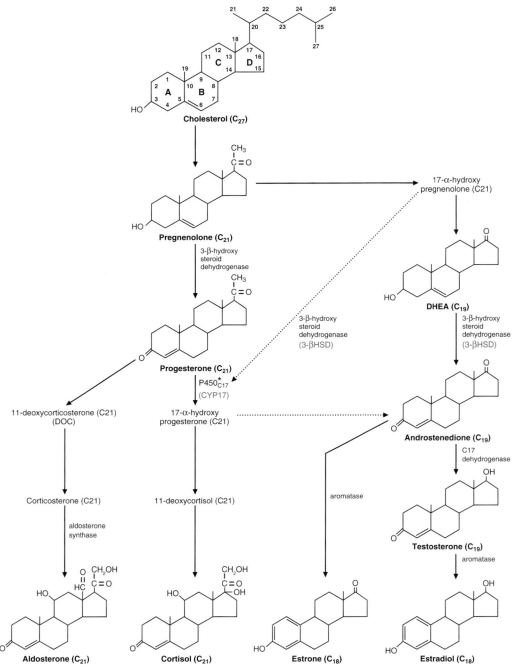

FIGURE 11-5 Synthesis of the steroid hormones. The rings of the precursor cholesterol are *lettered*. DHEA, dehydroepiandrosterone.

CLINICAL CORRELATES   **3-β-Hydroxysteroid dehydrogenase deficiency** is a disease resulting in decreased production of aldosterone, cortisol, and androgens (3-β-hydroxysteroid dehydrogenase is required for production of all three types of steroids). **Male infants** manifest with **ambiguous genitalia** (owing to lack of androgens), and both males and females show salt wasting (owing to lack of aldosterone).

17-α-hydroxylase deficiency is a disease resulting in decreased production of cortisol and androgens but increased production of aldosterone. Male and female teenagers are usually diagnosed during **puberty** with **lack of secondary sexual characteristics.** Increased aldosterone can cause excessive salt absorption.

F. **1,25-Dihydroxycholecalciferol** (1,25-DHC, or calcitriol) (Figure 11-6), the active form of vitamin D₃, can be produced by two hydroxylations of **dietary vitamin D₃** (cholecalciferol).
   1. The first hydroxylation occurs at position 25 (in the liver), and the second occurs at position 1 (in the kidney).
   2. In addition, 7-dehydrocholesterol, a precursor of cholesterol produced from acetyl CoA, can be converted by **ultraviolet light** in the **skin** to cholecalciferol and then hydroxylated to form 1,25-DHC.

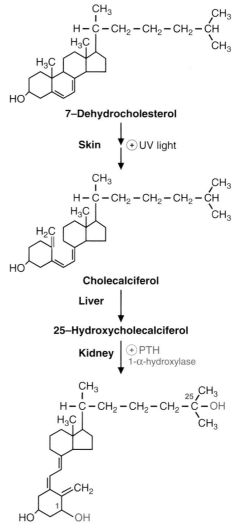

FIGURE 11-6 Synthesis of active vitamin D. PTH, parathyroid hormone; UV, ultraviolet.

Review Test

Directions: Each of the numbered questions or incomplete statements in this section is followed by answers or by completions of the statement. Select the **one** lettered answer or completion that is **best** in each case.

1. A 12-year-old boy presents with fatigue, polydipsia, polyuria, and polyphagia. A fingerstick glucose measurement shows a glucose level of 350 mg/dL in his serum. He is diagnosed with type 1 diabetes mellitus, a disease characterized by a deficiency of insulin. Which one of the following is most likely occurring in this patient?

(A) Increased fatty acid synthesis from glucose in liver
(B) Decreased conversion of fatty acids to ketone bodies
(C) Increased stores of triacylglycerol in adipose tissue
(D) Increased production of acetone
(E) Chronic pancreatitis

2. A 58-year-old woman is undergoing a myocardial infarct and is given 162 mg of aspirin, owing to the cardioprotective effects of aspirin during such an incident. Aspirin is a nonsteroidal anti-inflammatory drug that inhibits cyclooxygenase. Cyclooxygenase is required for which one of the following conversions?

(A) Thromboxanes from arachidonic acid
(B) Leukotrienes from arachidonic acid
(C) Phospholipids from arachidonic acid
(D) Arachidonic acid from linoleic acid
(E) HPETEs and subsequently hydroxyeicosatetraenoic acids (HETEs) from arachidonic acid

3. The cardioprotective effects of aspirin occur due to the inhibition of the synthesis of which one of the following?

(A) $PGF_{2\alpha}$
(B) PGE_2
(C) TXA_2
(D) PGA_2
(E) PGI_2

4. A 40-year-old woman has rheumatoid arthritis, a crippling disease causing severe pain and deformation in the joints of the fingers. She is prescribed prednisone, a steroid that exerts its beneficial effects through anti-inflammatory pathways. What is the mechanism of steroidal anti-inflammatory agents?

(A) Prevent conversion of arachidonic acid to epoxides
(B) Inhibit phospholipase A_2
(C) Promote activation of prostacyclins
(D) Degrade thromboxanes
(E) Promote leukotriene formation from HPETEs

5. An infant is born prematurely at 28 weeks and increasingly has significant difficulty breathing, taking rapid breaths with intercostal retractions. The child soon becomes cyanotic. He is diagnosed with respiratory distress syndrome due to a deficiency of surfactant. Which of the following is the phospholipid in highest concentration in surfactant?

(A) Dipalmitoyl phosphatidylcholine
(B) Dipalmitoyl phosphatidylethanolamine
(C) Dipalmitoyl phosphatidylglycerol
(D) Dipalmitoyl phosphatidylinositol
(E) Dipalmitoyl phosphatidylserine

6. An 11-year-old Ashkenazi Jewish girl presents with an enlarged liver and spleen, low white and red blood cell counts, bone pain, and bruising. She is diagnosed with Gaucher disease, a lysosomal storage disease. Which of the following compounds is accumulating in her lysosomes?

(A) Galactocerebroside
(B) Ceramide
(C) Glucocerebroside
(D) Sphingosine
(E) GM_1

7. A 4-month-old infant presents with muscular weakness that is progressing to paralysis. Examination of the back of the eye shows a cherry-red spot on the macula. An abnormally low level of hexosaminidase A is present, causing deposition of certain gangliosides in neurons. The accumulating material in this disorder is which of the following?

(A) GM_1
(B) GM_2
(C) GM_3
(D) GD_3
(E) GT_3

8. A male infant with 3-β-hydroxylase deficiency is born with ambiguous genitalia and severe salt wasting from lack of androgens and aldosterone, respectively. Testosterone, a major androgen, is produced by which of the following reactions?

(A) Oxidation of the A ring of pregnenolone
(B) Removal of the side chain of the D ring of progesterone

(C) Aromatization of the A ring of estradiol
(D) Cleavage of the side chain of progesterone
(E) Oxidation of aldosterone

9. A 2-year-old girl is failing to meet age-appropriate milestones, including a progressive difficulty in walking. An abnormally low level of arylsulfatase A is found in her cells, causing accumulation of sulfated glycolipids in neurons. Unfortunately, she dies 5 years later. Which one of the following is the most likely diagnosis for this disorder?

(A) Fabry disease
(B) Gaucher disease
(C) Niemann-Pick disease
(D) Tay-Sachs disease
(E) Metachromatic leukodystrophy

Answers and Explanations

1. **The answer is D.** A decreased insulin-to-glucagon ratio leads to a decrease in fatty acid synthesis and an increase in adipose triacylglycerol degradation, leading to fatty acid release into the circulation. The liver takes up the fatty acids, and within the mitochondria, fatty acids undergo β-oxidization. As acetyl CoA accumulates, the ketone bodies, acetoacetate and β-hydroxybutyrate, are formed and are released into the circulation. These ketone bodies are used to fuel the heart, brain, and muscle. Nonenzymatic decarboxylation of acetoacetate forms acetone, which can be smelled by some providers on the breath of patients in diabetic ketoacidosis. Because triglycerides are degraded under these conditions, there is not an increase in triglyceride storage. Pancreatitis does not result from an inability to produce insulin.

2. **The answer is A.** Prostaglandins, prostacyclins, and thromboxanes are synthesized from arachidonic acid by the action of cyclooxygenase. Inhibiting cyclooxygenase decreases the synthesis of prostaglandins. Leukotriene synthesis requires the enzyme lipoxygenase. Phospholipid synthesis does not require any oxygenase reaction. The conversion of linoleic acid to arachidonic acid involves fatty acid elongation and desaturation reactions, but not the participation of cyclooxygenase. HPETE and HETE synthesis is through the leukotriene pathway, or through a cytochrome P-450–mediated pathway.

3. **The answer is C.** Even though inhibition of cyclooxygenase leads to a decrease in synthesis of all the answers listed ($PGF_{2\alpha}$, PGE_2, TXA_2, PGA_2, and PGI_2), it is the inhibition of thromboxane A_2 that is cardioprotective. TXA_2 is a potent vasoconstrictor and a stimulator of platelet aggregation. The stimulation of platelet aggregation initiates thrombus formation at sites of vascular injury as well as in the vicinity of a ruptured atherosclerotic plaque in the lumen of vessels. Inhibition of TXA_2 synthesis reduces the risk for thrombus formation and occlusion of a vascular vessel.

4. **The answer is B.** Steroids such as cortisone and prednisone inhibit phospholipase A_2, which cleaves arachidonic acid from membrane phospholipids. In the absence of free arachidonic acid, the formation of prostaglandins and leukotrienes is reduced. Because these molecules are mediating the "pain" response, a reduction in their synthesis results in a feeling of less pain for the affected individual. Steroids do not prevent the conversion of arachidonic acid to epoxides, activate prostaglandins, degrade thromboxane, or stimulate leukotriene production.

5. **The answer is A.** Dipalmitoyl phosphatidylcholine (DPPC), also called *lecithin*, is the major phospholipid in surfactant. Surfactant is a protein and lipid mixture that is responsible for lowering surface tension at the alveolar air–fluid interface. DPPC contains a glycerol backbone, palmitic acid, esterified at positions 1 and 2, and phosphocholine esterified at position 3. The other phospholipids suggested as answers are present in nonappreciable levels in surfactant.

6. **The answer is C.** Patients with Gaucher disease have a deficiency of β-glucocerebrosidase, resulting in glucocerebroside accumulation in the lysosomes of cells of the liver, spleen, and bone marrow. Galactocerebroside accumulates in Krabbe disease. Ceramide accumulation is associated with Farber disease. Sphingosine accumulation is associated with Niemann-Pick disease. GM_1 accumulation is associated with generalized gangliosidosis.

7. **The answer is B.** This patient has either Tay-Sachs or Sandoff disease. Patients with these diseases have a deficiency of hexosaminidase A (Tay-Sachs), or hexosaminidase A and B (Sandhoff) activity, resulting in the buildup of GM_2 in neurons, which can result in neurodegeneration and early death. Hexosaminidase A (which is composed of proteins encoded by the *HexA* and *HexB* genes) removes *N*-acetylgalactosamine from GM_2, to form GM_3. The M series of gangliosides contain 1 sialic acid residue; the D series contain 2 sialic acid residues, and the T series contain 3 sialic acid residues.

8. The answer is B. 3-β-Hydroxylase deficiency is a disease resulting in decreased production of aldosterone, cortisol, and androgens (3-β-hydroxylase is required for production of all three types of steroids). Male infants manifest with ambiguous genitalia (owing to lack of androgens and testosterone), and both males and females show salt wasting (owing to lack of aldosterone). Testosterone is produced only by the removal of the side chain of the D ring of progesterone.

9. The answer is E. Metachromatic leukodystrophy is due to a deficiency in arylsulfatase A, a lysosomal enzyme that degrades sulfated glycolipids. These sulfatide compounds accumulate in neural tissue, causing demyelination of central nervous system and peripheral nerves, with resultant loss of cognitive and motor functions. Fabry disease is a result of a deficiency in α-galactosidase A; Niemann-Pick is a result of a deficiency in sphingomyelinase; Gaucher disease is a result of a deficiency in glucocerebrosidase; and Tay-Sachs is a result of a deficiency in hexosaminidase A.

chapter 12

Amino Acid Metabolism

I. ADDITION AND REMOVAL OF AMINO ACID NITROGEN

A. **Transamination reactions** (Figure 12-1)
   1. Transamination involves the **transfer of an amino group** from one amino acid (which is converted to its corresponding α-ketoacid) to an α-ketoacid (which is converted to its corresponding α-amino acid). Thus, the nitrogen from one amino acid appears in another amino acid.
   2. The enzymes that catalyze transamination reactions are known as **transaminases** or **aminotransferases.**
   3. **Glutamate** and **α-ketoglutarate** are often involved in transamination reactions, serving as one of the amino acid/α-ketoacid pairs (Figure 12-1B).
   4. Transamination reactions are readily reversible and can be used in the **synthesis** or the **degradation** of amino acids.
   5. Most amino acids participate in transamination reactions. **Lysine** is an exception; it **is not transaminated.**
   6. **Pyridoxal phosphate (PLP)** serves as the cofactor for transamination reactions. PLP is derived from vitamin B_6.

B. **Removal of amino acid nitrogen as ammonia**
   1. A number of amino acids undergo reactions in which their nitrogen is released as ammonia (NH_3) or ammonium ion (NH_4^+).
   2. **Glutamate dehydrogenase** catalyzes the oxidative deamination of glutamate (Figure 12-2). Ammonium ion is released, and α-ketoglutarate is formed. The glutamate dehydrogenase reaction, which is readily reversible, requires NAD or NADP.
   3. **Histidine** is deaminated by histidase to form NH_4^+ and urocanate.
   4. **Serine** and **threonine** are deaminated by serine dehydratase, which requires PLP. Serine is converted to pyruvate, and threonine is converted to α-ketobutyrate; NH_4^+ is released.
   5. The amide groups of **glutamine** and **asparagine** are released as ammonium ions by hydrolysis. Glutaminase converts glutamine to glutamate and NH_4^+. Asparaginase converts asparagine to aspartate and NH_4^+.
   6. The **purine nucleotide cycle** serves to release NH_4^+ from amino acids, particularly in muscle.
      a. Glutamate collects nitrogen from other amino acids and transfers it to aspartate by a transamination reaction.
      b. Aspartate reacts with inosine monophosphate (IMP) to form adenosine monophosphate (AMP) and generate fumarate.
      c. NH_4^+ is released from AMP, and IMP is re-formed.

C. **The role of glutamate** (Figure 12-3)
   1. **Glutamate provides nitrogen for synthesis** of many amino acids.
      a. NH_4^+ provides the nitrogen for amino acid synthesis by reacting with α-ketoglutarate to form glutamate in the glutamate dehydrogenase reaction.
      b. Glutamate transfers nitrogen by transamination reactions to α-ketoacids to form their corresponding α-amino acids.

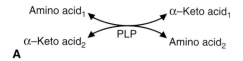

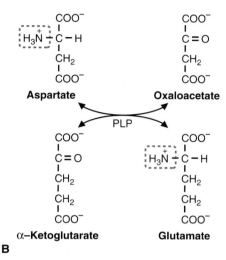

FIGURE 12-1 Transamination. The amino group from one amino acid is transferred to another. The enzymes mediating this reaction are termed *transaminases* or *aminotransferases*. **(A)** The generalized reaction uses pyridoxal phosphate (PLP) as a coenzyme. **(B)** The aspartyl transaminase reaction.

2. **Glutamate plays a key role in removing nitrogen** from amino acids.
   a. α-Ketoglutarate collects nitrogen from other amino acids by means of transamination reactions, forming glutamate.
   b. The nitrogen of glutamate is released as NH_4^+ via the glutamate dehydrogenase reaction.
   c. NH_4^+ and aspartate provide nitrogen for urea synthesis via the urea cycle. Aspartate obtains its nitrogen from glutamate by transamination of oxaloacetate.

II. UREA CYCLE

A. **Transport of nitrogen to the liver**
   1. **Ammonia** is **very toxic,** particularly to the central nervous system (CNS).
   2. The concentration of ammonia and ammonium ions in the blood is normally very low. Ammonia is in equilibrium with ammonium ion ($NH_3 + H^+ \leftrightarrow NH_4^+$), with a pK_a of 9.3. NH_3 is freely diffusible across membranes, but at physiologic pH, the concentration of ammonia is 1/100 the concentration of the NH_4^+ ion (remember the Henderson-Hasselbach equation).
   3. Ammonia travels to the **liver** from other tissues, mainly in the form of **alanine and glutamine.** It is released from amino acids in the liver by a series of transamination and deamination reactions.

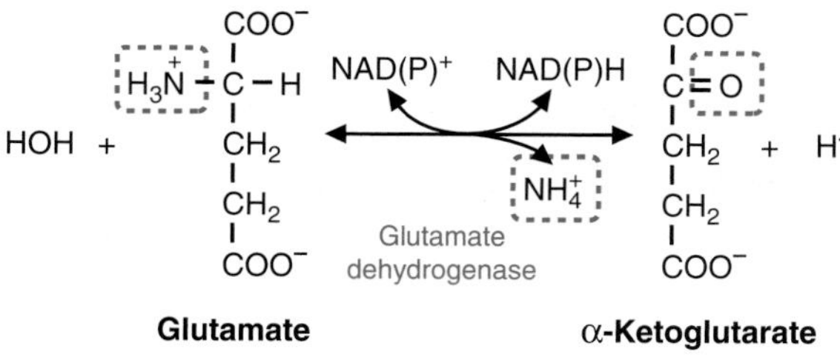

FIGURE 12-2 The glutamate dehydrogenase reaction. The reaction is readily reversible and uses NAD or NADP as a cofactor. The origin of the oxygen in α-ketoglutarate is H_2O.

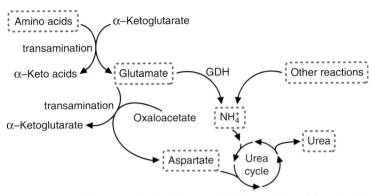

FIGURE 12-3 The role of glutamate in urea production. By transamination reactions, glutamate collects nitrogen from other amino acids. Nitrogen is released as NH_4^+ (ammonium ion) by glutamate dehydrogenase (GDH). NH_4^+ provides one nitrogen molecule for urea synthesis (the other is from glutamate via transamination of oxaloacetate).

4. Ammonia is also produced **by bacteria in the gut** and travels to the liver via the hepatic portal vein. The agent lactulose is used to treat this condition and is thought to work to reduce ammonia levels by either increasing bacterial assimilation of ammonia or reducing deamination of nitrogenous compounds. The use of lactulose for hepatic encephalopathy has become controversial, with recent studies indicating no benefit from lactulose administration.

B. **Reactions of the urea cycle** (Figure 12-4)
1. **NH_4^+** and **aspartate** provide the nitrogen that is used to produce **urea,** and CO_2 provides the carbon. Ornithine serves as a carrier that is regenerated by the cycle.
2. **Carbamoyl phosphate** is synthesized in the first reaction from NH_4^+, CO_2, and two adenosine triphosphate (ATP) molecules.
   a. Inorganic phosphate and two adenosine diphosphate (ADP) molecules are also produced.
   b. Enzyme: **carbamoyl phosphate synthetase I,** which is located in mitochondria and is activated by *N*-acetylglutamate. (Reaction 1)

> **CLINICAL CORRELATES**   Hereditary deficiency of **carbamoyl phosphate synthetase I (CPS I)** results in an inability for nitrogenous waste (ammonia) to be metabolized via the urea cycle. Ammonia levels in such patients rise, leading to brain damage, coma, or death, without strict dietary control.

3. **Ornithine** reacts with carbamoyl phosphate to form citrulline. Inorganic phosphate is released.
   a. Enzyme: **ornithine transcarbamoylase,** which is found in mitochondria. (Reaction 2)
   b. The product, citrulline, is transported to the cytosol in exchange for ornithine.

> **CLINICAL CORRELATES**   Deficiency of **ornithine transcarbamoylase, an X-linked trait,** results in similar neurologic sequelae as CPS I deficiency.

4. **Citrulline** combines with aspartate—using the enzyme **argininosuccinate synthetase** (Reaction 3)—to form argininosuccinate in a reaction that is driven by the hydrolysis of ATP to AMP and inorganic pyrophosphate.

> **CLINICAL CORRELATES**   Citrullinemia results from a deficiency of the enzyme **argininosuccinate synthetase,** causing an elevation in serum levels of citrulline. Again, without dietary management, the manifestations of this disease include lethargy, hypotonia, seizures, ataxia, and behavioral changes.

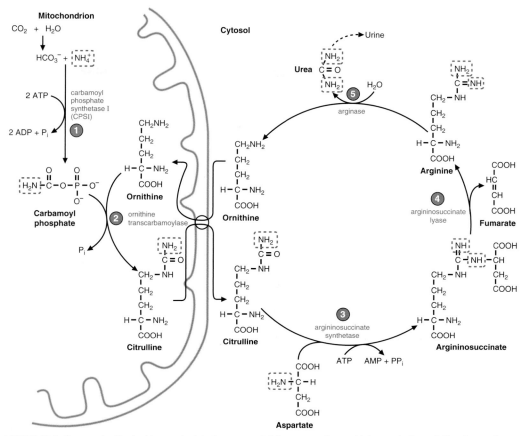

FIGURE 12-4 Urea cycle. *Dashed boxes* depict nitrogen-containing groups from which urea is formed. Numbers refer to reaction steps described in the text in section II.B. ADP, adenosine diphosphate; AMP, adenosine monophosphate; ATP, adenosine triphosphate; P_i, inorganic phosphate.

5. **Argininosuccinate** is cleaved to form arginine and fumarate.
   a. Enzyme: **argininosuccinate lyase.** (Reaction 4) This reaction occurs in the cytosol.

CLINICAL CORRELATES Argininosuccinate aciduria results from a deficiency of the enzyme **argininosuccinate lyase** in the urea cycle, resulting in hyperammonemia with grave effects on the CNS.

---

   b. The carbons of fumarate, which are derived from the aspartate added in reaction 3, can be converted to malate.
   c. In the fasting state in the liver, malate can be converted to glucose or to oxaloacetate, which is transaminated to regenerate the aspartate required for reaction 3.
6. **Arginine** is cleaved, with the help of the enzyme, **arginase,** to form urea and regenerate ornithine. (Reaction 5) **Arginase** is located primarily in the liver and is inhibited by ornithine.

CLINICAL CORRELATES Unlike deficiencies of other enzymes in the urea cycle, **arginase deficiency** does not result in severe hyperammonemia. The reason is twofold. First, the formed arginine, containing two "waste" nitrogen molecules, can be excreted in the urine. Second, there are two isozymes, and in the event that the predominant liver enzyme is dysfunctional, the peripheral isozyme is inducible, leading to adequate restoration of the pathway.

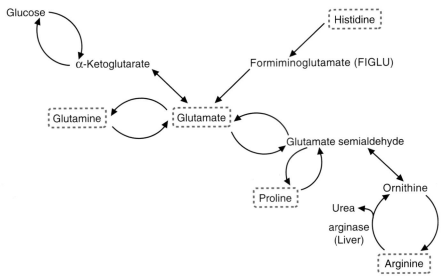

FIGURE 12-5 Amino acids related through glutamate. These amino acids contain carbons convertible to glutamate that can then be converted to glucose in the liver. Except for histidine, all these amino acids can be synthesized from glucose.

7. **Urea** passes into the blood and is excreted by the kidneys. The urea excreted each day by a healthy adult (about 30 g) accounts for about 90% of the nitrogenous excretory products.

8. **Ornithine** is transported back into the mitochondrion (in exchange for citrulline), where it can be used for another round of the cycle.
   a. When the cell requires additional **ornithine,** it is synthesized from glucose via glutamate (Figure 12-5).
   b. **Arginine** is a nonessential amino acid. It is synthesized from glucose via ornithine and the first four reactions of the urea cycle.

C. **Regulation of the urea cycle**
   1. *N*-**Acetylglutamate** is an activator of CPS I, the first enzyme of the urea cycle.
   2. **Arginine** stimulates the synthesis of *N*-acetylglutamate from acetyl coenzyme A (CoA) and glutamate.
   3. Although the liver normally has a great capacity for urea synthesis, the enzymes of the urea cycle are induced if a high-protein diet is consumed for 4 days or more.
   4. The key relationship between the urea cycle and the tricarboxylic acid (TCA) cycle is that one of the urea nitrogen molecules is supplied to the urea cycle as aspartic acid, which is formed from the TCA cycle intermediate oxaloacetic acid.

III. SYNTHESIS AND DEGRADATION OF AMINO ACIDS

A. **Synthesis of amino acids**
   1. Messenger RNA contains codons for 20 amino acids. Eleven of these amino acids can be synthesized in the body. The carbon skeletons of 10 of these amino acids can be derived from **glucose. These 10 are serine, glycine, cysteine, alanine, glutamic acid, glutamine, aspartic acid, asparagine, proline, and arginine. The essential amino acids derived from diet are histidine, isoleucine, leucine, lysine, methionine, phenylalanine, threonine, tryptophan,** and **valine. Note that tyrosine is derived from phenylalanine.**
   2. **Amino acids derived from intermediates of glycolysis** (Figure 12-6)
      a. Intermediates of glycolysis serve as precursors for serine, glycine, cysteine, and alanine.
      b. **Serine** can be synthesized from the glycolytic intermediate 3-phosphoglycerate, which is oxidized, transaminated by glutamate, and dephosphorylated.

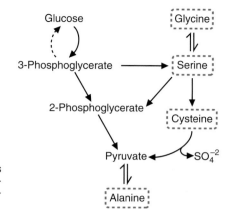

FIGURE 12-6 Amino acids derived from intermediates in glycolysis (synthesized from glucose). Their carbons can be reconverted to glucose in the liver. FH_4, tetrahydrofolate; SO_4^{-2}, sulfate anion; PLP, pyridoxal phosphate.

    c. Glycine and **cysteine** can be derived from serine.
        (1) Glycine can be produced from serine by a reaction in which a methylene group is transferred to tetrahydrofolate (FH_4).
        (2) Cysteine derives its carbon and nitrogen from serine. The essential amino acid **methionine** supplies the sulfur.
    d. Alanine can be derived by transamination of pyruvate.
  3. Amino acids derived from TCA cycle intermediates (Figure 12-7)
    a. Aspartate can be derived from oxaloacetate by transamination.
    b. Asparagine is produced from aspartate by amidation.
    c. Glutamate is derived from α-ketoglutarate by the addition of NH_4^+ via the glutamate dehydrogenase reaction or by transamination. **Glutamine, proline, and arginine** can be derived from glutamate (Figure 12-5).

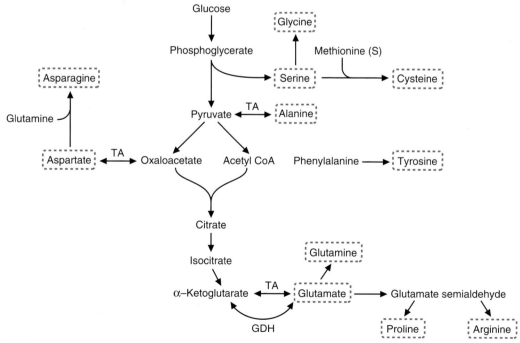

FIGURE 12-7 Overview of the synthesis of nonessential amino acids. Carbons of 10 amino acids can be produced from glucose via intermediates of glycolysis or the tricarboxylic acid (TCA) cycle. The 11th nonessential amino acid, tyrosine, is synthesized by hydroxylation of the essential amino acid, phenylalanine. The source of sulfur for cysteine is the essential amino acid methionine (the cysteines' carbon and nitrogen are derived from serine). CoA, coenzyme A; GDH, glutamate dehydrogenase; TA, transamination.

  (1) Glutamine is produced by amidation of glutamate.
  (2) Proline and arginine can be derived from **glutamate semialdehyde,** which is formed by reduction of glutamate.
  (3) Proline can be produced by cyclization of glutamate semialdehyde.
  (4) Arginine, via three reactions of the urea cycle, can be derived from ornithine, which is produced by transamination of glutamate semialdehyde.
 4. Tyrosine, the 11th nonessential amino acid, is synthesized by hydroxylation of the essential amino acid phenylalanine in a reaction that requires tetrahydrobiopterin.

B. Degradation of amino acids
 1. When the carbon skeletons of amino acids are degraded, the major products are **pyruvate,** intermediates of the TCA cycle, **acetyl CoA,** and **acetoacetate** (Figure 12-8).
  a. Amino acids that form pyruvate or intermediates of the TCA cycle in the liver are **glucogenic** (or gluconeogenic); that is, they provide carbon for the synthesis of glucose (Figure 12-8A).
  b. Amino acids that form acetyl CoA or acetoacetate are **ketogenic;** that is, they form ketone bodies (Figure 12-8B).

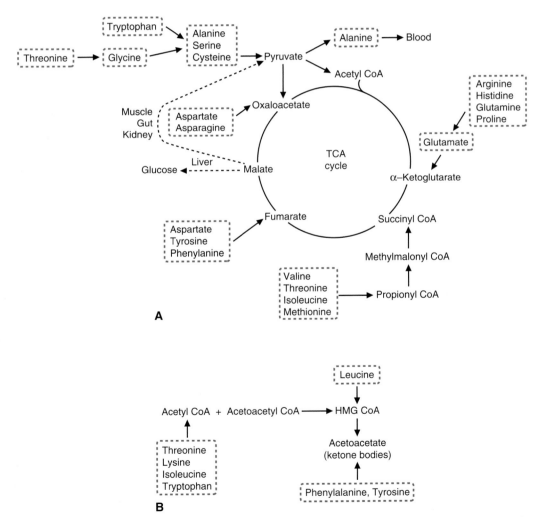

FIGURE 12-8 Degradation of amino acids. **(A)** Amino acids producing pyruvate or intermediates of the tricarboxylic acid (TCA) cycle. These amino acids are glucogenic, producing glucose in the liver. **(B)** Amino acids producing acetyl coenzyme A (CoA) or ketone bodies. These amino acids are ketogenic. HMG CoA, hydroxymethylglutaryl coenzyme A.

    c. Some amino acids (isoleucine, tryptophan, phenylalanine, and tyrosine) are both glucogenic and ketogenic.

2. Amino acids that are converted to pyruvate (Figure 12-6)

    a. The amino acids that are synthesized from intermediates of glycolysis (serine, glycine, cysteine, and alanine) are degraded to form pyruvate.

    b. Serine is converted to 2-phosphoglycerate, an intermediate of glycolysis, or directly to pyruvate and NH_4^+ by serine dehydratase, which is an enzyme that requires PLP.

    c. Glycine, in a reversal of the reaction used for its synthesis, reacts with methylene FH_4 to form serine.

        (1) Glycine also reacts with FH_4 and NAD^+ to produce CO_2 and NH_4^+.

        (2) Glycine can be converted to glyoxylate, which can be oxidized to CO_2 and H_2O, or converted to oxalate.

CLINICAL CORRELATES   **Type I primary oxaluria** results from the absence of a transaminase, which converts glyoxylate to glycine, resulting in renal failure due to excess oxalate in the kidney.

---

    d. Cysteine forms pyruvate. Its sulfur, which was derived from methionine, is converted to sulfuric acid (H_2SO_4), which is excreted by the kidneys.

    e. Alanine can be transaminated to pyruvate.

3. Amino acids that are converted to intermediates of the TCA cycle (Figure 12-8).

    a. Carbons from four groups of amino acids form the TCA cycle intermediates **α-ketoglutarate, succinyl CoA, fumarate,** and **oxaloacetate.**

    b. Amino acids that form α-ketoglutarate (Figure 12-5).

        (1) Glutamate can be deaminated by glutamate dehydrogenase or transaminated to form α-ketoglutarate.

        (2) Glutamine is converted by glutaminase to glutamate with the release of its amide nitrogen as NH_4^+.

        (3) Proline is oxidized so that its ring opens, forming glutamate semialdehyde, which is reduced to glutamate.

        (4) Arginine is cleaved by arginase in the liver to form urea and ornithine. Ornithine is transaminated to glutamate semialdehyde, which is oxidized to glutamate.

        (5) Histidine is converted to formiminoglutamate (FIGLU). The formimino group is transferred to FH_4, and the remaining five carbons form glutamate.

CLINICAL CORRELATES   In the rare hereditary metabolic disorder of **histidinemia,** histidase, which converts histidine to urocanate, is defective. Early cases were reported to be associated with mental retardation, but more recently, deleterious consequences have not been observed.

---

    c. Amino acids that form succinyl CoA (Figure 12-9)

        (1) Four amino acids (**threonine, methionine, valine,** and **isoleucine**) are converted to **propionyl CoA.**

           ■ Propionyl CoA is carboxylated in a biotin-requiring reaction to form methylmalonyl CoA.

           ■ Methylmalonyl CoA is rearranged to form succinyl CoA in a reaction that requires vitamin B_{12}.

CLINICAL CORRELATES   The hereditary deficiency of **methylmalonyl CoA mutase** results in failure to thrive, vomiting, dehydration, developmental delay, and seizures. Consequences of this deficiency are compounded by accumulation of propionyl CoA, a substrate for the TCA cycle enzyme citrate synthase, leading to the condensation of propionyl CoA with oxaloacetate, which leads to the accumulation of the TCA toxin, methyl citrate.

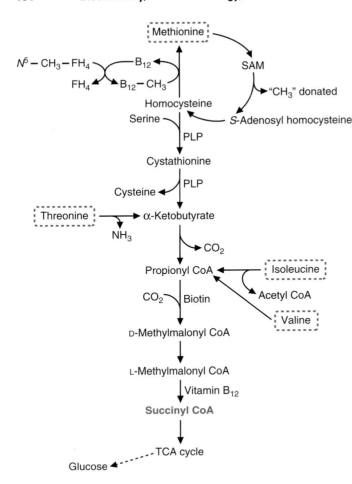

FIGURE 12-9 Amino acid conversion to succinyl coenzyme A (CoA). Methionine, threonine, isoleucine, and valine all form succinyl CoA via methylmalonyl CoA and are essential in the diet. Carbons of serine are converted to cysteine and thus do not form succinyl CoA by this pathway. PLP, pyridoxal phosphate; SAM, S-adenosylmethionine; TCA, tricarboxylic acid.

(2) **Threonine** is converted by a dehydratase to NH_4^+ and α-ketobutyrate, which is oxidatively decarboxylated to propionyl CoA. In a different set of reactions, threonine is converted to glycine and acetyl CoA.

(3) **Methionine** provides **methyl groups** for the synthesis of various compounds; its sulfur is incorporated into **cysteine;** and the remaining carbons form **succinyl CoA.**
   - Methionine and ATP form **S-adenosylmethionine (SAM),** which donates a methyl group and forms homocysteine.
   - **Homocysteine** is reconverted to methionine by accepting a methyl group from the FH_4 pool via vitamin B_{12}.
   - **Homocysteine** can also react with serine to form **cystathionine.** The cleavage of cystathionine produces cysteine, NH_4^+, and α-ketobutyrate, which is converted to propionyl CoA.

> **CLINICAL CORRELATES**   **Homocystinuria** is most often due to a defect in **cystathionine β-synthase,** leading to increased homocysteine and methionine. Patients present with dislocation of the lens, mental retardation, and skeletal and neurologic abnormalities.

(4) **Valine and isoleucine,** two of the three branched-chain amino acids, form succinyl CoA (Figure 12-9).
   - Degradation of all three branched-chain amino acids begins with a **transamination,** followed by an **oxidative decarboxylation** catalyzed by the branched-chain α-ketoacid

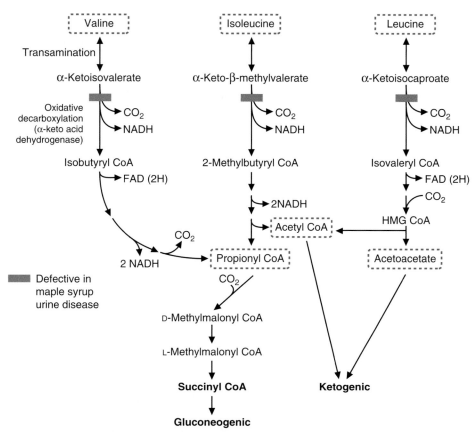

FIGURE 12-10 Degradation of branched-chain amino acids. Valine forms propionyl coenzyme A (CoA). Isoleucine forms propionyl CoA. Leucine forms acetoacetate and acetyl CoA. HMG CoA, hydroxymethylglutaryl coenzyme A; FAD, flavin adenine dinucleotide.

dehydrogenase complex (Figure 12-10). This enzyme, like pyruvate dehydrogenase and α-ketoglutarate dehydrogenase, requires thiamine pyrophosphate, lipoic acid, CoA, flavin adenine dinucleotide (FAD), and NAD⁺.

- **Valine** is eventually converted to succinyl CoA via propionyl CoA and methylmalonyl CoA.
- **Isoleucine** also forms succinyl CoA after two of its carbons are released as acetyl CoA.

CLINICAL CORRELATES   In **maple syrup urine disease,** the enzyme complex that decarboxylates the transamination products of the **branched-chain amino acids** (the α-ketoacid dehydrogenase) is defective (Figure 12-10). Valine, isoleucine, and leucine accumulate. **Urine has the odor of maple syrup. Mental retardation** and **poor myelination** of nerves occur. Dietary restrictions are difficult to implement because three essential amino acids are required.

d. Amino acids that form fumarate
  (1) Three amino acids (**phenylalanine, tyrosine,** and **aspartate**) are converted to fumarate (Figure 12-8A).
  (2) Phenylalanine is converted to **tyrosine** by phenylalanine hydroxylase in a reaction requiring tetrahydrobiopterin and O_2.

CLINICAL CORRELATES   In **phenylketonuria** (PKU), the conversion of phenylalanine to tyrosine is defective owing to defects in **phenylalanine hydroxylase.** A variant, nonclassic PKU, is a result of a defective enzyme in **tetrahydrobiopterin synthesis.** Phenylalanine accumulates in both disorders and is converted to compounds such as the phenylketones, which give the **urine a musty odor. Mental retardation** occurs. PKU is treated by restriction of phenylalanine in the diet.

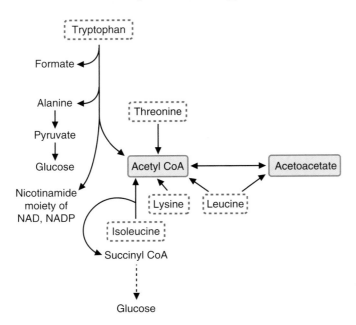

FIGURE 12-11 Ketogenic amino acids. Some of these amino acids (tryptophan, phenylalanine, and tyrosine) also contain carbons that can form glucose. Leucine and lysine are strictly ketogenic; they do not form glucose.

(3) **Tyrosine,** which is obtained from the diet or by hydroxylation of phenylalanine, is converted to homogentisic acid. The aromatic ring is opened and cleaved, forming **fumarate** and **acetoacetate.**

CLINICAL CORRELATES   In **alcaptonuria, homogentisic acid,** which is a product of phenylalanine and tyrosine metabolism, accumulates because **homogentisate oxidase** is defective. Homogentisic acid auto-oxidizes, and the products polymerize, **forming dark-colored pigments,** which accumulate in various tissues and are sometimes associated with a **degenerative arthritis.**

(4) **Aspartate** is converted to fumarate through reactions of the **urea cycle** and the **purine nucleotide cycle.** Aspartate reacts with IMP to form AMP and fumarate in the purine nucleotide cycle.
   e. **Amino acids that form oxaloacetate** (Figure 12-8A)
      (1) **Aspartate** is transaminated to form oxaloacetate.
      (2) **Asparagine** loses its amide nitrogen as NH_4^+, forming aspartate in a reaction catalyzed by asparaginase.
   4. **Amino acids that are converted to acetyl CoA or acetoacetate** (Figure 12-11)
      a. Four amino acids (**lysine, threonine, isoleucine,** and **tryptophan**) can form acetyl CoA.
      b. **Phenylalanine** and **tyrosine** form acetoacetate.
      c. **Leucine** is degraded to form both acetyl CoA and acetoacetate.

CLINICAL CORRELATES   **Isovaleric acidemia** results from a defect in **isovaleryl CoA dehydrogenase,** preventing the degradation of isovaleryl CoA during the **degradation of leucine.** The defect results in **neuromuscular irritability** and **mental retardation.** The patient has a distinctive odor of "**sweaty feet.**" Limiting the intake of leucine helps limit the progression of symptoms.

Review Test

Directions: Each of the numbered questions or incomplete statements in this section is followed by answers or by completions of the statement. Select the **one** lettered answer or completion that is **best** in each case.

1. A 5-year-old mentally retarded child is seen by an ophthalmologist for "blurry vision." Ocular examination demonstrates bilateral lens dislocations, and further workup is significant for osteoporosis and homocystinuria. Serum analysis would most likely show an elevation of which of the following substances?

(A) Cystathionine
(B) Valine
(C) Phenylalanine
(D) Tyrosine
(E) Methionine

2. A 3-month-old child presents with vomiting and convulsions. Notable findings include hepatomegaly and hyperammonemia. A deficiency in which of the following enzymes would most likely cause an elevation of blood ammonia levels?

(A) CPS II
(B) Glutaminase
(C) Argininosuccinate lyase
(D) Asparagine synthetase
(E) Urease

3. A 55-year-old man suffers from cirrhosis of the liver. He has been admitted to the hospital several times for hepatic encephalopathy. His damaged liver has compromised his ability to detoxify ammonia. Which of the following amino acids can be used to fix ammonia and thus transport and store ammonia in a nontoxic form?

(A) Aspartate
(B) Glutamate
(C) Serine
(D) Cysteine
(E) Histidine

4. A 27-year-old, semiprofessional tennis player seeks advice from a hospital-based nutritionist concerning his diet supplements. His coach had given him amino acid supplements consisting of phenylalanine and tyrosine. The rationale was that these neurotransmitter precursors would "help his brain focus" on his game. In reality, excess phenylalanine will be metabolized to provide energy. Phenylalanine will enter the TCA cycle as which one of the following TCA cycle intermediates?

(A) Oxaloacetate
(B) Citrate
(C) α-Ketoglutarate
(D) Fumarate
(E) Succinyl CoA

5. A 2-year-old girl was seen in the emergency room for vomiting and tremors. Laboratory tests revealed a plasma ammonium ion concentration of 195 μM (normal, 11- to 50 μM) and serum elevation of arginine. Two days later, after stabilization, ammonia and arginine levels were normal. You conclude that this patient may have a defect in which of the following enzymes?

(A) CPS I
(B) CPS II
(C) Ornithine transcarbamoylase
(D) Arginase
(E) Argininosuccinate lyase

6. A 23-year-old Golden Gloves boxing contender presents with assorted metabolic disorders, most notably ketosis. During the history and physical examination, he describes his training regimen, which is modeled after the Rocky films and involves consuming a dozen raw eggs a day for protein. Raw eggs contain a 70-kD protein called *avidin*, with an extremely high affinity for a cofactor required by propionyl CoA carboxylase, pyruvate carboxylase, and acetyl CoA carboxylase. The patient is functionally deficient in which one of the following cofactors?

(A) Tetrahydrobiopterin
(B) Tetrahydrofolate

(C) Biotin

(D) Methylcobalamin

(E) Pyridoxal phosphate

7. A new test is developed that can nonradioactively "label" compounds in the human body. As a physician with a background in the new field of metabolomics, you assess a 21-year-old with classic PKU. The patient is fed phenylalanine with a label in the phenyl ring, and a 24-hour urine sample is collected. Which of the following compounds would you expect to contain the greatest amount of label in this urine sample?

(A) Tyrosine

(B) Tryptophan

(C) Epinephrine

(D) Phenylketone

(E) Acetate

8. During a medical rotation, a medical student volunteered for a respiratory physiology examination that determines basal metabolic rate and the respiratory quotient. She followed the protocol for a resting individual in the postabsorptive state. Which of the following amino acids would be found in the highest concentration in serum?

(A) Alanine and glutamine

(B) Arginine and ornithine

(C) Glutamate and aspartate

(D) Branched chain amino acid

(E) Hydrophobic amino acids

Answers and Explanations

1. **The answer is E.** The child has homocystinuria, a deficiency of cystathionine β-synthase, which manifests with mental retardation, osteoporosis, and lens dislocations. This enzyme is responsible for the metabolism of sulfur-containing amino acids and normally catalyzes the conversion of homocysteine to cystathionine. When the enzyme is defective, homocysteine can dimerize via disulfide bond formation, generating homocystine. Another fate of homocysteine is remethylation to methionine, which can also accumulate in this disorder. Because cystathionine cannot be formed under these conditions, it will not accumulate. Valine, phenylalanine, and tyrosine are not associated with the defective pathway, and their blood levels remain normal.

2. **The answer is C.** There are two major types of hyperammonemia: acquired and hereditary. The hereditary type can result from deficiencies of any of the five enzymes of the urea cycle, which include CPS I, ornithine transcarbamoylase, argininosuccinate synthetase, argininosuccinate lyase, and arginase. CPS II is involved in pyrimidine synthesis and utilizes glutamine as a substrate (not ammonia). Glutaminase will generate (not fix) ammonia, and therefore a loss of glutaminase activity will not increase ammonia levels. Asparagine synthetase requires glutamine as a substrate (not ammonia). Urease is a bacterial and plant enzyme that can degrade urea into ammonia; it is not present in humans.

3. **The answer is B.** Three enzymes can fix ammonia into an organic molecule: glutamate dehydrogenase (α-ketoglutarate plus ammonia yield glutamate), CPS I (carbon dioxide, ammonia, and two ATP molecules yield carbamoyl phosphate), and glutamine synthetase (glutamate plus ammonia plus ATP yield glutamine). Thus, of the answer choices provided, glutamate is the correct answer. Aspartate is the precursor for asparagine synthesis, but glutamine is the nitrogen donor in that reaction, not ammonia. Serine, cysteine, and histidine are not utilized for nitrogen transport.

4. **The answer is D.** Although it is true (see Chapter 13) that tyrosine and phenylalanine are precursors for neurotransmitter synthesis, excess amino acid intake will lead to their degradation. Phenylalanine is converted directly to tyrosine and, through homogentisic acid, enters the TCA cycle as fumarate. Aspartate and asparagine enter through oxaloacetate; glutamate directly feeds into α-ketoglutarate; and valine, threonine, isoleucine, and methionine enter via propionyl CoA to succinyl CoA.

5. **The answer is D.** Arginase deficiency, the least common of the urea cycle defects, presents with episodic increases in serum ammonia and arginine, leading to the observed symptoms of vomiting and tremors. A defect in CPS I leads to constant hyperammonemia, without elevated arginine. A defect in CPS II would interfere with pyrimidine synthesis and does not alter blood ammonia levels. An ornithine transcarbamoylase deficiency leads to hyperammonemia and orotic aciduria. An argininosuccinate lyase deficiency leads to elevated argininosuccinate, not elevated arginine levels.

6. **The answer is C.** The cofactor required for propionyl CoA carboxylase, pyruvate carboxylase, and acetyl-CoA carboxylase is biotin. Avidin binds extremely tightly (hence the name avidin) to biotin, which can then no longer be used by these enzymes as a cofactor. Loss of pyruvate carboxylase activity reduces gluconeogenesis, so hypoglycemia and ketosis will result. Avidin does not bind to tetrahydrobiopterin, tetrahydrofolate, B_{12}, or pyridoxal phosphate.

7. **The answer is D.** PKU results from a defect in phenylalanine hydroxylase, resulting in a block in the conversion of phenylalanine to tyrosine. Phenylalanine accumulates in cells and is converted to phenylketones, which enter the blood and urine. Tyrosine is the product whose formation is blocked, and epinephrine, a product of tyrosine, would not be synthesized, so it would not

contain a "label." Acetate and tryptophan are not derived from labeled phenylalanine in a patient with PKU, so those compounds would not contain the label.

8. **The answer is A.** The postabsorptive state refers to after a meal, at a point at which excess amino acids for the meal are being degraded, with the carbons used for either glycogen or fatty acid synthesis and the nitrogen being used for urea synthesis. Amino acids, which carry nitrogen to the liver from outlying tissues, include alanine and glutamine. None of the other amino acids listed as potential answers (arginine, ornithine, aspartate, glutamate, branched-chain amino acids, hydrophobic amino acids) are utilized as nitrogen carriers in the body and would not be elevated in the blood in the postabsorptive state.

13 Products Derived from Amino Acids

I. SPECIAL PRODUCTS DERIVED FROM AMINO ACIDS

A. Creatine (Figure 13-1)

1. **Creatine** is produced from glycine, arginine, and *S*-adenosylmethionine (SAM). Glycine combines with arginine to form ornithine and guanidinoacetate, which is methylated by SAM to form creatine.

2. **Creatine** travels from the liver to other tissues, where it is converted to **creatine phosphate.** Adenosine triphosphate (ATP) phosphorylates creatine to form creatine phosphate in a reaction catalyzed by **creatine kinase (CK).**

   a. Muscle and brain contain large amounts of creatine phosphate.

   b. Creatine phosphate provides a small reservoir of high-energy phosphate that readily regenerates ATP from adenosine diphosphate (ADP). It plays a particularly important role during the early stages of exercise in muscle, where the largest quantities of creatine phosphate are found.

   c. Creatine also transports high-energy phosphate from mitochondria to actomyosin fibers.

3. Creatine phosphate spontaneously cyclizes, forming **creatinine,** which is **excreted by the kidney.**

CLINICAL CORRELATES   The amount of **creatinine** excreted per day depends on **body muscle mass** and **kidney function** and is constant at about 15 mmol for the average person. In cases of kidney failure, creatinine rises, as does the blood urea nitrogen (BUN).

B. Glutathione (GSH) (Figure 13-2)

1. **Structure**

   ▪ GSH is a tripeptide synthesized from glutamate, cysteine, and glycine. It contains an unusual linkage between the glutamate side-chain carboxylate group and the nitrogen of cysteine.

2. **Function**

   a. Involved in the transport of amino acids across the cell membranes (the **γ-glutamyl cycle**)

   b. Aids in the rearrangement of protein disulfide bonds under **oxidizing conditions** and **detoxification reactions** (Figure 13-2B)

      (1) The sulfhydryl groups of GSH are used to reduce oxidized proteins, resulting in the oxidation of two molecules of GSH to form **GSSG** (two glutathione molecules linked by a disulfide bond).

      (2) GSSG is reduced back to two molecules of GSH through the action of **glutathione reductase,** an NADPH-requiring enzyme.

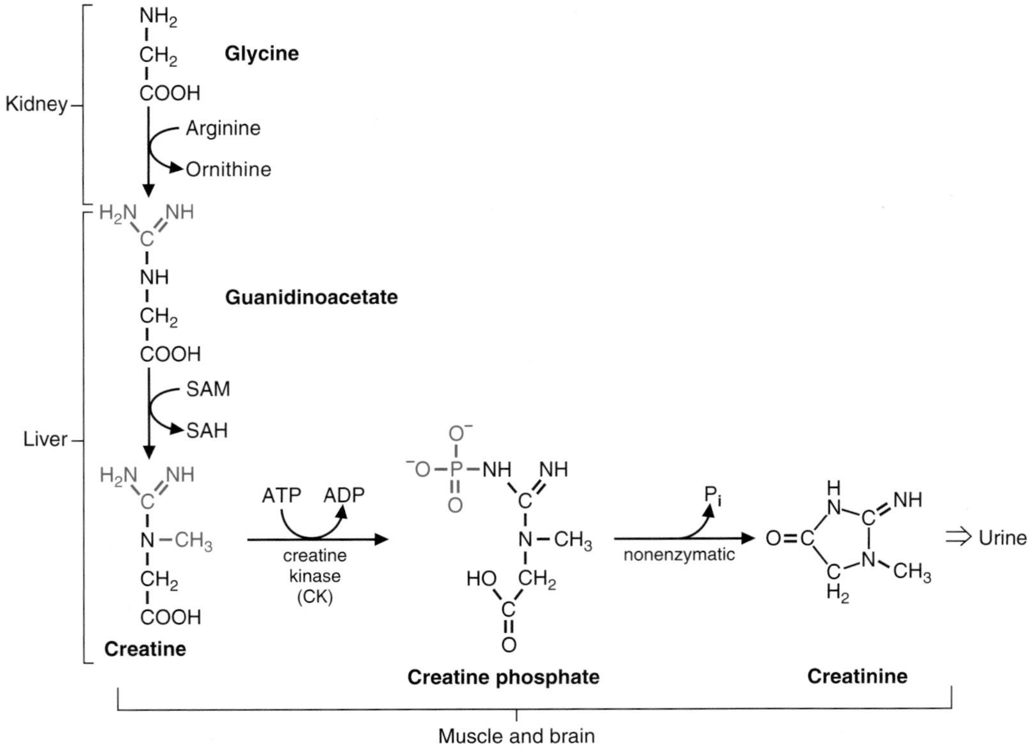

FIGURE 13-1 The synthesis of creatine phosphate and its spontaneous (nonenzymatic) conversion to creatinine. ADP, adenosine diphosphate; ATP, adenosine triphosphate; P_i, inorganic phosphate; SAH, S-adenosylhomocysteine; SAM, S-adenosylmethionine.

CLINICAL CORRELATES   **Acetaminophen** is the drug that is commonly ingested at an overdose level. **Glutathione** plays a major role in detoxifying this potential hepatotoxic and lethal agent. As stores of GSH dwindle, the patient moves from malaise and vomiting to **jaundice,** gastrointestinal bleeding, **encephalopathy,** and finally **death.** **N-Acetylcysteine (NAC)** is a medication that replenishes levels of GSH during acetaminophen toxicity.

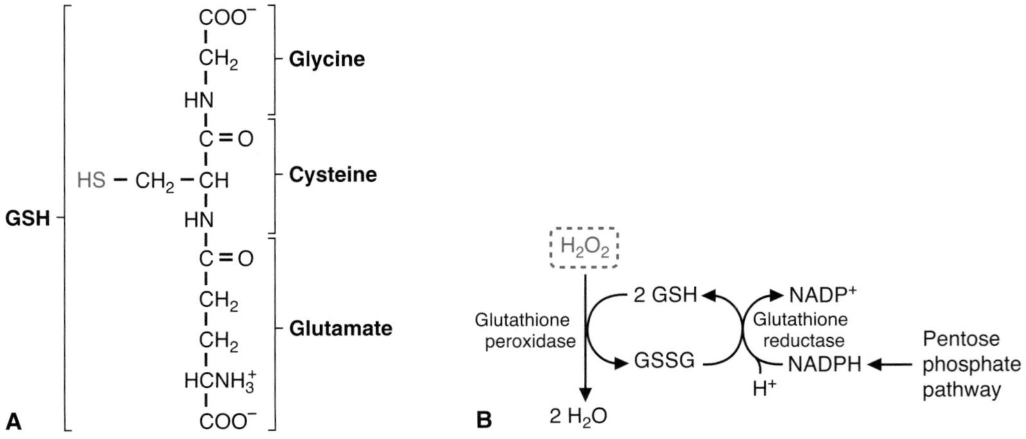

FIGURE 13-2 Glutathione (GSH) and the redox cycle. **(A)** The structure of glutathione. **(B)** The oxidation of glutathione by the oxidizing agent hydrogen peroxide (H_2O_2) and regeneration of reduced glutathione (GSSG).

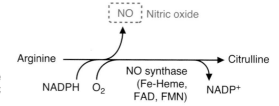

FIGURE 13-3 Nitric oxide (NO) synthase synthesizes the free radical nitric oxide. FAD, flavin adenine dinucleotide; Fe-Heme, iron hemoglobin; FMN, flavin mononucleotide.

C. Nitric Oxide (NO) (Figure 13-3)

1. Synthesis

a. Liberated in the conversion of L-arginine to citrulline

b. The enzyme **nitric oxide synthase (NOS)** is a complex enzyme requiring NADPH, flavin adenine dinucleotide (FAD), flavin mononucleotide (FMN), and tetrahydrobiopterin (BH_4).

c. NOS is found in three major isoforms.

(1) Neuronal NOS (nNOS or NOS-1).

(2) Macrophage or inducible NOS (iNOS or NOS-2).

(3) Endothelial NOS (eNOS or NOS-3).

2. Function

a. **iNOS** is important in **macrophages** for creating NO for the generation of free radicals, which are **bactericidal.**

b. NO stimulates the influx of Ca^{2+} into vascular endothelial cells, with the activation of **cyclic guanosine monophosphate** (cGMP) resulting in relaxation of vascular smooth muscle (NO is also known as **endothelium-derived relaxation factor [EDRF]**).

CLINICAL CORRELATES Numerous pharmacologic agents known as **nitrates** (i.e., **nitroglycerine, nitroprusside,** and **isosorbide dinitrate**) release NO once they are in the bloodstream and are used in the **control of blood pressure** in select patients.

D. Products formed by amino acid decarboxylations

1. Amines are produced by decarboxylation of amino acids in reactions that use pyridoxal phosphate (PLP) as a cofactor.

2. γ-Aminobutyric acid (**GABA**), an inhibitory neurotransmitter, is produced by decarboxylation of **glutamate** (Figure 13-4).

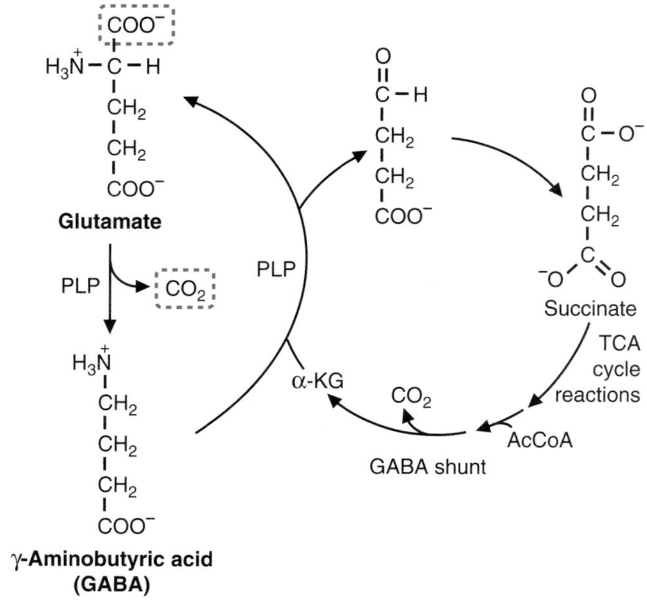

FIGURE 13-4 The decarboxylation of glutamate to form γ-aminobutyric acid (GABA). AcCoA, acetyl coenzyme A; α-KG, α-ketoglutarate; PLP, pyridoxal phosphate; TCA, tricarboxylic acid.

CLINICAL CORRELATES GABA promotes **neuron inhibition** by promoting entry of chloride into the neuron. Numerous pharmacologic agents (i.e., benzodiazepines, topiramate, lamotrigine, and tiagabine) **stimulate GABA** activity in the **treatment of seizures** and other hyperspastic disorders.

3. **Histamine** is produced by decarboxylation of **histidine.**
    a. Histamine causes vasodilation and bronchoconstriction.
    b. In the stomach, it stimulates the secretion of hydrochloric acid (HCl).

CLINICAL CORRELATES Histidine binds to H_1 **receptors** in the stomach, stimulating the release of gastric acid. Pharmacologic blockers of H_1 receptors are used in the treatment of **gastric reflux.** H_2 **receptors** are located on basophils and stimulate their degranulation during the allergic response. H_2 receptor blockers are used to treat **allergic conditions.**

4. The initial step in **ceramide** formation involves the condensation of **palmitoyl coenzyme A (CoA)** with **serine,** which undergoes a simultaneous decarboxylation. Ceramide forms the sphingolipids (e.g., sphingomyelin, cerebrosides, and gangliosides).
5. The production of **serotonin** from tryptophan and of **dopamine** from tyrosine involves decarboxylations of amino acids.

E. **Products derived from tryptophan**
    1. **Serotonin, melatonin,** and the nicotinamide moiety of **NAD** and **NADP** are formed from tryptophan (Figure 13-5).
    2. **Tryptophan** is hydroxylated in a BH_4-requiring reaction similar to the hydroxylation of phenylalanine. The product, 5-hydroxytryptophan, is decarboxylated to form **serotonin.**

CLINICAL CORRELATES **Serotonin** is an important stimulatory neurotransmitter involved in mood. **Selective serotonin reuptake inhibitors** (SSRIs) promote serotonin's actions and are first-line agents in **the treatment of depression.**

CLINICAL CORRELATES **Carcinoid tumors** overproduce the neurotransmitter **serotonin,** with the accumulation of the primary metabolite 5-hydroxyindole acetic acid (**5-HIAA**). When these tumors metastasize to the liver, they cause **carcinoid syndrome,** which is characterized by diarrhea, flushing, wheezing, and cardiac valve damage.

3. **Serotonin** undergoes acetylation by acetyl CoA and methylation by SAM to form **melatonin** in the pineal gland.
4. Tryptophan can be converted to the nicotinamide moiety of **NAD** and **NADP** (Figure 13-5), although the major precursor of nicotinamide is the vitamin niacin (nicotinic acid). Thus, to a limited extent, tryptophan can spare the dietary requirement for niacin.

F. **Products derived from phenylalanine and tyrosine**
    1. **Phenylalanine** can be hydroxylated to form **tyrosine** in a reaction that requires BH_4. Tyrosine can be hydroxylated to form **dopa** (3,4-dihydroxyphenylalanine) (Figure 13-6).
    2. **Thyroid hormones** (Figure 13-7)
        a. The follicular cells of the thyroid gland produce the protein **thyroglobulin,** which is secreted into the colloid.
        b. **Iodine,** which is concentrated in the follicular cells by a pump in the cell membrane, is oxidized by a peroxidase. Iodination of **tyrosine residues** in thyroglobulin produces

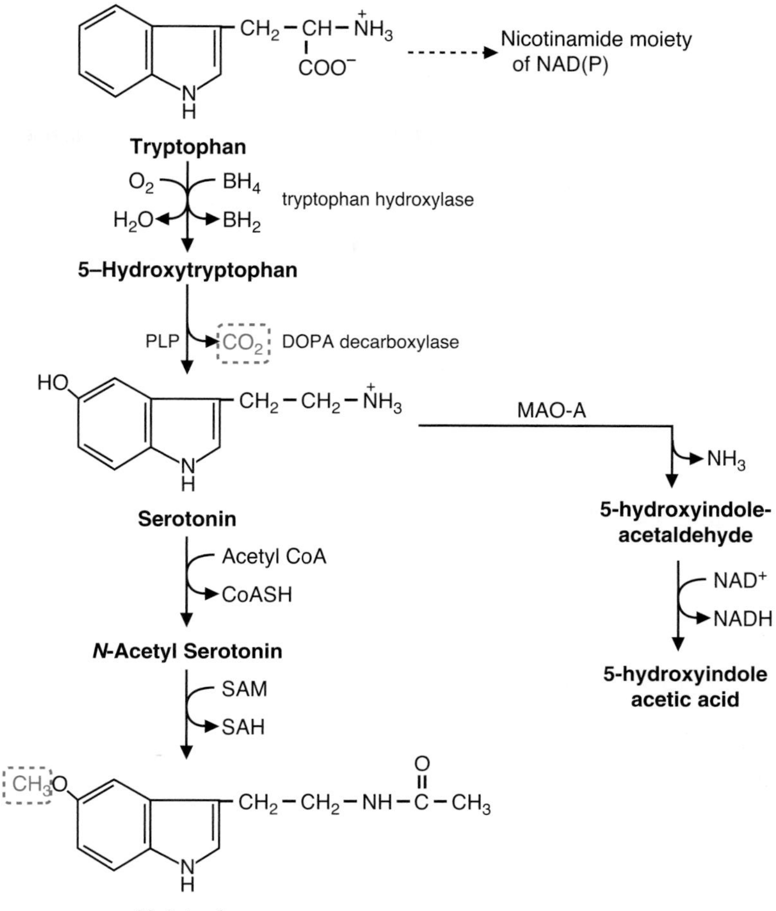

FIGURE 13-5 Synthesis and inactivation of serotonin. BH_4, tetrahydrobiopterin; BH_2, dihydrobiopterin; CoA, coenzyme A; CoASH, nonreacted coenzyme A; DOPA, dihydroxyphenylalanine; MAO-A, monoamine oxidase-A; PLP, pyridoxal phosphate; SAH, S-adenosylhomocysteine; SAM, S-adenosylmethionine.

monoiodotyrosine (MIT) and diiodotyrosine (DIT), which undergo **coupling reactions** to produce 3,5,3'-triiodothyronine (T_3) and 3,5,3',5'-tetraiodothyronine (T_4), which is also known as thyroxine.

CLINICAL CORRELATES   Agents used in the treatment of **hyperthyroidism** (i.e., **Graves disease**), such as **propylthiouracil** and **methimazole**, inhibit the iodination of tyrosine residues as well as the coupling reaction.

   c. Thyroid-stimulating hormone (**TSH**) stimulates **pinocytosis** of thyroglobulin, and **lysosomal proteases** cleave peptide bonds, releasing free T_3 and T_4 from thyroglobulin. These hormones enter the blood.
3. **Melanins,** which are pigments in skin and hair, are formed by polymerization of oxidation products (quinones) of **dopa.** In this case, dopa is formed by hydroxylation of tyrosine by an enzyme that uses copper rather than BH_4.

CLINICAL CORRELATES   **Albinism** results from a **defect in the conversion of tyrosine to melanin,** with partial or full absence of this pigment in the **hair, skin, or eye.** The disorder results from a deficiency of the enzyme **tyrosinase** (which converts tyrosine to melanin) or in defects in **tyrosine transport.** Lack of melanin **increases the risk** for developing **skin cancer.**

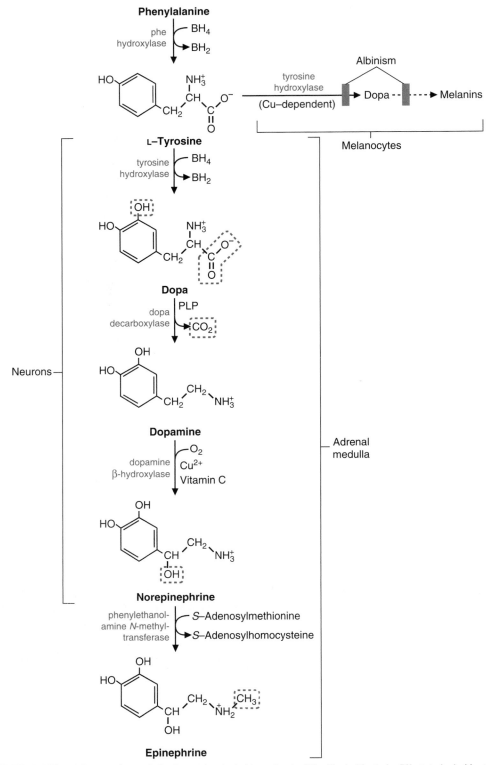

FIGURE 13-6 The pathways of catecholamine and melanin biosynthesis. BH_2, dihydrobiopterin; BH_4, tetrahydrobiopterin; Cu, copper; Dopa, dihydroxyphenylalanine.

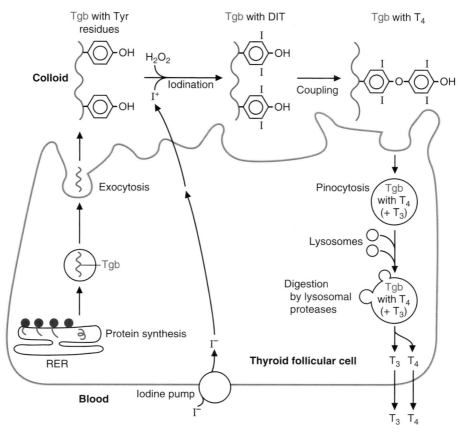

FIGURE 13-7 The synthesis of thyroid hormones. DIT, diiodotyrosine; H_2O_2, hydrogen peroxide; RER, rough endoplasmic reticulum; T_3, triiodothyronine; T_4, tetraiodothyronine; Tgb, thyroglobulin; Tyr, tyrosine.

4. **The catecholamines** (dopamine, norepinephrine, and epinephrine) are derived from tyrosine in a series of reactions (Figure 13-6).
   a. **Synthesis of the catecholamines**
      (1) Phenylalanine forms tyrosine, which forms **dopa**. In this case, both of these hydroxylation reactions require BH_4.
      (2) Decarboxylation of dopa forms the neurotransmitter **dopamine**.

CLINICAL CORRELATES   In **Parkinson disease,** dopamine levels are decreased because of a deficiency in conversion of dopa to dopamine. The common characteristics are **tremors,** difficulty initiating voluntary movement, a **masked face** with a staring expression, and a **shuffling gait. Infantile forms** of the disease have been found to be due to defects in **tyrosine hydroxylase.**

---

      (3) Hydroxylation of dopamine by an enzyme that requires copper and vitamin C yields the neurotransmitter **norepinephrine**.
      (4) Methylation of norepinephrine in the adrenal medulla by SAM forms the hormone **epinephrine**.
   b. **Inactivation of the catecholamines**
      (1) The catecholamines are inactivated by monoamine oxidase (**MAO**), which produces ammonium ion (NH_4^+) and hydrogen peroxide (H_2O_2) and converts the catecholamine to an aldehyde, and by catecholamine O-methyltransferase (**COMT**), which methylates the 3-hydroxy group.

> **CLINICAL CORRELATES**   Inhibition of **MAO** and **COMT** are both approaches in the treatment of neuropsychiatric disorders such as depression and **Parkinson disease.**

(2) The major urinary excretory product of the deaminated, methylated catecholamines is vanillylmandelic acid (**VMA**, or 3-methoxy-4-hydroxymandelic acid).

> **CLINICAL CORRELATES**   Patients with **pheochromocytomas** overproduce adrenally synthesized catecholamines and have increased levels of **VMA;** urinary levels of VMA are used to diagnose these tumors.

II. TETRAHYDROFOLATE AND *S*-ADENOSYLMETHIONINE: THE ONE-CARBON CARRIERS

A. Tetrahydrofolate
  1. **The nature of tetrahydrofolate (FH$_4$) and its derivatives**
     a. **FH$_4$** cannot be synthesized in the body; it is produced from the vitamin folate.
        (1) **NADPH (**2 moles**)** and **dihydrofolate reductase** convert folate to dihydrofolate (**FH$_2$**) and then **FH$_4$** (Figure 13-8). This reaction is reversible.
  2. **Sources of one-carbon groups carried by FH$_4$**
     a. Serine, glycine, formaldehyde, histidine, and formate transfer one-carbon groups to FH$_4$ (Figure 13-9, *top*), which are then transferred to other compounds (Figure 13-9, *bottom).*
     b. **Serine, glycine,** and **formaldehyde** produce N^5,N^{10}-methylene-FH$_4$.
        (1) **Serine** transfers a one-carbon group to FH$_4$ and is converted to glycine reversibly.
        (2) When **glycine** transfers a one-carbon unit to FH$_4$, NH$_4^+$ and CO$_2$ are produced.
        (3) **Formaldehyde** is produced from the –N–CH$_3$ of epinephrine.
     c. **Histidine** is degraded to formiminoglutamate (FIGLU), and the formimino group is transferred to FH$_4$.
     d. **Formate,** derived from tryptophan, produces N^{10}-formyl-FH$_4$.
  3. **Recipients of one-carbon groups**
     a. **Purine precursors** obtain carbons 2 and 8 from FH$_4$. Purines are required for DNA and RNA synthesis.
     b. **Deoxyuridine monophosphate (dUMP)** forms thymidine monophosphate (dTMP) by accepting a one-carbon group from FH$_4$ (Figure 13-10). This reaction produces the **thymine** required for **DNA synthesis.**

> **CLINICAL CORRELATES**   **Methotrexate** is a structural analog of folic acid that inhibits **dihydrofolate reductase.** It functions primarily by **inhibiting purine synthesis** and, therefore, slows down cell proliferation as in **cancer** or autoimmune diseases like **rheumatoid arthritis.**

> **CLINICAL CORRELATES**   **Trimethoprim** is a **folate analog** that binds specifically to **bacterial dihydrofolate reductase.** It is a potent antibacterial compound often used in conjunction with **sulfonamides,** which also inhibit the same pathway in bacteria.

> **CLINICAL CORRELATES**   **Spina bifida and anencephaly,** the most common neural tube defects, are reduced by **supplementation with folic acid** before conception and during the first trimester of pregnancy.

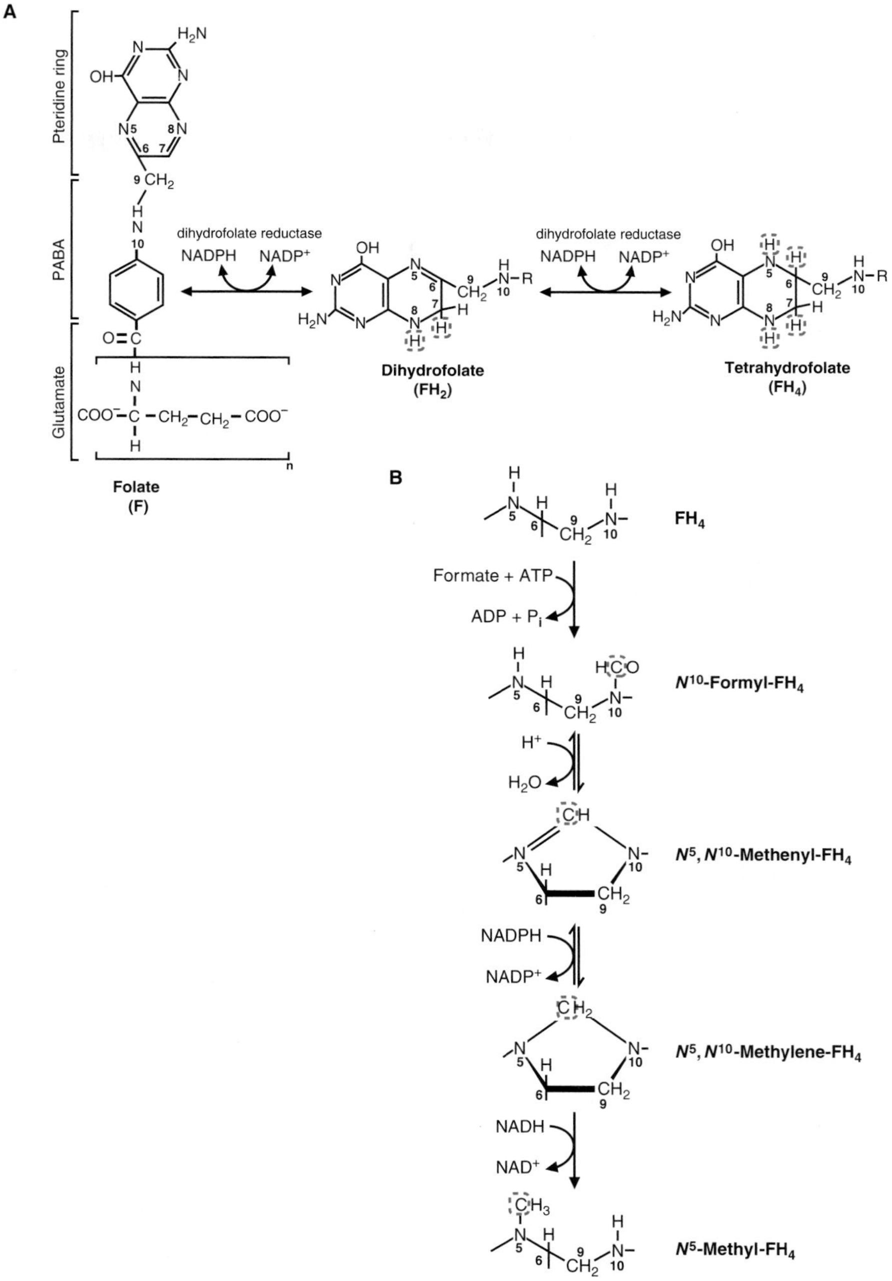

FIGURE 13-8 Tetrahydrofolate (FH_4). **(A)** Reduction of folate by dihydrofolate reductase. **(B)** The one-carbon groups carried by FH_4. The one-carbon groups are indicated by *dashed boxes.* Only atoms 5, 6, 9, and 10 of FH_4 are shown. The remainder of the structure is shown in **A.** ADP, adenosine diphosphate; ATP, adenosine triphosphate; PABA, para-aminobenzoic acid; P_i, inorganic phosphate.

   c. **Vitamin B_{12}** obtains a methyl group from 5-methyl-FH_4, transferring it to homocysteine to form **methionine** (Figure 13-9, *bottom*). This is the only fate of 5-methyl-FH_4.

B. *S*-Adenosylmethionine (SAM)
   1. SAM is synthesized from **methionine** and **ATP.**
   2. **Methyl groups** are supplied by SAM for the following conversions (Figure 13-9, *bottom*):
      a. Guanidinoacetate to **creatine**

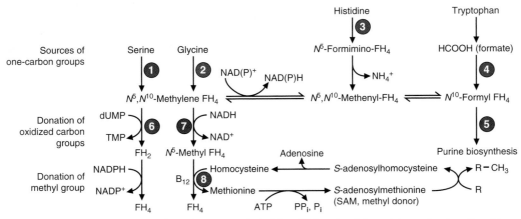

FIGURE 13-9 The sources of carbon (1 to 4) for the tetrahydrofolate (FH₄) pool and the recipients of carbon (5 to 8) from the pool. ATP, adenosine triphosphate; dUMP, deoxyuridine monophosphate; FH_2, dihydrofolate; P_i, inorganic phosphate; PP_i, inorganic pyrophosphate; SAH, S-adenosylhomocysteine; SAM, S-adenosylmethionine; TMP, thymidine monophosphate.

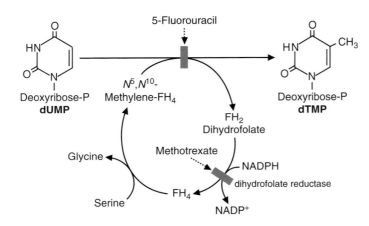

FIGURE 13-10 The transfer of a one-carbon unit from serine to deoxy-uridine monophosphate (dUMP) to form deoxythymidine monophosphate (dTMP). Tetrahydrofolate (FH₄) is oxidized to dihydrofolate (FH₂) in this reaction. FH₂ is reduced to FH₄ by dihydrofolate reductase. *Rectangles* indicate the steps at which the anti-metabolites methotrexate and 5-fluorouracil (5-FU) act.

    b. Phosphatidylethanolamine to **phosphatidylcholine**
    c. Norepinephrine to **epinephrine**
    d. Acetylserotonin to **melatonin**
    e. Polynucleotides to methylated polynucleotides
  3. When SAM transfers its methyl group to an acceptor, S-adenosylhomocysteine (SAH) is produced.
  4. SAH releases adenosine to form homocysteine, which obtains a methyl group from vitamin B_{12} to form methionine. Methionine reacts with ATP to regenerate SAM (Figure 13-9, *bottom*).

Review Test

Directions: Each of the numbered questions or incomplete statements in this section is followed by answers or by completions of the statement. Select the **one** lettered answer or completion that is **best** in each case.

1. A 56-year-old man with long-standing, poorly controlled diabetes visits his primary care physician for a follow-up after a recent hospitalization. The patient experienced an episode of acute renal failure while in the hospital, and his creatinine level rose to 3.4 (normal, 0.7 to 1.5). Creatinine, a marker of kidney function, is produced from which of the following precursors?

(A) Glutamine, aspartic acid, and CO_2
(B) Glutamine, cysteine, and glycine
(C) Serine and palmityl CoA
(D) Glycine and succinyl CoA
(E) Glycine, arginine, and SAM

2. A 75-year-old man experiences severe chest pain radiating down his left arm. He calls 911 and is transferred to the emergency room where an electrocardiogram indicates that he had a myocardial infarction. Serum levels of cardiac creatine kinase are found to be elevated. What is the biologic role of the product of this enzyme?

(A) An intracellular antioxidant
(B) A storage form of high-energy phosphate
(C) An inhibitory neurotransmitter
(D) Stimulates the release of hydrochloric acid from the stomach
(E) A bactericidal product produced by macrophages

3. A couple of African American descent gives birth to a boy after an otherwise uneventful pregnancy. The child is exceptionally fair-skinned and has almost white hair. Further examination reveals red pupils. A postnatal screen is likely to confirm the deficiency of which of the following enzymes in the child?

(A) Peroxidase
(B) Inducible nitric oxide synthase (iNOS)
(C) Glutathione reductase
(D) Tyrosinase
(E) Phenylalanine hydroxylase

4. A 40-year-old woman complains of decreased energy, significant weight gain, and cold intolerance. She is seen by her family physician, who has laboratory tests done that indicate she has a decreased level of thyroid hormone. Which of the following amino acids is iodinated in mature thyroid hormone?

(A) Serine
(B) Threonine
(C) Tryptophan
(D) Tyrosine
(E) Phenylalanine

Questions 5–11: Using answers (A) through (G) below, match the correct drug with its clinical effect.

5. Trimethoprim

6. Methotrexate

7. Propylthiouracil and methimazole

8. Diphenhydramine

9. Fluoxetine

10. Nitroprusside and isosorbide dinitrate

11. *N*-acetylcysteine

(A) Folic acid analog(s) that inhibit(s) dihydrofolate reductase, which leads to an inhibition of purine and deoxythymidine synthesis
(B) Folate analog(s) that bind(s) specifically to bacterial dihydrofolate reductase and used in conjunction with sulfonamides
(C) Histamine and basophil inhibitor(s) used to treat allergic reactions
(D) Increase(s) synaptic serotonin concentration in the treatment of depression
(E) Inhibitor(s) of tyrosine residue iodination
(F) Replenish(es) glutathione levels during acetaminophen toxicity
(G) Release(s) NO, create(s) smooth muscle relaxation, and very effective as antihypertensive

Answers and Explanations

1. **The answer is E.** Creatinine is formed from the cyclization of creatine phosphate, which is formed from glycine, arginine, and SAM. Glutamine, aspartic acid, and CO_2 are involved in the synthesis of purines and pyrimidines. Glutamine, cysteine, and glycine form the antioxidant molecule glutathione. Serine and palmityl CoA form sphingosine. Glycine and succinyl CoA are the precursors to the formation of heme.

2. **The answer is B.** Cardiac creatine kinase phosphorylates creatine to form creatine phosphate, a source of high-energy phosphate in muscle cells. Glutathione functions as an intracellular anti-oxidant. GABA is an example of an inhibitory neurotransmitter. Histamine, which is derived from histidine, stimulates the release of hydrochloric acid from the stomach. Nitric oxide is one of the bactericidal substances (free radicals) produced by macrophages.

3. **The answer is D.** Albinism results from a defect in the melanocyte isozyme of tyrosinase, which is required for the conversion of tyrosine to dihydroxyphenylalanine, on the pathway to melanin. Peroxidase is important in the formation of thyroid hormone. Glutathione reductase is an NADPH-requiring enzyme involved in regenerating oxidized glutathione. Phenylalanine hydroxylase converts phenylalanine to tyrosine; the absence of this enzyme leads to phenylketonuria.

4. **The answer is D.** Thyroid hormone is an iodinated molecule produced by several complex reactions in the follicular cells of the thyroid and the colloid. Certain tyrosine residues are iodinated in the precursor protein thyroglobulin. The side chains of serine, threonine, tryptophan, or phenylalanine are not substrates for iodination in thyroglobulin.

5. **The answer is B.** Trimethoprim is a folate analog that binds specifically to bacterial dihydrofolate reductase and is used in conjunction with sulfonamides, which block folate synthesis. A common formulation is trimethoprim-sulfamethoxazole (Bactrim).

6. **The answer is A.** Methotrexate is a structural folic acid analog that inhibits dihydrofolate reductase and blocks de novo purine and deoxythymidine synthesis. This reduces cell proliferation and is used in the treatment of cancer and rheumatoid arthritis.

7. **The answer is E.** Propylthiouracil and methimazole are used in the treatment of hyperthyroidism by inhibiting tyrosine residue iodination. This blocks the synthesis of mature and active thyroid hormone, alleviating hyperthyroidism.

8. **The answer is C.** Diphenhydramine blocks the effect of histamine at H_1 receptor sites and results in the reduction of smooth muscle contraction. It also prevents histamine release and mast cell degranulation. This drug is a mainstay in the treatment of allergic reactions.

9. **The answer is D.** Fluoxetine (Prozac) is a selective serotonin reuptake inhibitor that increases the extracellular serotonin concentration in the synapse. It is effective in the treatment of depression.

10. **The answer is G.** Nitroprusside and isosorbide dinitrate are compounds that decompose and release NO, which leads to smooth muscle relaxation. NO stimulates guanylate cyclase in smooth muscle cells, leading to an increase of cGMP levels. The elevated cGMP results in smooth muscle relaxation. This serves as an effective antihypertensive mechanism, and these medications are used in the treatment of hypertensive emergencies.

11. **The answer is F.** *N*-acetylcysteine is used as a precursor for glutathione synthesis. Increasing glutathione levels is essential to adequately treat acetaminophen overdose. Glutathione plays a major role in detoxifying excessive acetaminophen, and maintaining adequate levels is critical to avoid hepatotoxicity.

chapter 14

Nucleotide and Porphyrin Metabolism

I. PURINE AND PYRIMIDINE METABOLISM

A. Purine synthesis (Figure 14-1, *left*)

1. The **purine base** is synthesized on the **ribose moiety.**

   a. 5′-Phosphoribosyl-1′-pyrophosphate (**PRPP**) is the activated substrate in the synthesis of purine and pyrimidine synthesis. PRPP is formed from adenosine triphosphate (ATP) and ribose. The enzyme is **PRPP synthetase.**

CLINICAL CORRELATES   **Overactivity of PRPP synthetase,** owing to a lack of feedback inhibition, is an X-linked disorder resulting in **overproduction of nucleotides.** The condition leads to increased degradation as well, resulting in **hyperuricemia, gout,** and kidney stones.

---

   b. **PRPP** provides the ribose moiety, reacting with **glutamine** to form phosphoribosyl-amine, as catalyzed by amidophosphoribosyl transferase.

      (1) This first step in purine biosynthesis produces N9 of the purine ring.

      (2) The enzyme is inhibited by adenosine monophosphate (AMP) and guanosine monophosphate (GMP).

   c. A **glycine** molecule is added to the growing purine precursor.

      (1) Then, C8 is donated by **formyl tetrahydrofolate.**

      (2) N3 is donated by **glutamine.**

      (3) C6 is donated by CO_2.

      (4) N1 is donated by **aspartate.**

      (5) Finally, C2 is donated by **formyl tetrahydrofolate** (Figure 14-1, *bottom*).

   d. **Inosine monophosphate (IMP),** which contains the base hypoxanthine, is generated.

      (1) IMP can be converted in the liver to the free base, hypoxanthine, or to the nucleoside (by dephosphorylation).

      (2) Hypoxanthine, or inosine, travels to various tissues, where it is reconverted to the nucleotide.

2. **IMP** is the **precursor** of both **AMP** and **GMP.**

   a. In the formation of **GMP,** IMP is converted first to xanthosine monophosphate by the enzyme **IMP dehydrogenase** and finally to GMP by the action of GMP synthetase.

CLINICAL CORRELATES   **Mycophenolic acid** is a powerful immunosuppressant and a reversible inhibitor of **IMP dehydrogenase.** The drug limits the formation of nucleic acids in activated and **proliferating immune cells** and is used in treating **autoimmune disease** as well as to prevent **transplant rejection.**

---

   b. In the formation of **AMP,** IMP is converted first to adenylosuccinate by the enzyme **adenylosuccinate synthetase** and finally to AMP by the action of adenylosuccinase.

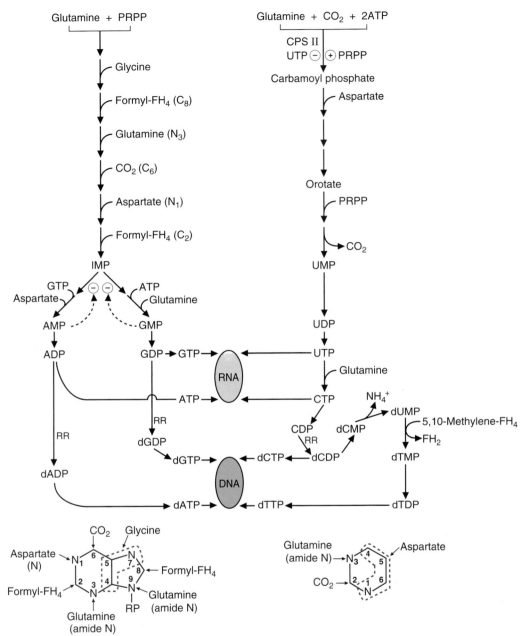

FIGURE 14-1 De novo synthesis of purines and pyrimidines. Ribonucleotide reductase (RR) catalyzes the reduction of the ribose moiety in adenosine diphosphate (ADP), guanosine diphosphate (GDP), and cytidine diphosphate (CDP) to deoxyribose. The source of each of the atoms is indicated in the *boxes* at the bottom of the figure. In hereditary orotic aciduria, the enzymes converting orotate to uridine monophosphate (UMP) are defective. AMP, adenosine monophosphate; CPS II, carbamoyl phosphate synthetase II; d before the phosphates, deoxy; FH4, tetrahydrofolate; GMP, guanosine monophosphate; GTP, guanosine triphosphate; IMP, inosine monophosphate; PRPP, 5′-phosphoribosyl-1′-pyrophosphate; TMP, thymidine monophosphate; TTP, thymidine triphosphate; UMP, uridine monophosphate.

    c. By feedback inhibition, each product regulates its own synthesis from the IMP branch point and also inhibits the initial step in the pathway.

    d. AMP and GMP can be phosphorylated to the triphosphate level.

    e. ATP and guanosine triphosphate (GTP) can be used for energy-requiring processes or for **RNA synthesis.**

3. **Reduction of the ribose moiety to deoxyribose** occurs at the diphosphate level and is catalyzed by **ribonucleotide reductase,** which requires the protein thioredoxin.
4. After the diphosphates are phosphorylated, deoxyadenosine triphosphate (dATP) and deoxy-guanosine triphosphate (dGTP) can be used for **DNA synthesis.**

CLINICAL CORRELATES The antineoplastic agent **hydroxyurea** is an inhibitor of **ribonucleotide reductase.** It is used in the treatment of **chronic myelogenous leukemia,** polycythemia vera, and essential thrombocytosis.

5. **Purine bases** can be salvaged by **reacting with PRPP** to re-form nucleotides (Figure 14-2). The purine-salvage enzymes are hypoxanthine-guanine phosphoribosyl transferase (**HGPRT**) and adenine phosphoribosyl transferase (**APRT**).

CLINICAL CORRELATES **Lesch-Nyhan syndrome,** an X-linked recessive disorder, is caused by a **defective HGPRT.** Purine bases cannot be salvaged (i.e., reconverted to nucleotides). The purines are converted instead to **uric acid,** which increases in the blood. **Mental retardation** and **self-mutilation** are characteristics of the disease.

CLINICAL CORRELATES Autosomal recessive mutations in **APRT** result in the inability of cells to salvage the purine base adenine. Patients develop **nephrolithiasis** with **renal colic,** hematuria, recurrent urinary tract infections, and **dysuria.**

B. **Purine degradation** (Figure 14-3)
1. In the degradation of the purine nucleotides, **phosphate** and **ribose** are removed first; then the nitrogenous base is oxidized.
2. **Degradation of GMP** (Figure 14-3, *left*)
   a. GMP is degraded to guanosine by the removal of the phosphate by a 5′-nucleotidase.
   b. Guanosine is degraded to guanine and ribose 1-phosphate by **purine nucleoside phosphorylase (PNP).**
   c. **Guanine** is then converted to xanthine.

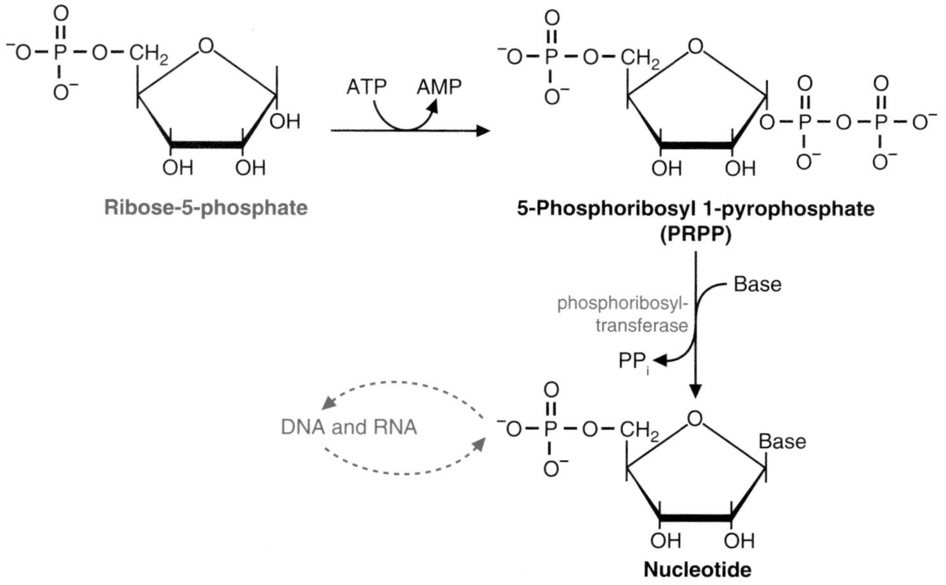

FIGURE 14-2 Salvage of the purine bases. Salvage of guanine, adenine, and hypoxanthine occurs in reactions catalyzed by phosphoribosyl transferases. AMP, adenosine monophosphate; ATP, adenosine triphosphate.

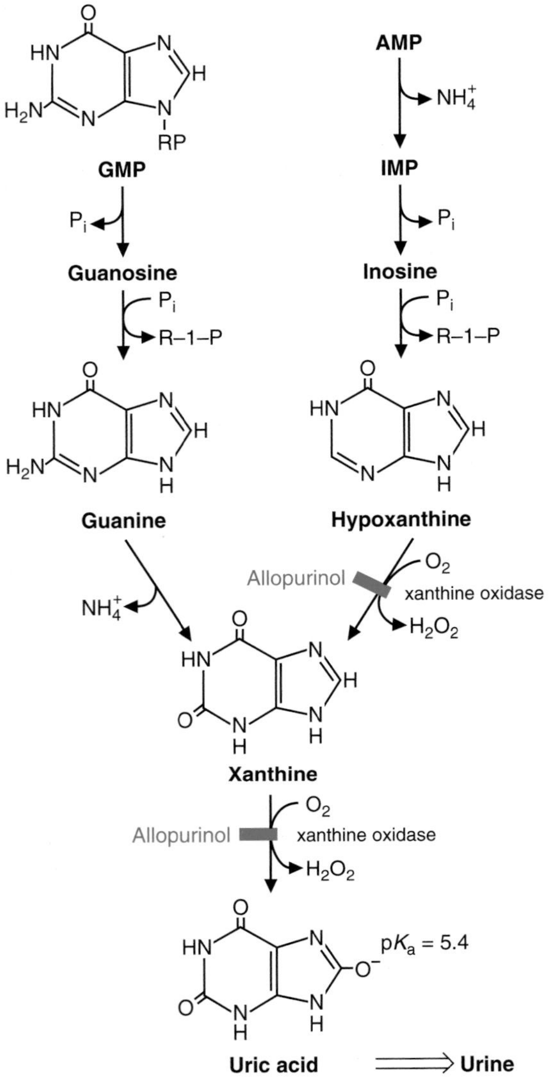

FIGURE 14-3 Purine degradation. Allopurinol (AP), which inhibits xanthine oxidase, is used to treat gout. Gout occurs when uric acid crystals precipitate in joints because of an increased concentration in the blood. AMP, adenosine monophosphate; GMP, guanosine monophosphate; H_2O_2, hydrogen peroxide; IMP, inosine monophosphate; P, phosphate; R-1-P, ribose 1-phosphate.

CLINICAL CORRELATES   Deficiency of **PNP** results in accumulation of both **dATP and dGTP** in lymphoid tissue, which is **toxic to immune cells.** Patients present with **decreased numbers of T cells** and **lymphopenia.** Neurologic symptoms, including **mental retardation** and muscle spasticity, and **autoimmune disease** are present.

3. **Degradation of AMP** (Figure 14-3, *right*)
   a. AMP is degraded to adenosine by the removal of the phosphate by a 5′-nucleotidase.
   b. Adenosine is converted to inosine by the enzyme **adenosine deaminase (ADA).**

CLINICAL CORRELATES   **ADA deficiency** leads to **severe combined immunodeficiency (SCID).** As in PNP deficiency, both **dATP and dGTP** accumulate. ADA deficiency results in a **T-, B-,** and **natural killer (NK)**-cell deficiency with marked lymphopenia.

    c. Degradation of inosine by **PNP** produces hypoxanthine and ribose 1-phosphate.

    d. Hypoxanthine is oxidized to xanthine by xanthine oxidase; this enzyme requires molybdenum.

  4. Xanthine is oxidized to **uric acid** by xanthine oxidase.

> **CLINICAL CORRELATES**   **Allopurinol,** an inhibitor of **xanthine oxidase,** is used in the treatment of gout. More recently, **febuxostat,** a novel **nonpurine analog** inhibitor of xanthine oxidase, has been used.

  5. Uric acid, which is not very water soluble, is **excreted** by the **kidneys.**

> **CLINICAL CORRELATES**   **Gout** results from accumulation of **uric acid** with the formation of uric acid crystals in the joints, especially the **first metatarsophalangeal joint (podagra).** This results in a **painful arthritis** that is treated with multiple agents like allopurinol.

C. Pyrimidine synthesis (Figure 14-1, *right*)

  1. The **pyrimidine base** is synthesized before addition of the ribose moiety.

    a. In the first reaction, **glutamine** reacts with CO_2 and **two ATP** molecules to form **carbamoyl phosphate.**

      (1) This reaction is analogous to the first reaction of the urea cycle.

      (2) However, for pyrimidine synthesis, glutamine provides the nitrogen, and the reaction occurs in the cytosol, where it is catalyzed by **carbamoyl phosphate synthetase II,** which is inhibited by uridine triphosphate (UTP).

    b. An **aspartate** molecule adds to carbamoyl phosphate. The molecule closes to yield a ring, which is oxidized, forming orotate.

    c. Orotate reacts with PRPP, producing orotidine 5′-phosphate (OMP), which is decarboxylated to form uridine monophosphate (UMP). Both reactions are catalyzed by **UMP synthase,** which functions both as orotate phosphoribosyl transferase and OMP decarboxylase.

> **CLINICAL CORRELATES**   In **hereditary orotic aciduria,** orotic acid is excreted in the urine because **UMP synthase is defective.** Pyrimidines cannot be synthesized, and therefore, **growth retardation occurs.** Oral administration of uridine bypasses the metabolic block and provides a source of pyrimidines.

  2. UMP is phosphorylated to UTP, which obtains an amino group from glutamine to form cytidine triphosphate (CTP). UTP and CTP are used for **RNA** synthesis.

  3. The ribose moiety of cytidine diphosphate (CDP) is reduced to **deoxyribose,** forming deoxycytidine diphosphate (dCDP). **Ribonucleotide reductase** is the enzyme.

    a. dCDP is dephosphorylated and deaminated to form **deoxyuridine monophosphate (dUMP).**

    b. dUMP is converted to **thymidine monophosphate (dTMP)** by **thymidylate synthase,** which requires methylene tetrahydrofolate.

> **CLINICAL CORRELATES**   **Thymidylate synthase** is inhibited by the antineoplastic agent **5-fluorouracil** (5-FU). 5-FU is converted by thymidylate synthase to 5-FdUMP, which remains bound to the enzyme, as a **suicide inhibitor.** 5-FU is an important agent in the treatment of cancers such as **breast** and **colon cancer.**

    c. Phosphorylations produce dCTP and deoxythymidine triphosphate (dTTP), which are precursors of **DNA.**

D. **Pyrimidine degradation.** In pyrimidine degradation, the carbons produce CO_2 and a variety of water-soluble products, and some nitrogens, released as ammonium ion, are used to produce urea.

II. HEME METABOLISM

A. Heme consists of a **porphyrin ring** coordinated with **iron** and is found mainly in **hemoglobin** but is also present in **myoglobin** and the **cytochromes.**

B. **Heme synthesis** (Figure 14-4)
   1. In the first step of heme synthesis, **glycine** and **succinyl coenzyme A (CoA)** condense to form δ-aminolevulinic acid (δ-ALA). **Pyridoxal phosphate** is the cofactor for δ-**aminolevulinic acid synthase.** Glycine is decarboxylated in this reaction.
   2. **Heme regulates** its own **production** by repressing the synthesis of δ-ALA synthase in the liver.
   3. Two molecules of δ-**ALA** condense to form the pyrrole porphobilinogen. This condensation reaction is mediated by δ-**aminolevulinic acid dehydrogenase.**

CLINICAL CORRELATES δ-**ALA dehydrogenase** is inhibited by heavy metal ions such as **lead.** This inhibition results in the **anemia** seen in patients with lead poisoning. Accumulation of lead leads to **abdominal pain** and **encephalopathy** with cognitive and motor impairment.

   4. Four **porphobilinogens** form the first in a series of porphyrins; these are hydroxymethylbilane, uroporphyrinogen III, coproporphyrinogen III, and protoporphyrinogen IX.
   5. The **porphyrins** are altered by decarboxylation and oxidation, and protoporphyrin IX is formed.
   6. **Protoporphyrin IX** binds **iron (Fe^{2+})**, forming **heme.**
      a. **Iron** obtained from the diet is transported via **transferrin** and is stored as **ferritin** in the bone marrow (Figure 14-4, *left*).
      b. **Vitamin C** increases the uptake of iron from the intestinal tract.
      c. **Ceruloplasmin,** a protein that contains copper, is involved in the oxidation of iron such that it can be carried by transferrin.
      d. **Excess iron** is stored as **hemosiderin.**
   7. **Erythropoietin** induces heme synthesis in bone marrow.
   8. **Heme stimulates** synthesis of the protein **globin** by maintaining the translational initiation complex on the ribosome in its active state (Figure 14-4, *middle*).
   9. Defects in the biosynthesis of heme result in a group of disorders known as **porphyrias** (Table 14-1).

C. **Heme degradation** (Figure 14-4, *middle*)
   1. After **red blood cells,** which contain hemoglobin, reach their life span of about 120 days, they are **phagocytosed** by cells of the reticuloendothelial system.
      a. Globin is released and converted to amino acids.
      b. Heme is degraded to **bilirubin,** which is excreted in the bile.

CLINICAL CORRELATES **Jaundice** results from a deficiency in the liver's ability to conjugate or transport bilirubin. Jaundice refers to the **yellow color** of **skin and eyes** that results from the deposition of bilirubin. Causes include **hemolytic anemia,** primary **liver disease, obstruction of the biliary system,** and **congenital deficiencies** of the enzymes responsible for the **metabolism of bilirubin.**

   2. **Heme** is oxidized and cleaved to produce carbon monoxide and biliverdin, a green pigment.
   3. **Iron** is released, oxidized, and returned by transferrin to the iron stores of the body.

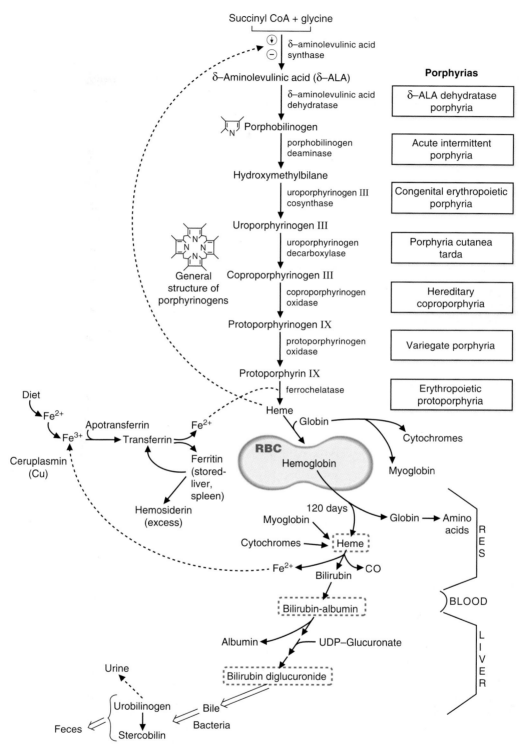

FIGURE 14-4 Hemoglobin synthesis and degradation. Regulation of heme synthesis occurs by repression of the synthesis of the enzyme δ-aminolevulinic acid (δ-ALA) synthase, by inhibition of this enzyme by heme in the liver, and by induction of this enzyme by erythropoietin in bone marrow. Bilirubin is converted to urobilinogens and stercobilins by bacterial flora in the intestine. CoA, coenzyme A; Cu, copper; RBC, red blood cell; RES, reticuloendothelial system; UDP, uridine diphosphate; ⊕, repression of enzyme synthesis; ⊖, inhibition.

table **14-1** Porphyrias

Disease	Enzyme Deficiency	Clinical Consequence
δ-ALA dehydrogenase porphyria	δ-ALA dehydrogenase	**Autosomal recessive** disorder characterized by acute attacks of **abdominal pain** and **neuropathy.**
Acute intermittent porphyria	Hydroxymethylbilane synthase (porphobilinogen deaminase)	**Autosomal dominant** disorder with **periodic attacks** of **abdominal colic,** peripheral **neuropathy, psychiatric disorders,** and tachycardia. Attacks are **precipitated by drugs** such as gonadal steroids, **barbiturates,** and alcohol.
Congenital erythropoietic porphyria	Uroporphyrinogen III cosynthase	**Autosomal recessive** disorder with **photosensitivity.** Sometimes it is almost immediate and **so severe** that the infant may scream when put in sunlight, with erythema, swelling, and **blistering occurring on exposed sites.** The patient may also have **hemolytic anemia** and **splenomegaly.**
Porphyria cutanea tarda	Uroporphyrinogen decarboxylase	This **autosomal dominant** disorder is the most common porphyria. It results in **photosensitivity** with vesicles and bullae on skin of exposed areas.
Hereditary coproporphyria	Coproporphyrinogen oxidase	An **autosomal dominant** disorder that presents with photosensitivity and **neurovisceral symptoms,** like **colic.**
Variegate porphyria	Protoporphyrinogen oxidase	An **autosomal dominant** disorder that presents with **photosensitivity** along with **neurologic symptoms** and **developmental delay** in children.
Erythropoietic protoporphyria	Ferrochelatase	**Autosomal dominant** disorder characterized by **photosensitivity** with skin lesions after brief sun exposure. Patients may also have **gallstones** and **mild liver dysfunction.**

δ-ALA, δ-aminolevulinic acid.

4. **Bilirubin,** which is produced by reduction of biliverdin, is carried by the protein albumin to the liver.
5. In the liver, bilirubin reacts with **uridine diphosphate (UDP)-glucuronate** to form bilirubin monoglucuronide, which is converted to the diglucuronide.

CLINICAL CORRELATES **Crigler-Najjar syndrome** results from a **deficiency of bilirubin uridine diphosphate gluconyl transferase** (UDP-GT). **Type I** results from a **complete absence of the gene,** with severe hyperbilirubinemia that accumulates in the brain of affected newborns, causing a toxic encephalopathy (kernicterus). **Type II,** a benign form, results from a mutation causing a **partial deficiency** of the gene.

CLINICAL CORRELATES **Gilbert syndrome** is a relatively **common** and benign disorder (2% to 10% of the population) that results from decreased activity of UDP-GT. Occasional bouts of mild jaundice with increased physiologic stress occur during hemolysis or hepatocellular injury.

6. Formation of the diglucuronide increases the solubility of the pigment, and **bilirubin diglucuronide** is **secreted** into the **bile.**
7. **Bacteria** in the intestine convert bilirubin to **urobilins** and **stercobilins,** which give feces its brown color.

Review Test

Directions: Each of the numbered questions or incomplete statements in this section is followed by answers or by completions of the statement. Select the **one** lettered answer or completion that is **best** in each case.

1. A 56-year-old diabetic patient with end-stage renal disease receives a kidney transplant from his son. His nephrologist is concerned about the possibility of transplant rejection and puts the patient on mycophenolic acid, which inhibits which important enzyme in the synthesis of nucleotides?

(A) PRPP synthetase
(B) IMP dehydrogenase
(C) Adenylosuccinate synthetase
(D) Ribonucleotide reductase
(E) Adenylosuccinate lyase

2. A physician evaluates a 42-year-old patient for fatigue. The patient is found to have an elevated white blood cell count and an enlarged spleen. A referral to an oncologist results in a diagnosis of chronic myelogenous leukemia. Treatment with hydroxyurea, a ribonucleotide reductase inhibitor, is begun. The normal function of ribonucleotide reductase is to catalyze which one of the following reactions?

(A) Form PRPP from adenosine diphosphate (ADP) and ribose
(B) Convert xanthine to uric acid
(C) Form carbamoyl phosphate from glutamine, CO_2, and two ATP molecules
(D) Convert ADP to dADP
(E) Convert guanosine to guanine and ribose 1-phosphate

3. A 4-day-old infant develops severe jaundice and is transferred to the neonatal intensive care unit for aggressive phototherapy. He is found to have a complete loss of UDP-GT activity. The loss of this enzyme activity leads to which of the following disorders?

(A) Crigler-Najjar syndrome
(B) Gilbert syndrome
(C) Dubin-Johnson syndrome
(D) Hereditary orotic aciduria
(E) Gout

4. A 3-year-old boy is brought to the emergency room with abdominal pain, mental status changes, and fatigue. On history, the physician finds that the patient lives in an older house and has been sucking on the paint chips that have crumbled in the windowsills, making the doctor suspicious for lead poisoning. Lead typically interferes with which of the following enzymes?

(A) Cytochrome oxidase
(B) Protoporphyrinogen oxidase
(C) UMP synthase
(D) δ-ALA dehydratase
(E) Porphobilinogen deaminase

5. A child is noted to have recurrent respiratory infections that necessitate hospitalization. His laboratory tests demonstrate a decrease in T cells, B cells, and NK cells. He has decreased levels of circulating antibodies and is diagnosed with severe combined immunodeficiency. The enzyme that is defective in this disorder is important in which one of the following processes?

(A) The conversion of ribonucleotides to deoxyribonucleotides
(B) The de novo synthesis of AMP
(C) The degradation of adenosine
(D) The de novo synthesis of UMP
(E) The conversion of dUMP to dTMP

6. A 7-year-old boy suffers from mental retardation and self-mutilation (e.g., biting through lip) and has an increased susceptibility to gout. These symptoms are characteristic of Lesch-Nyhan syndrome, which is due to a mutation in which of the following pathways?

(A) Salvage pathway for pyrimidines
(B) De novo biosynthesis of purines
(C) Pathway of uric acid synthesis
(D) Salvage pathway for purines
(E) De novo biosynthesis of pyrimidines

7. A 58-year-old man is awakened by a throbbing ache in his great toe. He has suffered these symptoms before, usually after indulging in a rich meal. On examination, he is noted to have a greatly inflamed great toe; also of note are several small nodules on the antihelix of his ear. Inhibition of which of the following proteins might prevent further occurrences of this man's ailments?

(A) Carbamoyl phosphate synthetase II
(B) HGPRT
(C) PRPP synthetase
(D) Xanthine oxidase
(E) Orotate phosphoribosyl transferase

8. An 8-year-old boy sees a dermatologist because he has developed vesicles and bullae on his face and arms that appeared after a week-long trip to Florida. His father has a similar condition. A diagnosis of porphyria cutanea tarda is confirmed by finding elevated levels of porphyrins in his serum, urine, and stool. His disease is due to a deficiency of which of the following enzymes?

(A) δ-ALA dehydratase
(B) Porphobilinogen deaminase
(C) Uroporphyrinogen III cosynthase
(D) Ferrochelatase
(E) Uroporphyrinogen decarboxylase

9. A 17-year-old woman who recently began taking birth control pills presents to the emergency room with cramping abdominal pain, anxiety, paranoia, and hallucinations. A surgical evaluation, including ultrasound and computed tomography scan, fails to demonstrate an acute abdominal process. A urinalysis reveals an increase in urine porphyrins. Which of the following is the most likely?

(A) Congenital erythropoietic porphyria
(B) Variegate porphyria
(C) Porphyria cutanea tarda
(D) Acute intermittent porphyria
(E) Erythropoietic protoporphyria

10. An otherwise healthy 19-year-old man recovering from a respiratory infection sees his family physician. His examination is unremarkable except for a slight degree of yellow discoloration to his skin and eyes. Laboratory tests are ordered that reveal a mild increase in unconjugated bilirubin but no other abnormalities. Which of the following is the most likely diagnosis in this patient?

(A) Crigler-Najjar syndrome, type I
(B) Crigler-Najjar syndrome, type II
(C) Gilbert syndrome
(D) Lead poisoning
(E) Erythropoietin deficiency

Answers and Explanations

1. **The answer is B.** Mycophenolic acid is a potent immunosuppressant and an inhibitor of IMP dehydrogenase, which normally converts IMP to xanthosine monophosphate. PRPP synthetase catalyses the initial step in nucleotide metabolism, forming PRPP from ATP and ribose. Adenylosuccinate synthetase and adenylosuccinate lyase are sequential enzymes in the synthesis of AMP and are not affected by mycophenolic acid.

2. **The answer is D.** Ribonucleotide reductase converts nucleoside diphosphates (NDPs) to deoxynucleoside diphosphates (dNDPs) for their use in DNA synthesis (an example is ADP to dADP). PRPP synthetase forms PRPP from ATP and ribose. Xanthine oxidase converts xanthine to uric acid. Carbamoyl phosphate is synthesized by carbamoyl phosphate synthetase II from glutamate, CO_2, and two ATP molecules (carbamoyl phosphate synthetase I utilizes ammonia, carbon dioxide, and two ATP molecules as substrates). Purine nucleoside phosphorylase degrades guanosine to guanine and ribose 1-phosphate (as well as inosine to hypoxanthine and ribose 1-phosphate).

3. **The answer is A.** Crigler-Najjar syndrome, type I, results from a complete lack of UDP-GT activity and is a lethal condition. Gilbert syndrome is a mild defect in bilirubin conjugation that is usually asymptomatic, although it is due to a subtle defect in the same enzyme. Dubin-Johnson syndrome is a transport defect in bilirubin and does not involve its conjugation with glucuronic acid. Hereditary orotic aciduria results from a defect in pyrimidine synthesis. Gout results from hyperuricemia, not hyperbilirubinemia.

4. **The answer is D.** Lead inhibits hemoglobin synthesis by inhibiting δ-ALA dehydratase. Cytochrome oxidase is a component of complex IV of the electron transport chain, which is inhibited by cyanide and carbon monoxide, but not by lead. Protoporphyrinogen oxidase is deficient in variegate porphyria, and is not sensitive to lead. UMP synthase is defective in the genetic condition of hereditary orotic aciduria. UMP synthase is not sensitive to the presence of lead. Patients with acute intermittent porphyria have a deficiency of porphobilinogen deaminase. Lead has no effect on this enzyme.

5. **The answer is C.** The enzyme deficiency in severe combined immunodeficiency disease (SCID) is likely adenosine deaminase, which normally degrades adenosine to inosine. The conversion of ribonucleotides to deoxyribonucleotides is performed by ribonucleotide reductase. AMP is formed from IMP through the action of adenylosuccinate synthetase, followed by the action of adenylosuccinate. UMP synthase is an important enzyme in the formation of UMP and, subsequently, cytidine triphosphate (CTP) and thymidine triphosphate (TTP). The conversion of dUMP to dTMP is mediated by thymidylate synthase. A second enzyme deficiency that can lead to SCID is the loss of a cytokine receptor subunit (the interleukin-2 receptor γ-chain). This is an X-linked form of SCID owing to the inability of immune cells to proliferate in response to interleukin-2.

6. **The answer is D.** Lesch-Nyhan syndrome results from a defect in HGPRT, an enzyme involved in the purine salvage pathway. HGPRT catalyzes the conversion of the free base (hypoxanthine of guanine) to a nucleotide (IMP or GMP). HGPRT is not required for de novo purine synthesis, or urate synthesis, or for either the de novo or salvage pathways of pyrimidine metabolism.

7. **The answer is D.** Gout is caused by either the increased production or reduced excretion of uric acid, leading to the deposition of urate crystals. Allopurinol, a xanthine oxidase inhibitor, decreases the production of urate from hypoxanthine and xanthine. Carbamoyl phosphate synthetase II is an enzyme in pyrimidine biosynthesis and is not involved in urate formation. HGPRT is an enzyme in the pathway for purine salvage. Inhibition of HGPRT activity would increase urate production. Orotate phosphoribosyl transferase is important in the synthesis of

pyrimidines. PRPP synthetase is an important enzyme in the biosynthesis of purines; loss of its activity would reduce urate production.

8. **The answer is E.** Porphyria cutanea tarda is the most common of the porphyrias and results from a deficiency of uroporphyrinogen decarboxylase. Deficiency of δ-ALA dehydratase results in δ-ALA dehydratase porphyria. Acute intermittent porphyria is due to a deficiency of porphobilinogen deaminase (also known as hydroxymethylbilane synthase). Deficiency of uroporphyrinogen III cosynthase results in congenital erythropoietic porphyria. Finally, ferrochelatase deficiency results in erythropoietic protoporphyria.

9. **The answer is D.** Acute intermittent porphyria is an autosomal dominant disease resulting from the deficiency of porphobilinogen deaminase (also known as *hydroxymethylbilane synthase*). Often these intermittent attacks are provoked by drugs such as gonadal steroids, barbiturates, or alcohol. These drugs are metabolized by cytochrome P-450 systems, which contain heme. The presence of these drugs induces cytochrome P-450 synthesis (which includes an increase in heme biosynthesis). The induction of heme biosynthesis is the event that leads to an accumulation of the toxic intermediate. The other choices, including congenital erythropoietic porphyria, porphyria cutanea tarda, variegate porphyria, and erythropoietic protoporphyria, are considered erythropoietic porphyries, which are characterized by photosensitivity and rarely exhibit abdominal pain.

10. **The answer is C.** This patient has Gilbert syndrome, which is a common disorder that manifests with mild jaundice as a result of decreased bilirubin UDP-GT activity. Crigler-Najjar syndrome also results from a deficiency of the same enzyme, although it is far rarer and, in the case of type I disease, is lethal. Lead poisoning would lead to anemia, not jaundice. Erythropoietin deficiency is seen in patients with renal failure because erythropoietin is normally produced by the kidney.

chapter **15** | # Integrative Metabolism and Nutrition

I. METABOLIC FUELS AND DIETARY REQUIREMENTS

A. Fuels
1. When **fuels** are metabolized (via **catabolism**) in the body, **heat** is generated to maintain body temperature, and adenosine triphosphate (**ATP**) is synthesized for energy reactions.
2. **Energy** is produced by oxidizing fuels to the final products CO_2 and H_2O.
    a. **Carbohydrates** produce about 4 kcal/g.
    b. **Proteins** produce about 4 kcal/g.
    c. **Fats** produce more than twice as much energy (**9 kcal/g**) as proteins and carbohydrates.
    d. **Alcohol,** present in many diets, produces about **7 kcal/g.**

B. The **Recommended Daily Allowance (RDA)** is the average daily dietary intake level that is sufficient to meet the nutritional requirement of nearly all individuals.
1. The distribution of food intake is based on a **Food Pyramid** (Figure 15-1). Exercise is also recommended.
2. The **basal metabolic rate (BMR)** is an estimate of the rate of metabolism determined by measuring the volume of respiratory gases generated during a period of time. An estimate of **BMR = 24 kcal/kg body weight per day (about 1680** for an average 70-kg man). **Add 50%** for the **average calorie expenditure.**

> **CLINICAL CORRELATES** Anorexia nervosa is characterized by **self-induced weight loss.** Individuals frequently affected include young, affluent, white women, who despite an emaciated appearance, often claim to be "fat." It is partially a behavioral problem; those afflicted are obsessed with losing weight.

C. Carbohydrates
1. **Carbohydrates** should constitute between **45% and 65%** of daily caloric intake.
2. Dietary carbohydrate intake in the form of simple and refined sugars and starches should be limited.
3. Consuming a high-fiber diet provides bulk without the addition of significant calories.

D. Lipids
1. **Fat** should constitute less than 30% total calories—10% each of polyunsaturated, monounsaturated, and saturated fatty acids.
2. **Cholesterol** intake should be no more than 300 mg/day.
3. **Essential fatty acids** such as **linoleic** and α**-linolenic acids** cannot be synthesized by humans and are required in the diet. These polyunsaturated fatty acids are required for the **synthesis of prostaglandins and other eicosanoids.**

E. Protein
1. The recommended protein intake is 0.8 g/kg body weight per day.

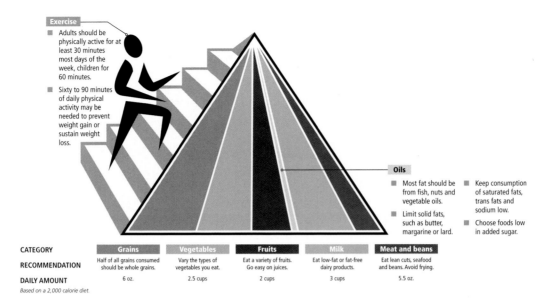

■ Adults should be physically active for at least 30 minutes most days of the week, children for 60 minutes.

■ Sixty to 90 minutes of daily physical activity may be needed to prevent weight gain or sustain weight loss.

Oils

■ Most fat should be from fish, nuts and vegetable oils.

■ Limit solid fats, such as butter, margarine or lard.

■ Keep consumption of saturated fats, trans fats and sodium low.

■ Choose foods low in added sugar.

CATEGORY	Grains	Vegetables	Fruits	Milk	Meat and beans
RECOMMENDATION	Half of all grains consumed should be whole grains.	Vary the types of vegetables you eat.	Eat a variety of fruits. Go easy on juices.	Eat low-fat or fat-free dairy products.	Eat lean cuts, seafood and beans. Avoid frying.
DAILY AMOUNT	6 oz.	2.5 cups	2 cups	3 cups	5.5 oz.

Based on a 2,000 calorie diet.

FIGURE 15-1 A version of the Food Pyramid. (From U.S. Department of Agriculture, Center for Nutrition Policy and Promotion. Available www.mypyramid.gov.)

2. **Essential amino acids**
   a. **Nine** amino acids cannot be synthesized in the body and are required in the diet: **histidine, isoleucine, leucine, lysine, methionine, phenylalanine, threonine, tryptophan,** and **valine.**
   b. Only a small amount of **histidine** is required in the diet; however, **larger amounts** are required for **growth** (e.g., children, pregnant women, people recovering from injuries).
   c. **Arginine** can be synthesized in limited amounts and is required in the diet for **growth.**

CLINICAL CORRELATES Kwashiorkor commonly occurs in children in developing countries where the **diet, adequate in calories,** is **low in protein.** A deficiency of dietary protein causes a decrease in protein synthesis and eventually inhibits regeneration of intestinal epithelial cells, further compounded by **malabsorption.** Hepatomegaly and a **distended abdomen** are often observed.

CLINICAL CORRELATES **Marasmus** results from a **diet deficient** in both **protein and calories.** Persistent starvation ultimately results in death.

F. **Water-soluble vitamins** (Table 15-1)
   ● Vitamins and minerals are required in the diet. Many serve as cofactors for enzymes.
   1. **Thiamine pyrophosphate**
      a. Thiamine pyrophosphate is involved in the **oxidative decarboxylation of α-keto acids.**
      b. The α-carbon of the α-ketoacid becomes covalently attached to thiamine pyrophosphate, and the carboxyl group is released as CO_2.
      c. Thiamine pyrophosphate is the cofactor for **transketolase** of the pentose-phosphate pathway.
      d. Thiamine pyrophosphate is formed from ATP and the vitamin **thiamine.**
   2. **Lipoic acid**
      a. Lipoic acid is not derived from a vitamin and is involved in oxidative decarboxylation reactions.
      b. Lipoic acid participates in the oxidation of the keto group of a decarboxylated α-ketoacid

table 15-1 Water-Soluble Vitamin Deficiencies

Vitamin	Biochemical Function	Clinical Consequence of Vitamin Deficiency
Thiamine (B_1)	Cofactor for pyruvate and α-ketoglutarate dehydrogenase	**Beriberi:** high-output **heart failure** (wet beriberi) and **peripheral neuropathy** (dry beriberi) **Wernicke-Korsakoff syndrome:** deficiency in chronic **alcoholics** manifesting with **ataxia, ophthalmoplegia**, confusion, and **confabulation**
Riboflavin (B_2)	Precursor to the coenzymes flavin mononucleotide (**FMN**) and flavin adenine dinucleotide (**FAD**)	Rare deficiency because **grain and cereal products are fortified with riboflavin.** Deficiency is associated with atrophy of the tongue (**glossitis**), fissures of the corner of the mouth (**cheilosis**), dermatitis, and corneal ulceration.
Niacin (B_3)	Required for the production of **NAD$^+$** and **NADP$^+$** as well as numerous **dehydrogenases**	Deficiency results in **pellagra,** characterized by **diarrhea, dementia,** and **dermatitis.** Deficiency can result from the antituberculoid medication **isoniazid, Hartnup disease,** or **carcinoid syndrome.**
Pyridoxine (B_6)	Required for several **transaminase** and **decarboxylation reactions**	Most severe symptoms due to the requirement for **decarboxylating glutamic acid to the inhibitory neurotransmitter GABA,** resulting in **seizures.** Deficiency can be associated with **isoniazid** or penicillamine use.
Biotin	Required for some **carboxylation reactions**	Deficiency is rare because biotin is **synthesized by gastrointestinal bacteria,** although deficiency may be associated with long-term antibiotic use. Deficiency is also associated with the **consumption of raw eggs,** containing **avidin,** that binds and inhibits absorption of biotin.
Cobalamin (B_{12})	Required by **methylmalonyl CoA mutase** and **methionine synthase**	Deficiency associated with **lack of intrinsic factor,** produced by **parietal cells of the stomach.** Deficiency results in a block in **purine and thymidine biosynthesis,** resulting in **megaloblastic anemia** and **subacute combined degeneration** of the spinal cord. It also causes a functional **deficiency of folate.**
Folate	Reduced by dihydrofolate reductase to tetrahydrofolate (THF), which functions as a **one-carbon donor** in many biosynthetic pathways	Lack of folate results in **impaired thymidine monophosphate (dTMP) synthesis,** with **arrest of DNA synthesis** in rapidly dividing cells, like hematopoietic cells, resulting in **megaloblastic anemia. Pregnant patients** require more folate; deficiency results in **neurotubule defects,** such as **spina bifida,** in the developing fetus.
Vitamin C	**Hydroxylation of proline residues in collagen** and aids in iron absorption	Deficiency can result in **scurvy,** which is characterized by **easy bruising, muscular fatigue, soft swollen gums, hemorrhage,** and anemia.

    c. After an α-ketoacid is decarboxylated, the remainder of the compound is oxidized as it is transferred from thiamine pyrophosphate to lipoic acid, forming a thioester with lipoate. The compound is then transferred to the sulfur of coenzyme A.

    d. Lipoate is limiting in the cell, so reduced lipoate is reoxidized for reuse. It is reoxidized by flavin adenine dinucleotide (FAD), which generates $FADH_2$. The $FADH_2$ is reoxidized by NAD^+, generating NADH.

3. NADPH (the reduced form of $NADP^+$) is identical to NADH except for an extra phosphate on the ribose attached to adenine.

    a. NADPH provides reducing equivalents for the synthesis of **fatty acids** and other compounds and for the reduction of **glutathione.**

4. Biotin

    a. Biotin is involved in the **carboxylation** of **pyruvate** (which forms oxaloacetate), **acetyl coenzyme A (CoA)** (which forms malonyl CoA), and **propionyl CoA** (which forms methylmalonyl CoA).

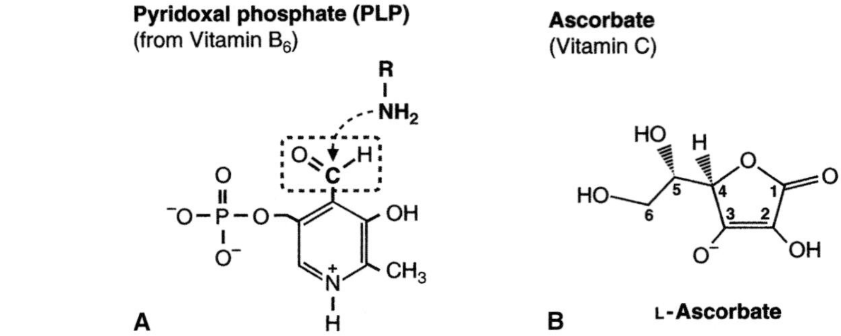

FIGURE 15-2 The structures of pyridoxal phosphate **(A)** and ascorbate **(B)**. The *arrow* in panel A indicates the reactive site of pyridoxal phosphate.

5. **Pyridoxal phosphate** (Figure 15-2A)
   a. **Pyridoxal phosphate,** an aldehyde, interacts with an amino acid to form a Schiff base.
   b. Amino acids are **transaminated, decarboxylated,** or **deaminated** in pyridoxal phosphate–requiring reactions.
   c. Pyridoxal phosphate is derived from **vitamin B_6** (pyridoxine).
6. **Tetrahydrofolate**
   a. Tetrahydrofolate is synthesized from the **vitamin folate and transfers one-carbon units** (that are more reduced than CO_2) from compounds such as serine to compounds such as deoxyuridine monophosphate (dUMP) to form thymidine monophosphate (dTMP).
7. **Vitamin B_{12}** (Figure 15-3)
   a. **Sources of vitamin B_{12}**
      (1) Vitamin B_{12} is produced by microorganisms but not by plants.
      (2) Animals obtain vitamin B_{12} from their intestinal flora, from bacteria in their food supply, or by consuming the tissues of other animals.

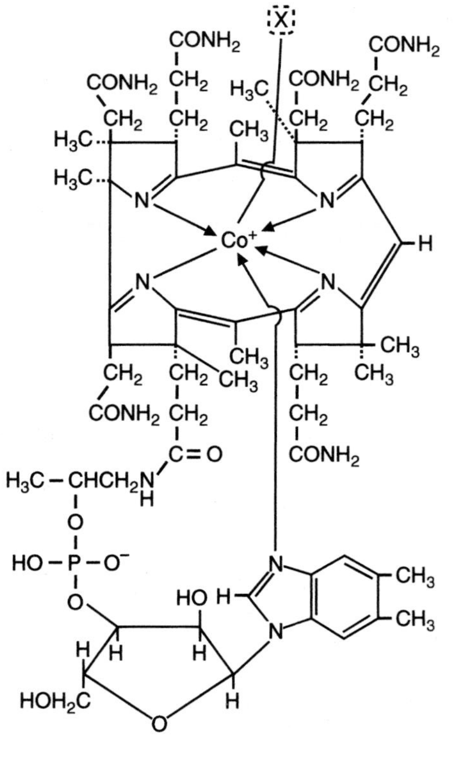

FIGURE 15-3 Vitamin B_{12}. X (in the *dashed box*) can be an adenosyl moiety or a methyl group in the coenzyme forms of the vitamin. Adenosylcobalamin is the cofactor for the conversion of methylmalonyl coenzyme A (CoA) to succinyl CoA, and methyl-cobalamin is the cofactor for the conversion of homocysteine to methionine.

(3) **Intrinsic factor,** produced by gastric parietal cells, is required for absorption of vitamin B_{12} by the intestine.

(4) Vitamin B_{12} is stored and efficiently recycled in the body.

b. **Functions of vitamin B_{12}**

(1) Vitamin B_{12} contains **cobalt** in a corrin ring that resembles a porphyrin.

(2) **Vitamin B_{12}** is the cofactor for methylmalonyl CoA mutase, which catalyzes the rearrangement of **methylmalonyl CoA to succinyl CoA.** Amino acids whose degradation pathways lead to succinyl CoA (such as valine, isoleucine, threonine, and methionine) do so by forming methylmalonyl CoA. Propionyl CoA is formed by the oxidation of fatty acids with an odd number of carbons, and the propionyl CoA is converted to methylmalonyl CoA by propionyl CoA carboxylase, a biotin requiring enzyme.

(3) **Vitamin B_{12}** facilitates the transfer of methyl groups from FH_4 to **homocysteine to form methionine.**

8. **Vitamin C** (ascorbic acid) (Figure 15-2B)

a. It is involved in **hydroxylation reactions,** such as the hydroxylation of prolyl residues in the precursor of collagen.

b. It functions in the **absorption of iron.**

c. It is an **antioxidant.**

G. **Fat-soluble vitamins** (Figure 15-4 and Table 15-2)

1. **Vitamin K** activates precursors of prothrombin and other **clotting factors** by carboxylation of glutamate residues.

2. **Vitamin A** is necessary for **vision,** for normal **growth** and **reproduction,** and for differentiation and maintenance of **epithelial tissues.**

a. Δ^{11}-*cis*-Retinal binds to the protein opsin, forming rhodopsin. Light causes conversion of Δ^{11}-*cis*-retinal to **all-*trans*-retinal,** which dissociates from opsin, causing changes allowing light to be perceived by the brain.

b. Retinoic acid, the most oxidized form of vitamin A, acts like a steroid hormone.

3. **Vitamin E** serves as an **antioxidant.**

a. It prevents free radicals from oxidizing compounds such as polyunsaturated fatty acids.

b. Maintains integrity of membranes by preventing free radical–induced oxidation of the fatty acid residues in phospholipids.

4. **Vitamin D** (as 1,25-dihydroxycholecalciferol) is involved in **calcium metabolism.**

H. Minerals required in large amounts include **calcium and phosphate** for structural components of bone. Trace minerals include **iron,** a component of heme (Table 15-3).

II. METABOLISM DURING THE FED OR ABSORPTIVE STATE (FIGURE 15-5)

A. **The fate of glucose in the liver**

1. **Glucose** is **oxidized** to CO_2 and H_2O to meet the immediate energy needs of the liver.

2. **Excess glucose** is **stored** in the liver as **glycogen,** which is used during periods of fasting to maintain blood glucose.

3. **Excess glucose** can be **converted to fatty acids** and a **glycerol** moiety, which combine to form **triacylglycerols,** which are released from the liver into the blood as **very-low-density lipoprotein (VLDL).**

B. **The fate of glucose in other tissues**

1. The **brain,** which depends on glucose for its energy, **oxidizes glucose to CO_2 and H_2O,** producing ATP.

2. **Red blood cells,** lacking mitochondria, oxidize glucose to **pyruvate** and **lactate,** which are released into the blood.

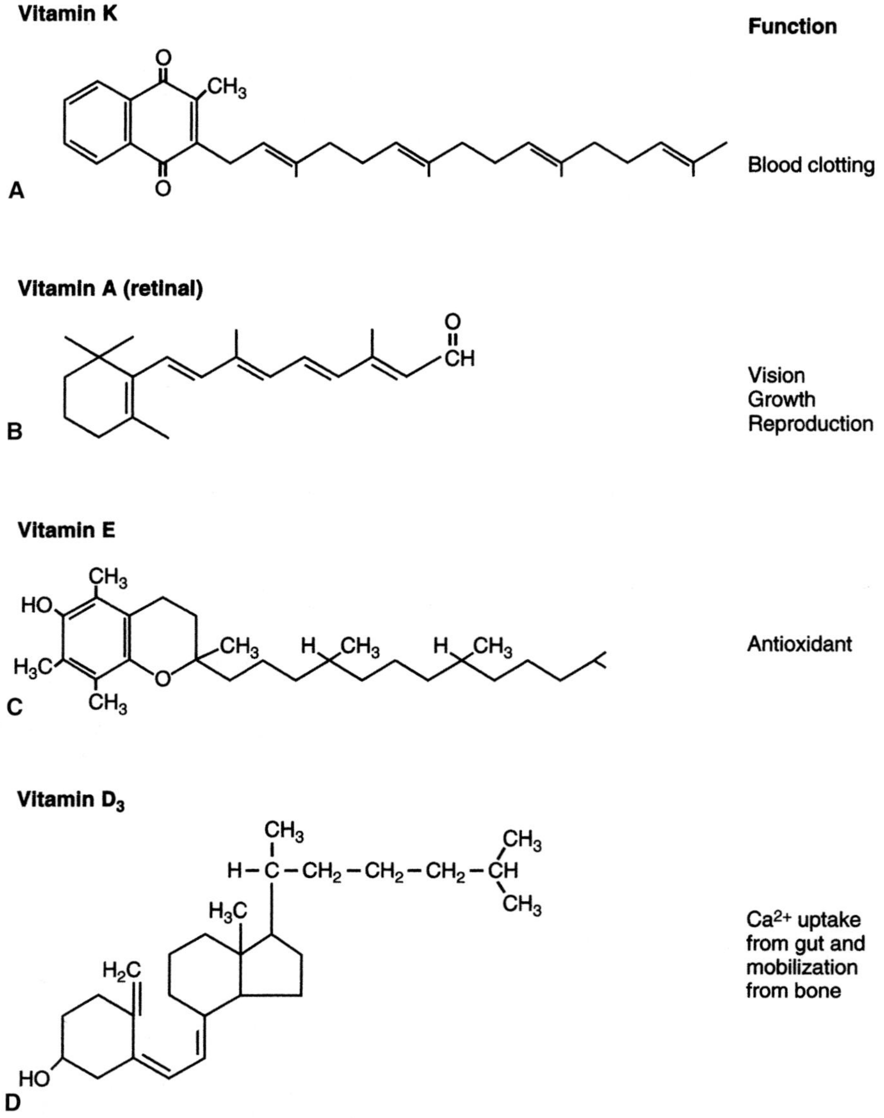

Vitamin K

Function

A

Blood clotting

Vitamin A (retinal)

B

Vision
Growth
Reproduction

Vitamin E

C

Antioxidant

Vitamin D₃

D

Ca²⁺ uptake
from gut and
mobilization
from bone

FIGURE 15-4 The fat-soluble vitamins.

3. **Muscle cells** take up glucose by an **insulin-stimulated transport** process and **oxidize glucose** to CO_2 and H_2O to generate ATP for contraction. Muscle **stores** glucose as **glycogen** for use during contraction.
4. **Adipose cells** take up glucose by an **insulin-stimulated transport** process and oxidize glucose to produce energy and convert it to the glycerol moiety used to produce triacylglycerol stores.

C. **The fate of lipoproteins in the fed state**
   1. The triacylglycerols of **chylomicrons** (produced from dietary fat) and **VLDL** (produced from glucose by the liver) are **substrates** in capillaries for **lipoprotein lipase** to form fatty acids and glycerol.
   2. The **fatty acids** are taken up by **adipose tissue,** converted to **triacylglycerols,** and stored.

D. **The fate of amino acids from dietary proteins in the fed state.** The amino acids enter cells and are:
   1. Used for **protein synthesis** (which occurs on ribosomes and requires mRNA). Proteins are constantly being synthesized and degraded.

table **15-2** Lipid-Soluble Vitamin Deficiencies

Vitamin	Biochemical Function	Clinical Consequence of Vitamin Deficiency
Vitamin A	Required for **growth and differentiation;** required for the production of the light-absorbing vision protein **rhodopsin**	Deficiency results in **night blindness,** dry eyes leading to **corneal damage,** and **urinary stones**
Vitamin D	**Regulation of gene expression** for the **absorption of calcium** from the gastrointestinal tract	**Rickets** in **children** results in **defective bone mineralization** with a "squared" head, chest deformity, spine abnormalities, and **bowing of the legs.** In **adults, osteomalacia** can occur, with **weakening of bone** and increased incidence of **fracture.**
Vitamin E	Functions as an **antioxidant** and free radical scavenger	Rare; however, lack of vitamin E can contribute to the development of **atherosclerosis** and **cardiovascular disease.**
Vitamin K	Required for the γ-**carboxylation of coagulation factors II, VII, IX, and X**	Deficiency is seen in **newborns** because vitamin K is **produced by the yet undeveloped gastrointestinal flora,** resulting in **hemorrhage and bleeding diathesis.** The blood thinner **warfarin,** used to treat **blood clots, antagonizes** the vitamin's actions.

2. Used to make **nitrogenous compounds** such as heme, creatine phosphate, epinephrine, and the bases of DNA and RNA.
3. Oxidized to generate **ATP.**

III. FASTING (FIGURE 15-6)

A. Energy reserves: fasting versus starvation (long-term)
   1. The **principal energy reserves** used for long-term food deprivation are triglycerides (stored **in adipose tissue [fat])** for *both lean and obese individuals.*
   2. The contribution of **carbohydrate to total energy reserves is very small,** yet it is the **energy source called on *first* with heavy energy expenditures.**

CLINICAL CORRELATES A normal person (Table 15-4) refers to a 70-kg individual with a fuel reserve of 30% by weight. The **increased reserve of the obese individual is mostly fat. Complete fasts** indicate one can live without food, but with water, **for about 60 days** (theoretically, a 70-kg person has 21 kg of fuel reserve, divided as 15 kg of fat and 6 kg of protein. This approximates 165,840 calories of energy. The daily metabolic need of such a person is about 2620 calories per day, for a survival time of 63 days). Death ensues when essential proteins (e.g., from brain, heart) start to be used for energy.

table **15-3** Important Mineral Deficiencies

Mineral	Biochemical Function	Clinical Consequence of Mineral Deficiency
Copper	Component of many **oxidases** in **oxidative metabolism,** neurotransmitter synthesis, and **collagen synthesis**	Deficiency results in muscle weakness, **neurologic defects,** and **abnormal collagen** cross-linking.
Iodine	Essential component of thyroid hormone	Deficiency results in **goiter** and hypothyroidism; uncommon with the advent of **iodized salt.**
Iron	Essential component of **hemoglobin** as well as other metalloenzymes	Deficiency results in defective hemoglobin production and developing **hypochromic, microcytic anemia.**
Selenium	Component of **glutathione peroxidase**	Deficiency results in cardiomyopathy (**Keshan disease**).
Zinc	Component of many **oxidases**	Deficiency results in growth retardation and impaired wound healing.

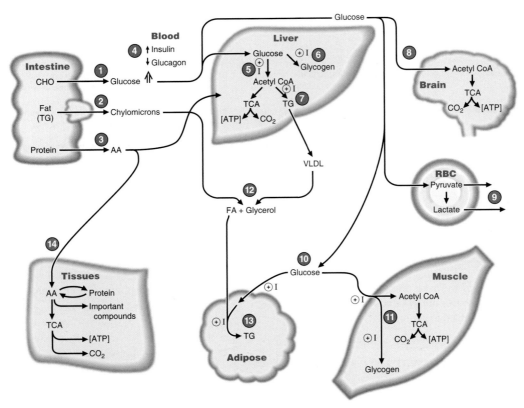

FIGURE 15-5 The fed state. The *circled numbers* serve as a guide, indicating the approximate order in which the processes begin to occur. AA, amino acid; ATP, adenosine triphosphate; CoA, coenzyme A; FA, fatty acid; I, insulin; RBC, red blood cells; TCA, tricarboxylic acid; TG, triacylglycerols; VLDL, very-low-density lipoprotein; ⊕, stimulated by.

B. The liver during fasting

1. The liver produces **glucose** and **ketone bodies** that are released into the blood and serve as sources of energy for other tissues.
2. **Production of glucose by the liver**
   a. The liver must **maintain blood glucose levels.** Glucose is required by the brain and red blood cells. The brain oxidizes glucose to CO_2 and H_2O, whereas red blood cells oxidize glucose to pyruvate and lactate.
   b. **Glycogenolysis**
      (1) About 2 to 3 hours after a meal, the liver breaks down its glycogen stores by glycogenolysis, and free glucose is released into the blood.
      (2) Glucose is then taken up by tissues and oxidized.
   c. **Gluconeogenesis**
      (1) After about 4 to 6 hours of fasting, the **liver** begins the process of gluconeogenesis. Within 30 hours, liver glycogen stores are depleted, leaving gluconeogenesis as the major process responsible for maintaining blood glucose.
      (2) **Carbon sources** for gluconeogenesis are:
         (a) **Lactate** produced by tissues like red blood cells or exercising muscle
         (b) **Glycerol** from breakdown of triacylglycerols in adipose tissue
         (c) **Amino acids,** particularly alanine, from muscle protein
         (d) **Propionate** from oxidation of odd-chain fatty acids (minor source)
3. Production of ketone bodies by the liver
   a. As glucagon levels rise, adipose tissue breaks down its **triacylglycerol stores** into fatty acids and glycerol, which are released into the blood.
   b. Through β-**oxidation,** the liver converts fatty acids to acetyl CoA.

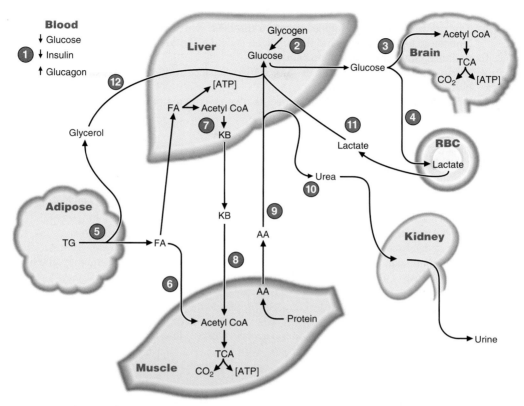

FIGURE 15-6 The fasting (basal) state. This state occurs after an overnight (12-hour) fast. The *circled numbers* serve as a guide, indicating the approximate order in which the processes begin to occur. KB, ketone bodies. For other abbreviations, see Figure 15-5.

   c. **Acetyl CoA** is used by the liver for ketone body synthesis. The ketone bodies are **acetoacetate and β-hydroxybutyrate.** The **liver cannot oxidize** ketone bodies and releases them into the blood.

C. **Adipose tissue during fasting**
   1. As glucagon levels rise, adipose **triacylglycerol stores** are **mobilized.** The liver converts the fatty acids to ketone bodies and the glycerol to glucose.
   2. Tissues such as muscle oxidize the fatty acids to CO_2 and H_2O.

D. **Muscle during fasting**
   1. **Degradation of muscle protein**
      a. During fasting, muscle protein is degraded, producing amino acids that are partially metabolized by muscle and released into the blood, mainly as **alanine** and **glutamine.**

t a b l e 15-4 Fuels Available in the Human Body for Long-Term Fasting

Fuel Reserve	Normal Man		Obese Man	
	kg	kcal	kg	kcal
Fat (adipose triglycerides)	15.0	141,000 (85%)	80.0	752,000 (96%)
Protein (mainly muscle)	6.0	24,000 (14%)	8.0	32,000 (4%)
Glycogen: muscle	0.120	480	0.160	640
Glycogen: liver	0.070	280	0.070	280
Glucose (extracellular fluid)	0.020	80	0.025	100
Total available energy	165,840		785,020	

   b. Tissues, such as **gut** and **kidney,** metabolize the glutamine.
   c. The products (mainly **alanine**) travel to the **liver,** where the carbons are converted to glucose or ketone bodies and the nitrogen is converted to urea.
2. **Oxidation of fatty acids and ketone bodies**
   a. During **fasting,** muscle oxidizes fatty acids released from adipose tissue, and ketone bodies produced by the liver.
   b. During **exercise,** muscle can also use its own glycogen stores as well as glucose, fatty acids, and ketone bodies from the blood.

IV. PROLONGED FASTING (STARVATION) (FIGURE 15-7)

A. **Metabolic changes in starvation.** When the body enters the **starved state,** after **3 to 5 days of fasting,** changes occur in the use of fuel stores.
   1. Muscle decreases use of ketone bodies and oxidizes fatty acids as its energy source.
   2. Because of decreased use by muscle, **blood ketone body levels rise.**
   3. The **brain** then takes up and **oxidizes ketone bodies** to derive energy. Consequently, the brain decreases its use of glucose, although glucose is still a major fuel for the brain.
   4. Liver **gluconeogenesis decreases.**
   5. **Muscle protein is spared** (i.e., less muscle protein is degraded to provide amino acids for gluconeogenesis).
   6. Because of decreased conversion of amino acids to glucose, **less urea is produced** from amino acid nitrogen in starvation than after an overnight fast.

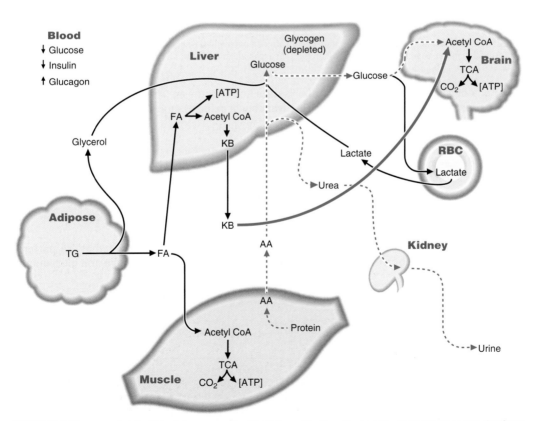

FIGURE 15-7 The starved state. This state occurs after 3 to 5 days of fasting. *Dashed lines* indicate processes that have decreased, and the *heavy solid line* indicates a process that has increased relative to the fasting state. For abbreviations, see Figures 15-6 and 15-7.

B. Fat: the primary fuel (see section III.A)
1. The body uses its fat stores as its primary source of energy during starvation, conserving functional protein.
2. Overall, fats are quantitatively the most important fuel in the body.
3. The length of time that a person can survive without food depends mainly on the amount of fat stored in adipose tissue.

V. BIOCHEMICAL FUNCTIONS OF TISSUES

A. Stomach
1. **Chief cells** produce the proteolytic enzyme **pepsin** as its inactive precursor pepsinogen. Pepsin digests proteins.
2. **Parietal cells** produce hydrochloric acid (**HCl**) and **intrinsic factor.**
   a. **HCl** causes pepsinogen (the precursor of pepsin) to cleave itself (autocatalysis), producing active **pepsin.**
   b. **Intrinsic factor** binds dietary **vitamin B$_{12}$** and aids in its absorption.

B. Gallbladder
1. **Bile salts,** synthesized in the liver from cholesterol, pass through the gallbladder into the intestine, where they aid in lipid digestion.
2. **Bilirubin diglucuronide,** produced in the liver from bilirubin (the excretory product of heme degradation), passes through the gallbladder into the intestine.

C. Pancreas
1. **Produces bicarbonate (HCO$_3^-$),** which neutralizes stomach acid as it enters the intestinal lumen. The subsequent increase in pH allows more extensive **ionization of bile salts** (making them better detergents) and increases **digestive enzyme activity**.
2. Produces **digestive enzymes** (e.g., trypsin, chymotrypsin, carboxypeptidases, elastase, α-amylase, lipase).
3. The B (or β) cells of the endocrine pancreas produce **insulin** (the hormone that stimulates the storage of fuels in the fed state), and the A (or α) cells produce **glucagon** (the hormone that stimulates the release of stored fuels during fasting).

D. Intestine
1. **Enzymes** from the **exocrine pancreas digest food** in the intestinal lumen.
2. **Digestive enzymes** are bound to the brush borders of **intestinal epithelial cells** (aminopeptidases, dipeptidases, tripeptidases, lactase, sucrase, maltases, and isomaltases).
3. **Absorption** of digestive products occurs through intestinal epithelial cells.
4. Intestinal epithelial cells produce **chylomicrons** from the digestive products of dietary fat (fatty acids and 2-monoacylglycerols) and secrete the chylomicrons into the lymph.
5. Most **bile salts** are **resorbed** in the ileum and **recycled** by the liver. Only **5% are excreted** in the feces.

E. Liver functions
1. **Under normal conditions**
   a. Storage of **glycogen** is produced from dietary carbohydrate.
   b. Synthesis of **VLDL** occurs, mainly from dietary carbohydrate.
   c. Production of high-density lipoprotein (**HDL**) transfers C-II and E apoproteins to chylomicrons and VLDL, converts cholesterol to cholesterol esters (via lecithin-cholesterol acyl transferase [LCAT]), and reduces blood cholesterol levels by transporting cholesterol and cholesterol esters from tissues to the liver.
   d. **Maintenance of blood glucose** during fasting occurs via glycogenolysis and gluconeogenesis.

   e. Production of **urea** from nitrogen is derived, in part, from amino acids converted to glucose (via gluconeogenesis) during fasting.
   f. Production of **ketone bodies** from fatty acids is derived from lipolysis of adipose triacylglycerols during fasting.
   g. Synthesis of **cholesterol** (also made in other tissues) and conversion to bile salts occur.
   h. Many **blood proteins** (e.g., albumin, blood-clotting proteins) are produced.
   i. **Purines** and **pyrimidines** are produced and transported to other tissues via red blood cells.
   j. **Degradation of purines** (to uric acid) and **pyrimidines** (to water-soluble products) occurs.
   k. **Oxidation of drugs** and other **toxic compounds** occurs via the cytochrome P-450 system.
   l. **Conjugation of bilirubin** occurs, with excretion of bilirubin diglucuronide into the bile.
   m. **Oxidation of alcohol** occurs via alcohol and acetaldehyde dehydrogenases and the microsomal ethanol–oxidizing system (MEOS).
   n. Synthesis of **creatine** (from guanidinoacetate), which is used to produce creatine phosphate, mainly in muscle and brain.
   o. Conversion of **dietary fructose** to glycolytic intermediates.
  2. **Altered liver cell function** (e.g., in viral hepatitis or alcoholic cirrhosis):
   a. Toxic **NH_4^+** (particularly to the central nervous system) **increases** in blood.

CLINICAL CORRELATES Patients with severe liver disease cannot detoxify ammonia and thus develop **hepatic encephalopathy** from the accumulation of **ammonia in the CNS.** **Lactulose** is used to treat this condition and **reduces ammonia** by either increasing bacterial assimilation of ammonia or reducing deamination of nitrogenous compounds.

   b. The **blood urea nitrogen (BUN) decreases** because of the liver's decreased capacity to produce urea. BUN measures the kidney's ability to excrete nitrogenous waste.
   c. **Blood glucose decreases** because of decreased glycogenolysis and gluconeogenesis.
   d. Blood **cholesterol** levels **decrease**.
   e. Production of **bile salts decreases.**
   f. **Bilirubin** levels **increase** in the body (causing jaundice).
   g. Lysis of damaged liver cells allows **enzymes** to **leak** into the blood.

CLINICAL CORRELATES Transaminases are common diagnostic markers of liver damage found in serum. The cytosolic **alanine aminotransferase (ALT)** and **aspartate aminotransferase (AST)** are released from dying cells upon insult.

   h. **Chronic** liver problems result in **decreased protein synthesis.**
    (1) **Serum proteins** (e.g., albumin) decrease.
    (2) **VLDL** production decreases because of decreased apoprotein B-100, and triacylglycerols accumulate in the liver. A fatty liver results.
  3. **Specific diseases** that affect the liver are as follows.
   a. **Glycogen storage diseases**
   b. **Alcoholism**
    (1) Oxidation of ethanol **produces NADH** by reactions that occur in the liver.
    (2) Ingestion of ethanol without food intake results in a high [NADH]/[NAD$^+$] ratio, which can cause:
     (a) Increased conversion of pyruvate to lactate, producing a **lactic acidosis**
     (b) Inhibition of gluconeogenesis, leading to **hypoglycemia**
     (c) Increased levels of glycerol 3-phosphate, which combines with fatty acids from adipose triacylglycerols to form VLDL. Increased VLDL produces **hyperlipidemia.**
    (3) In **chronic alcoholism, protein synthesis decreases** in the liver. Thus, VLDL secretion decreases, leading to a **fatty liver** (the accumulation of triacylglycerol).

c. **Diabetes mellitus (DM)**

(1) Low insulin (type 1) or insulin insensitivity (type 2) results in increased glycogenolysis and gluconeogenesis, which contribute to the clinical finding of **elevated blood glucose.**

(2) Increased ketone body production can lead to **diabetic ketoacidosis** (DKA), particularly in type 1 diabetes mellitus. Ketone body synthesis increases because of increased release of fatty acids from adipose triacylglycerols, but because there is adequate glucose in the circulation, the brain does not use the ketone bodies for energy. The accumulation of ketone bodies in the blood then leads to an acidosis as the buffering capacity of the blood is exceeded.

F. Brain

1. **Glucose** is the major fuel for the brain.
2. The brain uses **ketone bodies after 3 to 5 days of fasting when blood ketones are elevated.**
3. The brain needs energy to **think** (i.e., memory involves RNA synthesis), conduct **nerve impulses,** and synthesize **neurotransmitters.**
   a. Abrupt decreases in blood glucose can result in **coma** from **lack of ATP.**
   b. Very elevated blood glucose levels can cause a **hyperosmolar coma.**

G. Red blood cells

1. **Lack mitochondria,** with no tricarboxylic acid (TCA) cycle, β-oxidation of fatty acids, electron transport chain, and other pathways that occur in mitochondria.
2. **Glucose** is the **major fuel** and is converted to pyruvate and lactate.
3. Red blood cells **carry nucleotide bases** and **nucleosides** from the liver to other tissues.
4. The major function of red blood cells is to **carry O_2** from the lungs to the tissues and to aid in the **return** of CO_2 from the tissues to the lungs.

H. Adipose tissue

1. The **major fuel** is **glucose.**
2. **Insulin** stimulates the **transport of glucose** into adipose cells.
3. Adipose tissue **stores triacylglycerol** in the fed state and releases free fatty acids and glycerol (via **lipolysis**) during fasting.
   a. **In the fed state,** insulin stimulates the synthesis and secretion of lipoprotein lipase (LPL) which degrades the triacylglycerols of chylomicrons and VLDL in the capillaries. Fatty acids enter adipose cells and are converted to triacylglycerols and stored. Glucose provides the glycerol moiety. (Glycerol is *not used* because adipose cells lack glycerol kinase.)
   b. **During fasting,** hormone-sensitive lipase (phosphorylated and activated via protein kinase A) initiates lipolysis in adipose cells.
   c. **In diabetes mellitus,** low insulin (type 1) or insulin resistance (type 2) results in the decreased degradation of triacylglycerols within chylomicrons and VLDL (due to decreased LPL secretion).

I. Muscle

1. Muscle uses **all available fuels** from blood (glycogen stores and fatty acids, glucose, ketone bodies, lactate, and amino acids) to obtain energy for contraction.
2. During fasting, muscle protein is degraded to provide **amino acids** (particularly alanine) for **gluconeogenesis.**
3. **Creatine phosphate** transports high-energy phosphate from the mitochondria to actinomyosin fibers and provides ATP for muscle contraction.
4. **Creatinine** is produced from the spontaneous cyclization of creatine phosphate at a constant rate. A **constant amount** (dependent on body muscle mass) of creatinine is released into blood each day and excreted by the kidneys.
5. **Muscle glycogen phosphorylase** differs from liver phosphorylase but catalyzes the same reaction (glycogen + P_i ↔ glucose 1-phosphate).
6. **Insulin** stimulates the **transport of glucose** into muscle cells.

J. Heart

1. The heart is a specialized muscle using **all fuels available** from the blood.
2. The muscle-brain **(MB) isozyme** of creatine kinase (CK) is found in heart muscle. Its release can be used to monitor a heart attack.
3. **Heart disease**
   a. **Atherosclerotic plaques** can occlude blood vessels, blocking nutrients and O_2. Muscle tissue distal to the block suffers from a lack of energy and can die. **Heart failure** occurs when the remaining cardiac tissue is insufficient to pump blood through the body at a normal rate.
   b. **Hypercholesterolemia is** associated with increased risk for a heart attack (or stroke, a similar process in the brain). Cholesterol is carried on lipoproteins and is elevated in **hyperlipidemias.**

K. Kidney

1. The kidney **excretes substances** via the urine, including **urea** (produced by the urea cycle in the liver), **uric acid** (from purine degradation), **creatinine** (from creatine phosphate), NH_4, (from glutamine via glutaminase), H_2SO_4 (produced from the sulfur of cysteine and methionine), and **phosphoric acid.**

> **CLINICAL CORRELATES**
> The **BUN** is a widely used measure of the kidney's functional ability to excrete the nitrogenous waste produced by the body.

2. Daily **creatinine** excretion is **constant** and depends on body muscle mass. It is used as a measure of kidney function (the creatinine clearance rate).
3. **Glutaminase** increases during **acidosis** producing NH_3, which enters the urine and reacts with H^+ to form NH_4^+. NH_4^+ buffers the urine and removes acid (H).
4. **Uric acid** excretion is inhibited by lead (Pb) and metabolic acids (ketone bodies and lactic acid). High blood uric acid can result in **gout** by increased production or decreased excretion of uric acid.
5. **Kidney dysfunction** can lead to increased BUN, creatinine, and uric acid in the blood and decreased levels of these compounds in the urine.
6. During ketoacidosis, **ketone bodies** are excreted by the kidney, and during lactic acidosis, **lactic acid** is excreted.
7. Elevated blood glucose (>180 mg/dL) in diabetes mellitus results in urinary **excretion of glucose.**
8. The kidney produces the hormone **erythropoietin (EPO)**, important in producing red blood cells.

> **CLINICAL CORRELATES**
> **EPO**, produced by **recombinant DNA technology,** is used in the management of anemia resulting from kidney failure, hemolytic anemia, or anemia associated with chemotherapy. It is also a **blood doping** agent in endurance sports such as cycling, rowing, and long-distance running.

Review Test

Directions: Each of the numbered questions or incomplete statements in this section is followed by answers or by completions of the statement. Select the **one** lettered answer or completion that is **best** in each case.

Questions 1–4: Using answers choices (A) through (D) below, match the appropriate vitamin with the clinical vignette.

(A) A postpartum woman from a rural Appalachian community recently gave birth to a baby boy with the aid of a midwife at home. She now brings the baby to the hospital because of continued bleeding and oozing from the umbilical stump.
(B) A child with bowing of the long bones and growth in the lowest fifth percentile
(C) A child with dark, purplish spots on the legs, bleeding gums and gingivitis with tooth loss, epistaxis, and profuse diarrhea
(D) A child from a developing country with visual impairment and poor skin healing

1. Vitamin A

(A)
(B)
(C)
(D)

2. Vitamin C

(A)
(B)
(C)
(D)

3. Vitamin D

(A)
(B)
(C)
(D)

4. Vitamin K

(A)
(B)
(C)
(D)

5. A 57-year-old alcoholic man with chronic pancreatitis is admitted to the hospital for treatment. The absorption of which one of the following vitamins may be affected with pancreatitis?

(A) Vitamin B_{12} (cobalamin)
(B) Folic acid
(C) Vitamin B_2 (riboflavin)
(D) Vitamin B_6 (pyridoxine)
(E) Vitamin D

6. A 54-year-old Native American living on an Indian reservation in southwest Arizona is brought into the clinic by a family member. They are concerned because of impaired memory, diarrhea, and a rash on the face, neck, and dorsum of the hands. Which vitamin deficiency do these symptoms represent?

(A) Niacin
(B) Cobalamin
(C) Folic acid
(D) Vitamin C
(E) Vitamin E

7. A 32-year-old woman presents to the physician with extreme fatigue and vague neurologic complaints. On examination, it is found that she has decreased positional and vibrational sense, and her complete blood count reveals a megaloblastic anemia. She relates a history of gastric resection 4 years ago for severe stomach ulcers. Which vitamin deficiency does this represent?

(A) Vitamin C
(B) Vitamin D
(C) Vitamin K
(D) Vitamin B_{12}
(E) Folate

8. A 75-year-old chronic alcoholic man presents to the emergency room after being found unconscious on the floor of his home. On examination, he is found to have a distended abdomen consistent with ascites. Which of the following functions of the liver has been compromised to lead to the finding of abdominal ascites?

(A) Lipid metabolism
(B) Albumin synthesis
(C) Estrogen metabolism
(D) Alcohol detoxification
(E) Decreased production of coagulation factors

9. A 45-year-old alcoholic man walks into the emergency room with a clumsy, wide-based gait and appears confused. He has pronounced nystagmus, and laboratory tests are significant for a metabolic acidosis and a serum blood alcohol level of 0.13. This patient should most probably be treated with IV fluids containing which of the following?

(A) Thiamine
(B) Riboflavin
(C) Niacin
(D) Pantothenic acid
(E) Biotin

10. A fourth-year medical student does an international rotation in Sub-Saharan Africa. While immunizing children against polio, he sees hundreds of malnourished children in refugee camps with bloated-appearing abdomens. He learns that they are severely protein deficient because they are fed a diet of cornmeal that is provided by international relief agencies. These children likely suffer from which of the following?

(A) Marasmus
(B) Anorexia nervosa
(C) Bulimia
(D) Kwashiorkor
(E) Cachexia

Answers and Explanations

1. **The answer is D.** Vitamin A is required for formation of the visual pigments and maintenance of epithelial tissues. The child described in this answer choice is exhibiting the symptoms of vitamin A deficiency.

2. **The answer is C.** Vitamin C is required for the hydroxylation of proline and lysine residues in collagen. The lack of hydroxylation leads to altered connective tissue formation. Vitamin C deficiency results in scurvy, which is depicted in the clinical vignette of answer choice C.

3. **The answer is B.** Vitamin D stimulates calcium uptake from the intestine and resorption from bone and urine. The lack of vitamin D will lead to rickets. The child described in the vignette has rickets as evidenced by the poor skeletal development and growth.

4. **The answer is A.** Vitamin K is required for the γ-carboxylation of coagulation factors II, VII, IX, and X. In the absence of this modification, the clotting factors cannot bind to developing clots. Bleeding problems result from vitamin K deficiency, as described in the clinical vignette.

5. **The answer is E.** Although alcoholics are often malnourished with various nutrient deficiencies, pancreatitis will affect the role of the exocrine pancreas in the absorption of fat-soluble vitamins. Vitamin D is the only vitamin listed that is fat soluble; the other vitamins listed are water soluble. With the lack of pancreatic lipase dietary fat cannot be digested, and the fat-soluble vitamins cannot be released from the lipids. The vitamins thus pass through the intestine, nonabsorbed. The other fat-soluble vitamins are vitamins E, K, and A.

6. **The answer is A.** The patient presents with the classic presentation of pellagra, or niacin deficiency, with diarrhea, dementia, and dermatitis. Niacin is synthesized from the essential amino acid tryptophan, which is particularly deficient in corn-based diets. However, niacin is still required in the diet because the amount of niacin derived from tryptophan is insufficient for daily needs. A cobalamin deficiency (vitamin B_{12}) will lead to megaloblastic anemia along with methylmalonic acidemia. Folic acid deficiency often manifests with megaloblastic anemia. Vitamin C deficiency results in scurvy. Vitamin E deficiency is rare and can result in neurologic symptoms.

7. **The answer is D.** Both folate and vitamin B_{12} deficiency lead to a megaloblastic anemia secondary to a reduction in DNA synthesis. Only vitamin B_{12} deficiency causes neurologic dysfunction associated with damage to the dorsal spinal columns. The history of gastric resection is consistent with a deficiency of intrinsic factor required for reabsorption of vitamin B_{12} in the terminal ileum. Vitamin C, D, and K deficiencies will not lead to megaloblastic anemia.

8. **The answer is B.** Cirrhosis results in several complications, including ascites, caused by decreased oncotic pressure causing extravasation of intravascular fluid. Albumin is the primary protein that maintains oncotic pressure within the vessels. Albumin is synthesized by the liver, and in malnourished or chronic disease states, such as chronic alcoholism, the liver synthesizes reduced levels of albumin, and hypoalbuminemia results. Decreased production of coagulation factors leads to bleeding problems, not ascites production. Ascites production is not due to problems in lipid metabolism, estrogen metabolism, or alcohol detoxification.

9. **The answer is A.** Wernicke encephalopathy, with the classic triad of ataxia, confusion, and ophthalmoplegia (and nystagmus), is due to thiamine deficiency. Thiamine is an essential coenzyme in carbohydrate metabolism, including the pentose-phosphate pathway (transketolase) and the TCA cycle (pyruvate dehydrogenase and α-ketoglutarate dehydrogenase). Riboflavin deficiency is possible in malnourished alcoholics, causing cheilosis, glossitis, and corneal changes. Niacin deficiency causes diarrhea, dementia, and dermatitis. Deficiencies of

pantothenic acid and biotin are rare, although a biotin deficiency will lead to hypoglycemia and mild ketosis.

10. **The answer is D.** Protein deficiency (but not overall calorie deficiency), as in kwashiorkor, results in a deficiency of visceral proteins, including those in the blood that normally provide oncotic pressure to retain fluid within vessels. As such, patients with kwashiorkor have abdominal bloating secondary to edema. Marasmus is a deficiency of calories and protein; the children in this question are presumably receiving carbohydrate calories through the cornmeal. Anorexia nervosa and bulimia are disorders of self-induced weight loss that are found mostly in developed countries. Cachexia is weight loss associated with cancer.

I. GENERAL MECHANISMS OF HORMONE ACTION

A. Hormones that bind to cell membrane receptors

  1. Hormones that activate tyrosine kinases (Figure 16-1)

    a. Insulin binds to a receptor on the cell surface, causing the β subunits of the receptor (that extend through the membrane) to **phosphorylate** themselves on **tyrosine residues** located on the inner surface.

    b. The phosphorylated receptor acts as a **kinase,** phosphorylating an intracellular protein known as **insulin receptor substrate-1** (IRS-1).

    c. Phosphorylated IRS-1 then activates other signal transduction proteins, **initiating a sequence of events** that ultimately produce the intracellular effects of insulin.

  2. Hormones that act through cyclic nucleotides (refer to Figure 6-5 later in this chapter)

    a. Epinephrine and certain polypeptide hormones, such as glucagon, bind to **receptors on the external surface** of the cell membrane.

    (1) These hormone–receptor complexes interact with **G proteins** (so-called because they bind guanine nucleotides) (Figure 16-2) and activate **adenylate cyclase,** which **converts adenosine triphosphate (ATP) to cyclic adenosine monophosphate (cAMP).**

    (2) cAMP activates **protein kinase A,** which subsequently **phosphorylates** certain intracellular proteins, altering their activity.

    (3) The activity of these proteins can be returned to their previous state by **phosphatases** that **dephosphorylate** these proteins. The activity of the phosphatases is controlled by hormones such as insulin, which opposes the action of glucagon.

    b. Some of these hormone–receptor complexes **lower cAMP** levels, either by inhibiting adenylate cyclase or by activating the **phosphodiesterase** that cleaves cAMP to adenosine monophosphate (AMP).

> **CLINICAL CORRELATES** Caffeine, theophylline, and other members of the **methylxanthine** group of compounds **inhibit phosphodiesterase,** leading to increased cellular levels of cAMP.

    c. At least one hormone, **atrial natriuretic peptide (ANP),** activates guanylate cyclase, which produces cyclic guanosine monophosphate (cGMP).

    (1) cGMP activates **protein kinase G.**

    (2) ANP is released from atrial cells of the heart and produces effects that include increased urine volume, excretion of sodium ions, and vasodilation.

  3. Hormones that act through calcium (Ca^{2+}) and the phosphatidylinositol bisphosphate (PIP_2) system (Figure 16-3)

    a. Some hormones (e.g., thyrotropin-releasing hormone [TRH] and oxytocin [OT]) interact with G proteins to alter the amount and distribution of calcium ions within the cell and activate **protein kinase C.**

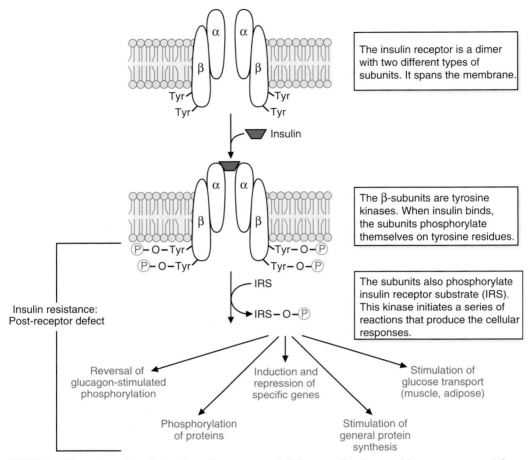

FIGURE 16-1 The actions of insulin. Insulin resistance or type 2 diabetes mellitus is caused by a post-receptor defect. IRS, insulin receptor substrate; Ⓟ, phosphate; Tyr, tyrosine.

   b. Hormone–G protein complexes **open calcium channels** within the cell membrane, allowing extracellular calcium to move into the cell.

   c. Some complexes **activate phospholipase C,** which cleaves phosphatidylinositol bisphosphate (PIP_2) in the cell membrane to produce two messengers, diacylglycerol (DAG) and inositol 1, 4, 5 trisphosphate (IP_3) (Figure 16-4).

     (1) **DAG activates protein kinase C,** which phosphorylates certain proteins, altering their activity.

     (2) Inositol 1,4,5-trisphosphate **(IP_3) causes Ca^{2+} to be released** from intracellular stores, such as those in the endoplasmic reticulum.

     (3) Ca^{2+}, either directly or complexed with calmodulin, interacts with proteins, altering their activity.

B. **Hormones that bind to intracellular receptors and activate genes** (Figure 16-5)

   1. **Steroid** and **thyroid** hormones, 1,25-dihydroxycholecalciferol **(1,25-DHC),** and **retinoic acid** cross the cell membrane and bind to **intracellular receptors.**

CLINICAL CORRELATES   Androgen insensitivity syndrome (formerly know as *testicular feminization*) results in **mutations in the steroid receptor for androgens.** This disorder is an **X-linked disease** resulting in the lack of masculinization of genitalia of chromosomally male individuals, giving them the **phenotypic appearance of females.**

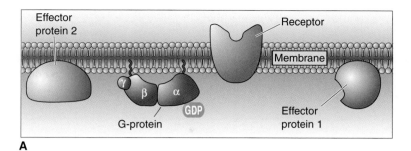

A

B

C

D

FIGURE 16-2 The basic mode of operation of G proteins. **(A)** In its inactive state, the α subunit of the G protein binds guanosine diphosphate (GDP). **(B)** When activated by a G-protein-coupled receptor, the GDP is exchanged for GTP. **(C)** The activated G protein splits, and both the α (guanosine triphosphate [GTP]) subunit and the $\beta\gamma$ subunits become available to activate effector proteins. **(D)** The α subunit slowly removes phosphate (PO_4) from its bound GTP, converting GTP to GDP and terminating its own activity.

2. **Intracellular receptors** contain domains that bind the hormone and domains that bind to **regulatory elements** (i.e., hormone response elements [HRE]) **on DNA** that stimulate or inhibit the synthesis of messenger RNA (mRNA) (Figure 16-5). Translation of this mRNA produces **proteins** that are responsible for the physiologic effects of the hormone.

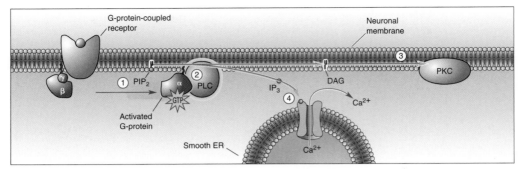

FIGURE 16-3 Second messengers generated by the breakdown of phosphatidylinositol bisphosphate (PIP$_2$), a membrane phospholipid. (1) Activated G proteins (G) stimulate ($\oplus$) the enzyme phospholipase C (PLC). (2) PLC splits PIP$_2$ into diacylglycerol (DAG) and inositol 1,4,5-trisphosphate (IP$_3$). (3) DAG stimulates the downstream enzyme protein kinase C (PKC). (4) IP$_3$ stimulates the release of Ca^{2+} from intracellular stores. The Ca^{2+} can go on to stimulate various downstream enzymes.

II. REGULATION OF HORMONE LEVELS

A. **Regulation of hormone synthesis and secretion**
  1. The **release of hormones** is stimulated by changes in the environment or physiologic state or by a stimulatory hormone from another tissue that acts on the cells that release the hormone. For example:
     a. A **decrease** in **blood pressure** initiates a sequence of events that ultimately causes the adrenal gland to release **aldosterone.**
     b. In response to **stress,** the hypothalamus releases corticotropin-releasing hormone **(CRH),** which stimulates the anterior pituitary to release **adrenocorticotropic hormone (ACTH).** ACTH stimulates the adrenal gland to release **cortisol** (Figure 16-6).

CLINICAL CORRELATES   The **cosyntropin test** is used to evaluate **the hypothalamic-pituitary-adrenal (HPA) axis.** Cosyntropin, a synthetic form of ACTH, is administered, and serum cortisol levels are measured at 30 and 60 minutes. Abnormal results suggest **adrenal insufficiency,** requiring the administration of **exogenous corticosteroids.**

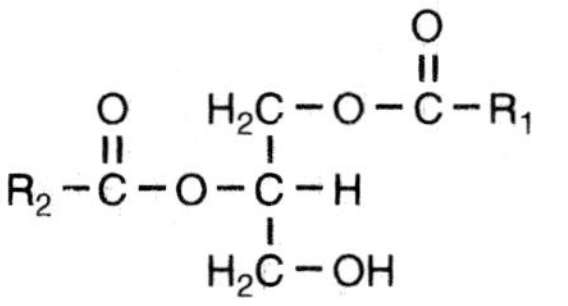

Diacylglycerol (DAG)

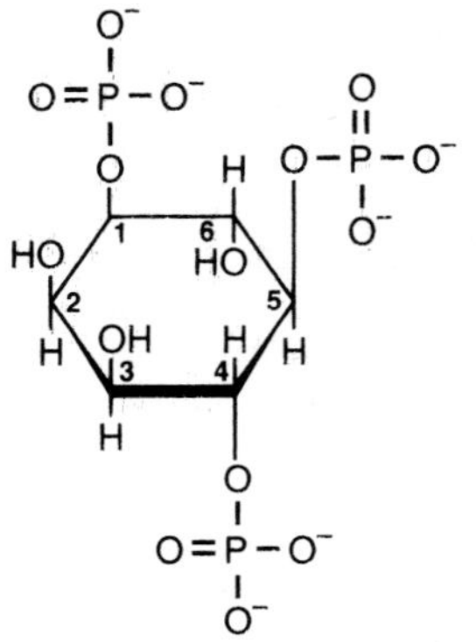

Inositol 1,4,5–trisphosphate (IP$_3$)

FIGURE 16-4 Structures of diacylglycerol and inositol triphosphate.

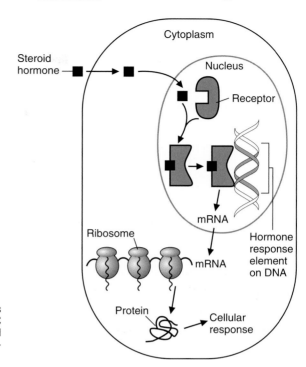

FIGURE 16-5 The mechanism of action of hormones of the steroid-thyroid family. 1,25-dihydroxyvitamin C (the active form of vitamin D_3) and retinoic acid (produced from vitamin A) are members of this family of hormones. mRNA, messenger RNA.

2. The physiologic effect of the hormone or the hormone itself causes a **decrease in the signal** that initially promoted the synthesis and release of the hormone. For example:
    a. Aldosterone causes an increased resorption from the kidney tubule of sodium (Na^+) and, consequently, of water, increasing blood pressure.
    b. Cortisol feeds back on the hypothalamus and the anterior pituitary, inhibiting the release of CRH and ACTH (Figure 16-6).

B. Hormone inactivation
    1. After hormones exert their physiologic effects, they are inactivated and excreted or degraded.
    2. Some hormones are converted to compounds that are no longer active and may be readily **excreted** from the body. For example, cortisol, a steroid hormone, is reduced and conjugated with glucuronide or sulfate and excreted in the urine and the feces.
    3. Some hormones, particularly the polypeptides, are taken up by cells via the process of endocytosis and subsequently **degraded by lysosomal enzymes.**
    4. The **receptor,** which is internalized along with the hormone, can be **degraded** by lysosomal proteases or **recycled** to the cell membrane.

III. ACTIONS OF SPECIFIC HORMONES

A. Hypothalamic hormones (Figure 16-7)
    1. The hypothalamus produces **vasopressin (VP)** and **OT.**
    2. It also produces **other hormones** (mainly peptides and polypeptides) that regulate the synthesis and release of hormones from the anterior pituitary.

B. Hormones of the posterior pituitary (Figure 16-7, *top*)
    1. VP (also called antidiuretic hormone [ADH]) and **OT** are synthesized in the hypothalamus and travel through nerve axons to the posterior pituitary where they are stored, each complexed with a neurophysin. They are released into the blood in response to the appropriate stimulation.
    2. VP, in response to decreased blood volume or increased Na^+ concentration, **stimulates** the **resorption of water** by kidney tubules.

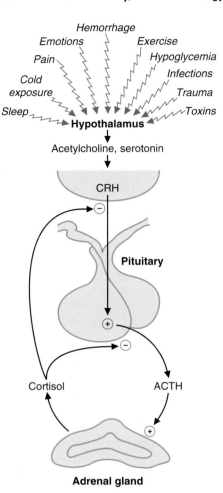

FIGURE 16-6 Hormone feedback regulation. ACTH, adrenocortico-tropic hormone; CRH, corticotropin-releasing hormone; ⊕, acti-vates; ⊖, inhibits.

CLINICAL CORRELATES   Overproduction of ADH results in the **syndrome of inappropriate ADH (SIADH)**. SIADH manifests with dilutional **hyponatremia, reduced serum osmolarity,** and an inability to dilute the urine. It can be caused by **trauma to the head** or, more likely, from the **ectopic** production of ADH by **lung tumors**.

---

   3. **Oxytocin promotes** the **ejection of milk** from the mammary gland in response to suckling and the **contraction of the uterus** during childbirth.

C. **Hormones of the anterior pituitary** (Figure 16-7)
   1. **Prolactin (PRL),** released in response to prolactin-releasing hormone (PRH) from the hypothal-amus caused by suckling of an infant, stimulates the **synthesis of milk proteins** during lacta-tion. Dopamine from the hypothalamus inhibits PRL release.

CLINICAL CORRELATES   The **most common tumor of the pituitary is a prolactinoma.** Patients present with **double vision,** owing to compression of the optic chiasm, as well as **amenorrhea** and **galactorrhea.** Hyperprolactinemia can also result from **drugs that inhibit dopamine's action,** including some of the **antipsychotic medications** used for schizophrenia.

---

   2. **Growth hormone (GH)** stimulates the **release of insulin-like growth factors** (IGFs) and **antago-nizes** the **effects of insulin on carbohydrate and fat metabolism.** The release of GH is stimu-lated by growth hormone–releasing hormone (GHRH) and inhibited by somatostatin from the hypothalamus.

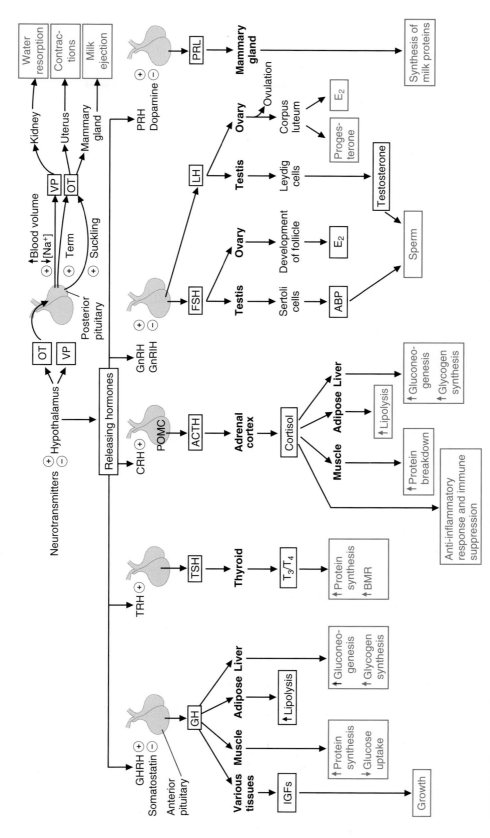

FIGURE 16-7 The actions of hypothalamic and pituitary hormones on their target cells. BMR, basal metabolic rate. The abbreviations are defined in the text.

3. **Thyroid-stimulating hormone (TSH),** which is produced in response to thyrotropin-releasing hormone (TRH) from the hypothalamus, **stimulates** the release of triiodothyronine (T_3) and tetraiodothyronine (T_4) from the thyroid gland.

CLINICAL CORRELATES   TSH is used to screen patients for thyroid disease. **Elevated levels of TSH** suggest low levels of thyroid hormone, that is, **hypothyroidism,** whereas **low levels** suggest increased thyroid hormone, that is, **hyperthyroidism.**

4. Luteinizing hormone (**LH**) and follicle-stimulating hormone (**FSH**) **stimulate** the **gonads** to release hormones that are involved in reproduction. The release of LH and FSH is stimulated by gonadotropin-releasing hormone (GnRH) and inhibited by gonadotropin inhibitory hormone (GnIH) from the hypothalamus.
5. The protein product of the **pro-opiomelanocortin (*POMC*)** gene, produced in response to CRH from the hypothalamus, is cleaved to generate a number of polypeptides.
   a. **ACTH** stimulates the production of cortisol and has a permissive effect on the production of aldosterone by the adrenal cortex.
   b. **Lipotropin (LPH)** may be cleaved to form melanocyte-stimulating hormone and endorphins.
   c. **Melanocyte-stimulating hormone (MSH),** which is part of ACTH and LPH, stimulates the production of the pigment melanin by the melanocytes in the skin.
   d. **Endorphins** produce analgesic effects.

CLINICAL CORRELATES   **Opioids** are pharmacologic agents that mimic the effects of endogenous endorphins. Several opioid derivatives, such as **morphine,** are used for **pain control**; however, they have significant **addictive potential.**

D. **Thyroid hormone**
   1. T_3 is much more active metabolically than T_4.
      a. Although the thyroid secretes some T_3, most is produced by **deiodination of T_4,** a process that occurs in nonthyroidal tissue.
      b. During starvation, T_4 is converted to reverse T_3 (rT_3), which is not active.
   2. **Thyroid hormone** binds to nuclear receptors and **regulates the expression of many genes.**
   3. Thyroid hormone is necessary for **growth, development,** and **maintenance** of almost all tissues of the body. It **stimulates** oxidative metabolism and causes the **basal metabolic rate** (BMR) to increase.

CLINICAL CORRELATES   In patients with hypothyroidism, the stimulatory effect of thyroid hormone on the oxidation of fuels is diminished. As a consequence, the generation of ATP is reduced, causing a sense of **weakness, fatigue,** and **hypokinesis.** The **reduced BMR** is associated with diminished heat production, causing **cold intolerance** and **decreased sweating.** With less demand for the delivery of fuels and oxygen to peripheral tissues, the circulation is slowed, causing a reduction in heart rate and, when far advanced, a reduction in blood pressure.

CLINICAL CORRELATES   When the thyroid gland secretes excessive quantities of thyroid hormone, the rate of oxidation of fuels by muscle and other tissues is increased (i.e., the **BMR** is **increased**). With enhanced oxidative metabolism, heat production is increased, leading to a sense of **heat intolerance** and the need to dissipate heat through **increased sweating.** Thyroid hormone excess raises the tone of the sympathetic (adrenergic) nervous system, **raising** the **heart rate** and **systolic blood pressure.** In addition, **tremulousness,** a sense of **restlessness,** and **insomnia** often occur. Because stored fuels in muscle and fat tissue are being used at an excessive rate, **weight loss** occurs despite increased caloric intake.

E. Hormones that stimulate growth

1. **Insulin** and **GH** stimulate growth and promote protein synthesis.
2. However, **GH antagonizes** many of the metabolic actions of **insulin,** stimulating gluconeogenesis and promoting lipolysis. The result is that alternative fuels are made available so that muscle protein (i.e., growth) can be preserved.

> **CLINICAL CORRELATES** Excessive secretion of GH occurs as a result of a **benign tumor** of the **anterior pituitary gland.** If the hypersecretion begins before closure of the growth centers in the long bones, excessive height (**gigantism**) occurs. If hypersecretion begins after the growth centers have closed, the bones grow in bulk and width, leading to a condition called **acromegaly.** Soft tissue overgrowth occurs as well, leading to **organomegaly, thickness of the skin, and coarseness of the facial features.**

F. Hormones that mediate the response to stress

1. **Glucocorticoids** (particularly cortisol) and **epinephrine** act in concert to supply fuels to the blood so that energy can be produced to combat stressful situations.
2. **Glucocorticoids** (Figure 16-8)
   a. In response to ACTH, the adrenal cortex produces glucocorticoids. **Cortisol** is the major glucocorticoid in humans.
   b. Glucocorticoids have **anti-inflammatory effects.** They induce the synthesis of **lipocortin,** a protein that inhibits phospholipase A_2, the rate-limiting enzyme in prostaglandin, thromboxane, and leukotriene synthesis.
   c. Glucocorticoids **suppress the immune response** by causing the lysis of lymphocytes.
   d. Glucocorticoids **influence metabolism** by causing the movement of fuels from peripheral tissues to the liver, where gluconeogenesis and glycogen synthesis are stimulated (Figures 16-7 and 16-8).
      (1) **Amino acids** are released from muscle protein.
      (2) **Lipolysis** occurs in adipose tissue.

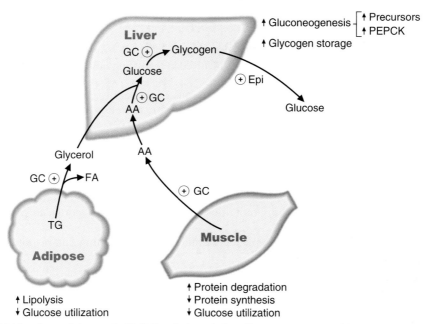

FIGURE 16-8 The effects of glucocorticoids (GC) on fuel metabolism. Chronic stress causes GC to stimulate the breakdown of fuels in peripheral tissues, and gluconeogenic precursors are converted to glycogen in the liver. Acute stress causes the release of epinephrine (Epi), which stimulates the breakdown of liver glycogen to produce blood glucose as fuel for "fight or flight." Epinephrine also stimulates glycogen breakdown in muscle to produce adenosine triphosphate (ATP) for muscle contraction, and it stimulates lipolysis in adipose tissue and gluconeogenesis in the liver. AA, amino acid; FA, fatty acid; PEPCK, phosphoenolpyruvate carboxykinase.

(3) In addition to providing amino acids and glycerol as carbon sources, **glucocorticoids promote gluconeogenesis** by **inducing** synthesis of the enzyme phosphoenolpyruvate carboxykinase (**PEPCK**).

(4) **Glucose,** which is produced by gluconeogenesis promoted by glucocorticoids, is **stored as glycogen** in the liver.

(5) Glucocorticoids prepare the body during stressful conditions so that fuel stores are ready for the "alarm" reaction mediated by epinephrine.

CLINICAL CORRELATES   **Hypercortisolemia** has an adverse effect on virtually every tissue of the body. Central nervous system effects range from **hyperirritability** to **depression.** The catabolic effect on protein-containing tissues leads to a reduction in the ground substance of bone and, eventually, to **osteoporosis;** loss of muscle protein, which causes **weakness;** and thinning and tearing of dermal and epidermal structures, which is manifest as reddish stripes, or **striae,** over the lower abdomen. Increased vascular fragility also results with **easy bruising.** A suppressive effect on immunocompetence may increase the likelihood of infection. The diabetogenic actions of cortisol may lead to **glucose intolerance** or overt **diabetes mellitus.** A peculiar tendency for the disposition of fat in the face (**moon facies**), posterior neck (**buffalo hump**), thorax, and abdomen, while sparing the distal extremities, causes a distinct "**central obesity.**" This constellation of clinical signs and symptoms resulting from chronic hypercortisolemia is referred to as **Cushing syndrome** if the condition is caused by excessive production of **cortisol** by an **adrenal tumor** or by intake of **exogenous glucocorticoids. Cushing disease** refers to hypercortisolemia caused by excessive secretion of **ACTH** by a **pituitary tumor.**

3. Epinephrine
  a. Epinephrine increases blood glucose by **stimulating liver glycogenolysis** (Figure 16-8).
  b. It also **stimulates lipolysis** in adipose tissue and **glycogen degradation in muscle.**
  c. Overall, it makes fuels available for "fight or flight."

G. Hormones that regulate salt and water balance
  1. In addition to **VP** and **ANP, aldosterone** is involved in regulating salt and water balance.
  2. Synthesis of aldosterone
    a. Renin (produced by the juxtaglomerular cells of the kidney in response to decreased blood pressure, blood volume, or sodium ion concentration) **cleaves angiotensinogen to angiotensin I.**
    b. Angiotensin I is **cleaved** to **angiotensin II** by angiotensin-converting enzyme (**ACE**), which is made in the lung. Further cleavage to angiotensin III occurs.
    c. Angiotensin II acts directly on vascular smooth muscle cells, causing **vasoconstriction,** which increases blood pressure.
    d. Angiotensin II and III (and also decreased serum sodium [Na^+] and increased serum potassium [K^+]) **stimulate** the glomerulosa cells of the adrenal cortex to produce and secrete **aldosterone.**
    e. ACTH has a permissive effect (i.e., it maintains cells so that they can respond to angiotensin II).
  3. Action of aldosterone
    a. Aldosterone causes the production of proteins in cells of the distal tubule and the collecting ducts of the kidney.
      (1) A **permease** is **produced** that allows Na^+ to enter cells from the lumen.
      (2) **Citrate synthase** is **induced,** which increases the capacity of the tricarboxylic acid (TCA) cycle for the generation of ATP.
      (3) Energy is thus provided to drive the **Na^+-K^+ ATPase pump,** which may also be induced.
    b. Overall, K^+ and hydrogen ions (H^+) are lost; Na^+ is retained; water is resorbed; and blood volume and pressure are increased.

CLINICAL CORRELATES **Primary hyperaldosteronism** is most often the result of an aldosterone-secreting tumor of one of the adrenal glands (**Conn syndrome**). This disorder manifests with sodium retention and potassium secretion, with **resultant hypertension** and **hypokalemia.**

CLINICAL CORRELATES A deficiency of adrenocortical secretion of aldosterone is usually accompanied by a reduction in the secretion of other adrenal steroid hormones. The loss of adrenocortical steroids is known as **Addison disease.** The mineralocorticoid deficiency leads to a net loss of sodium ions and water in the urine with a reciprocal retention of potassium ions (**hyperkalemia**) and hydrogen ions (**mild metabolic acidosis**). The subsequent contraction of the effective plasma volume may lead to a **reduction in blood pressure.** If volume loss is profound, perfusion of vital tissues, such as the brain, could lead to lightheadedness and possibly loss of consciousness.

H. **Hormones that control reproduction** (Figure 16-7, *right*)
  1. The hypothalamus produces **GnRH,** which causes the anterior pituitary to release **FSH** and **LH,** which act on both the **ovary** and the **testis.**
  2. **The action of FSH and LH on the ovary**
    a. **The menstrual cycle**
      (1) Initially, **FSH acts on** the **follicles** to promote maturation of the ovum and to stimulate estradiol (E_2) production and secretion.
      (2) **Estradiol acts on** the uterine **endometrium,** causing it to thicken and vascularize in preparation for implantation of a fertilized egg.
      (3) A **surge of LH** at the midpoint of the menstrual cycle **stimulates** the ripe **follicle to ovulate,** leaving the residual follicle, which forms the **corpus luteum** and **secretes** both **progesterone and estradiol.**
      (4) **Progesterone** causes the endometrium to continue to thicken and vascularize and increase its secretory capacity.
    b. **Events in the absence of fertilization**
      (1) The **corpus luteum regresses** because of declining LH levels. It produces diminishing amounts of progesterone and estradiol.
      (2) Because of the low steroid hormone levels, the cells die, and the degenerating **endometrium is sloughed** into the uterine cavity and excreted (**menstruation**).
      (3) The low levels of estradiol and progesterone cause feedback inhibition to be relieved, and the hypothalamus releases GnRH, initiating a new menstrual cycle.

CLINICAL CORRELATES Combination **oral contraceptive pills** (OCPs) contain **low levels of estrogen and progestin** derivatives, which **reduce both LH and FSH** levels. Decreased levels of these pituitary hormones destroy the **normal cyclicity** of hormones and result in a **failure to ovulate,** thus preventing conception.

    c. **Events following fertilization**
      (1) The **corpus luteum is maintained** initially by **human chorionic gonadotropin (hCG)** produced by the cells of the developing embryo (trophoblast).

CLINICAL CORRELATES Over-the-counter **pregnancy tests** detect the presence **of hCG in the urine.** Serum quantitation of hCG levels can be used to differentiate a normal intrauterine pregnancy from an ectopic pregnancy.

      (2) Subsequently, the **placenta produces hCG and progesterone.**
      (3) After the corpus luteum dies, the **placenta** continues to produce large amounts of **progesterone.**

(4) Near **term,** hCG and, subsequently, **progesterone, levels fall.** Fetal cortisol may cause the decline in progesterone.

(5) Prostaglandin F$_{2\alpha}$ (PGF$_{2\alpha}$) and **OT** (released from both maternal and fetal pituitaries) stimulate uterine contractions, and the infant is delivered.

CLINICAL CORRELATES **Pitocin** is a synthetic form of **OT** that can be **administered during labor** to **initiate contractions** or **augment labor** in the event of failure of the normal progression of labor.

---

3. **The action of FSH and LH on the testis**
   a. **LH stimulates Leydig cells** to produce and secrete testosterone.
   b. **FSH** acts on **Sertoli cells** of the seminiferous tubule to promote the synthesis of androgen-binding protein **(ABP).**
   c. **ABP binds testosterone** and transports it to the site of spermatogenesis, where **testosterone is converted by 5-α-reductase** to the more potent androgen, dihydrotestosterone **(DHT).**

CLINICAL CORRELATES **5-α-reductase** is required for **normal male development,** and genetic deficiency of this enzyme results in a **phenotype similar to androgen insensitivity syndrome.** In addition, pharmacologic agents that inhibit this enzyme (i.e., **finasteride**) are used to inhibit some of the effects of DHT in normal men, including **male pattern baldness** and **benign prostatic hyperplasia** (BPH).

---

   d. **Testosterone** plays a role in **spermatogenesis** in the adult male.
      (1) Testosterone is responsible for **masculinization** during early development.
      (2) At puberty, testosterone promotes **sexual maturation** of the male.

I. **Hormones that promote lactation** (Figure 16-7, *far right*)
   1. Many hormones are necessary for development of the mammary glands during adolescence.
   2. **Preparation of the mammary gland for lactation**
      a. During pregnancy, **prolactin, glucocorticoids, and insulin** are the major hormones responsible for differentiation of mammary alveolar cells into secretory cells capable of producing milk.
      b. **PRL stimulates** the **synthesis of the milk proteins,** particularly casein and α-lactalbumin.
         (1) α-**Lactalbumin,** the major protein in human milk, serves as a **nutrient.**
         (2) α-Lactalbumin binds to galactosyl transferase, decreasing its K$_m$ for glucose and, thus, **stimulating synthesis** of the milk sugar **lactose.**
      c. **Progesterone inhibits milk protein production** and secretion during pregnancy.
      d. At term, when progesterone levels fall, the inhibition of milk protein synthesis is relieved.
   3. **Regulation of milk secretion during lactation**
      a. **PRL causes milk proteins to be produced** and secreted into the alveolar lumen.
      b. **Oxytocin causes contraction** of the myoepithelial cells surrounding the alveolar cells and the lumen, and **milk is ejected** through the nipple.
      c. The **secretion** of both PRL and OT by the pituitary is stimulated by **suckling** of the infant and by other factors.

J. **Hormones involved in growth and differentiation**
   1. **Retinoids are produced** in the body from dietary **vitamin A.** The major dietary source, β-carotene, is cleaved to two molecules of retinal.
   2. **Retinal** (an aldehyde) and **retinol** (an alcohol) are interconverted by oxidation and reduction reactions. **Retinoic acid** is produced by oxidation of retinal and cannot be reduced.
   3. **Retinol,** the **transport** form, is stored as retinyl esters.
   4. **Retinal** is a functional component of the reactions of the **visual cycle.**
   5. **Retinoic acid** is involved in **growth** and also in **differentiation** and **maintenance** of **epithelial tissue.** The functions of **retinoic acid** result from its ability to **activate genes** (i.e., it acts like a steroid hormone).

K. **Hormones that regulate Ca^{2+} metabolism**
   1. **Calcium** has many important functions. It is involved in blood coagulation, activation of muscle phosphorylase kinase, and secretory processes. It combines with phosphate to form the hydroxyapatite of bone. Parathyroid hormone (**PTH**), **1,25-DHC**, and **calcitonin** are the major regulators of Ca^{2+} metabolism.
   2. **PTH,** produced in response to low calcium levels, acts to **increase Ca^{2+}** levels in the extracellular fluid.
      a. PTH promotes Ca^{2+} and phosphate mobilization from **bone.**
      b. PTH acts on **renal tubules** to resorb Ca^{2+} and excrete phosphate.
      c. PTH stimulates the **hydroxylation of 25-hydroxycholecalciferol** to form 1,25-DHC, the active hormone.

> **CLINICAL CORRELATES** Hyperparathyroidism can be either the result of a **tumor of the parathyroid** gland **(primary hyperparathyroidism)** or **renal failure (secondary hyperparathyroidism).** Patients can present with **fractures of long bones,** renal **stones,** gastrointestinal disturbance, lethargy (**moans**), and weakness.

> **CLINICAL CORRELATES** Hypoparathyroidism is most often the result of **trauma** to the parathyroids during **surgical excision of the thyroid.** Patients complain of **neuromuscular excitability** and lethargy.

   3. **1,25-DHC** stimulates the synthesis of a protein involved in **Ca^{2+} absorption** by **intestinal** epithelial cells. 1,25-DHC acts synergistically with PTH in **bone resorption** and promotes resorption of Ca^{2+} by **renal tubular cells.**
   4. **Calcitonin lowers Ca^{2+}** levels by inhibiting its release from bone and stimulating its excretion in the urine.

L. **Hormones that regulate the utilization of nutrients**
   1. **Gut hormones**
      a. **Gastrin** from the gastric antrum and the duodenum stimulates gastric acid and pepsin secretion.

> **CLINICAL CORRELATES** Gastrinomas, which are gastrin-secreting endocrine tumors, are associated with **Zollinger-Ellison syndrome.** Hypergastrinemia results in increased hydrochloric acid (HCl) production with resultant **recurrent peptic ulcers.**

      b. **Cholecystokinin (CCK)** from the duodenum and jejunum stimulates contraction of the gallbladder and the secretion of pancreatic enzymes.
      c. **Secretin** from the duodenum and jejunum stimulates the secretion of bicarbonate by the pancreas.
      d. **Gastric inhibitory polypeptide (GIP)** from the small bowel enhances insulin release and inhibits secretion of gastric acid.
      e. **Vasoactive intestinal polypeptide (VIP)** from the pancreas relaxes smooth muscles and stimulates bicarbonate secretion by the pancreas.

> **CLINICAL CORRELATES** VIPomas are rare tumors that secrete vasoactive intestinal peptide. This condition is associated with **watery diarrhea, hypokalemia,** and **achlorhydria.**

---

t a b l e   16-1   Actions of Insulin and Glucagon

Insulin	Glucagon
Is elevated in the fed state	Elevated during fasting
Promotes the storage of fuels: glycogen and triacylglycerol	Increases the availability of fuels (glucose and fatty acids) in the blood
Stimulates:	
Glycogen synthesis in liver and muscle	Glycogen degradation in liver, but *not* in muscle
Triacylglycerol synthesis in liver and conversion to very-low-density lipoprotein	Gluconeogenesis
Triacylglycerol storage in adipose tissue	Lipolysis (breakdown of triacylglycerols) in adipose tissue
Glucose transport into muscle and adipose cells	
Protein synthesis and growth	

2. **Insulin and glucagon**
   a. The two major hormones that **regulate fuel metabolism,** insulin and glucagon, are produced by the pancreas.
   b. Their actions are summarized in Table 16-1.

Review Test

Directions: Each of the numbered questions or incomplete statements in this section is followed by answers or by completions of the statement. Select the **one** lettered answer or completion that is **best** in each case.

1. A 73-year-old woman is admitted to the intensive care unit for septic shock from a urinary tract infection. The critical care fellow is concerned she may not have an appropriate stress response and orders a cosyntropin test. Which hormone does this test evaluate?

(A) Oxytocin
(B) Vasopressin
(C) Cortisol
(D) Corticotropin-releasing hormone (CRH)
(E) Adrenocorticotropic hormone (ACTH)

2. A 56-year-old woman with a 60-pack year history of smoking is recently found to have a large neoplastic pulmonary mass. Laboratory tests demonstrate a sodium of 127 mmol/L (normal, 135 to 145 mmol/L) and reduced urine osmolality. She likely has which of the following endocrine abnormalities?

(A) Cushing disease
(B) SIADH
(C) Cushing syndrome
(D) Acromegaly
(E) Prolactinoma

3. A 75-year-old woman with osteoporosis complains of back pain. A computed tomographic scan of her back confirms a compression fracture of the L3 vertebra. The attending physician begins treating the patient with morphine for pain control. Morphine is an analgesic that works similarly to which of the following endogenously produced substances?

(A) ACTH
(B) POMC
(C) Lipotropin
(D) MSH
(E) Endorphin

4. A 13-year-old boy has developed polydipsia, polyphagia, and weight loss over the past few weeks. He was brought to the emergency room by his parents because he woke up this morning very lethargic. His blood glucose was found to be 600 mg/dL, and he was immediately placed on an insulin drip. Insulin works primarily by which one of the following mechanisms?

(A) Activating adenylate cyclase
(B) Binding to an intracellular receptor
(C) Activating caspases
(D) Producing cGMP
(E) Causing phosphorylation of tyrosine residues

5. A 43-year-old man presents to the neurologist with headache and double vision. He also complains of a milky discharge from his breast. An MRI of his head confirms the diagnosis of a prolactinoma. Which of the following substances could inhibit the release of prolactin from the pituitary?

(A) Dopamine
(B) Caffeine
(C) Endorphins
(D) Renin
(E) $PGF_{2\alpha}$

6. A 50-year-old woman complains of feeling warm all of the time. Her eyes appear as though they are "bulging out of their sockets" (proptosis). She sees a family physician to evaluate her condition. Laboratory tests demonstrate a decreased level of TSH. Which of the following would you expect in this patient?

(A) Reduced blood pressure
(B) Weight gain
(C) Increased basal metabolic rate
(D) Reduced heart rate
(E) Excess sleep

7. A 43-year-old man comes to the emergency room with a headache and blurred vision. He complains that his wedding ring no longer fits him, and that his favorite hat no longer fits on his head. His wife feels that his nose has become wider, and he is diagnosed with acromegaly. Which of the following metabolic effects would you expect in this patient?

(A) Decreased protein synthesis
(B) Inhibition of gluconeogenesis
(C) Inhibition of lipolysis
(D) Increased protein synthesis
(E) Gigantism

8. A 23-year-old woman is referred to an endocrinologist for weight gain, especially around the waist. She also has striae over the abdomen and a rounded appearance to her face. She is found to have Cushing disease. Which of the following would most likely be found in this patient, compared with someone who does not have Cushing disease?

(A) Increased synthesis of immunoglobulins
(B) Increased protein synthesis
(C) Inhibition of lipolysis
(D) Increased gluconeogenesis
(E) Reduced liver glycogen stores

9. A 56-year-old woman with no known medical conditions presents to the emergency room with pain in the upper arm. She denies any trauma; however, a fracture of the humerus is found on radiograph. She is found to have an elevated PTH level. Which of the following statements best describes PTH?

(A) It lowers serum calcium.
(B) It directly promotes the absorption of calcium from the intestine.
(C) It stimulates the conversion of vitamin D to the active form.
(D) It promotes the reabsorption of phosphate from the kidney.
(E) It promotes the excretion of calcium from the kidney.

10. A 75-year-old man complains of increased urinary frequency, especially at night. He has difficulty starting his stream (hesitancy) and often dribbles urine when he finishes. His urologist suspects BPH and places him on a 5-α-reductase inhibitor. This drug would decrease which of the following?

(A) Conversion of cAMP to AMP
(B) Release of calcium from the endoplasmic reticulum
(C) Prostaglandin synthesis
(D) Conversion of angiotensin I to angiotensin II
(E) Conversion of testosterone to DHT

Answers and Explanations

1. **The answer is C.** The primary stress hormone in the body is cortisol. Normally, CRH from the hypothalamus stimulates the release of ACTH from the anterior pituitary. ACTH then acts on the adrenal gland to produce cortisol. Cosyntropin is a synthetic ACTH injected to stimulate the release of cortisol to evaluate an appropriate stress response. Thus, a cosyntropin test is measuring the release of cortisol. Oxytocin is involved in labor during birth and milk ejection afterward. Vasopressin comes from the posterior pituitary and controls overall volume status and blood pressure.

2. **The answer is B.** This patient has a metabolic derangement consistent with SIADH secondary to a paraneoplastic syndrome associated with lung tumors. Head trauma, strokes, and intracranial tumors can disrupt the hypothalamus-pituitary axis and cause SIADH. The inappropriate release of antidiuretic hormone leads to hyponatremia and fluid overload. Cushing syndrome is a result of increased cortisol, which, when due to a pituitary adenoma secreting tumor, is referred to as Cushing disease. Acromegaly results from growth hormone excess, and a prolactinoma would cause amenorrhea and galactorrhea in a female.

3. **The answer is E.** Morphine and other opioids are agonists of the endorphin receptors and mimic the action of naturally occurring endorphins. Endorphins result from the proteolytic cleavage of POMC. The two main peptides produced from POMC are ACTH, which stimulates cortisol production, and lipotropin. Lipotropin is further processed to MSH and the endorphins.

4. **The answer is E.** Insulin binds to extracellular receptors, promoting dimerization and subsequent phosphorylation of tyrosine residues on the intracellular portion of the receptor. This leads to increased tyrosine phosphorylation of other proteins, which mediate the intracellular effects of insulin action, including glucose uptake and storage. Hormones like epinephrine bind to G protein–coupled receptors with activation of adenylate cyclase. Insulin's primary effect is not achieved via activation of adenylate cyclase. Steroid hormones are lipid soluble and diffuse through the cell membrane, binding intracellular receptors that activate gene transcription. Caspases are involved in apoptosis, a process that is antagonized by insulin. ANP activates guanylate cyclase, which produces cGMP.

5. **The answer is A.** Dopamine normally inhibits the release of prolactin from the anterior pituitary. When there is damage to the dopamine-producing neurons of the hypothalamus, or drugs inhibiting dopamine release are given, prolactin levels increase, resulting in galactorrhea. Caffeine inhibits phosphodiesterase and, therefore, the conversion of cAMP to AMP. Caffeine does not affect prolactin release. Endorphins are produced by proteolytic processing of POMC from the anterior pituitary and do not play a role in prolactin release. Renin is produced by the kidney and cleaves angiotensinogen to angiotensin I. $PGF_{2\alpha}$ is important in stimulating uterine contractions during delivery but does not play a role in regulating prolactin levels.

6. **The answer is C.** This patient presents with the symptoms and laboratory results consistent with hyperthyroidism. Thyroid hormone increases the basal metabolic rate, and if excess thyroid hormone is released, weight loss and an increase in body temperature will result. Thyroid hormone release is regulated by TSH (thyrotropin) secretion from the pituitary gland. Low TSH would occur by feedback inhibition of its release by thyroid hormone. The other answer choices, such as reduced blood pressure, weight gain, and excess sleep, are all observed with hypothyroidism, not hyperthyroidism.

7. **The answer is D.** Acromegaly results from a growth hormone–producing tumor of the anterior pituitary. GH is an important metabolic regulator, stimulating primarily anabolic pathways. As such, increased GH levels result in increased protein synthesis, increased gluconeogenesis, and

increased lipolysis. GH excess in children before the closing of the growth plates of bones results in gigantism, but would not have this effect in a grown man.

8. **The answer is D.** Cushing disease leads to excessive cortisol release due to an adenoma in the pituitary gland, leading to the release of ACTH, which stimulates cortisol release from the adrenal gland. Excess levels of cortisol lead to a variety of debilitating symptoms, which include central obesity, a "buffalo hump," a round face (often referred to as a "moon face"), excessive sweating, dilation of capillaries (telangiectasia), thinning of the skin with purple or red striae, hirsutism, sexual dysfunction, and mental changes. Cortisol is a "stress" hormone and is preparing the tissues for survival during the stressful period. This includes an increase in lipolysis and gluconeogenesis, and glycogen storage. Steroids, including cortisol, suppress the immune response and are often administered exogenously to control autoimmune diseases. Thus, immunoglobulin synthesis would not be increased. Protein synthesis is also not increased in response to cortisol.

9. **The answer is C.** This patient likely has a PTH-producing tumor of the parathyroid. PTH is an important regulator of calcium homeostasis. It stimulates the conversion of vitamin D to the active form, which, in turn, promotes the absorption of calcium from the intestine as well as reabsorption of calcium (not phosphate) from the kidney filtrate. PTH functions to increase serum calcium by liberating calcium phosphate from bone, making it weaker and prone to fracture. PTH prevents accumulation of phosphate by promoting its excretion from the kidneys. PTH does not promote the excretion of calcium from the kidney.

10. **The answer is E.** DHT is a stimulatory growth factor for prostate cells, and a 5-α-reductase inhibitor would decrease the conversion of testosterone to DHT. Reducing DHT levels shrinks the prostate, thereby reducing the patient's symptoms. Caffeine inhibits cAMP phosphodiesterase, which converts cAMP to AMP. IP_3, derived from the cleavage of PIP_2 by phospholipase C, is the signal that releases calcium from the endoplasmic reticulum to the cytoplasm. 5-α-Reductase inhibitors do not interfere with the phospholipase C pathway. Prostaglandin synthesis can be blocked by cyclooxygenase inhibitors (such as aspirin), or by lipocortin, an inhibitor of phospholipase A_2. ACE inhibitors, which are used in the control of blood pressure, are used to inhibit the conversion of angiotensin I to angiotensin II.

17 DNA Replication and Transcription

I. NUCLEIC ACID STRUCTURE

A. The structure of DNA

1. **Chemical components of DNA**
   a. Each polynucleotide chain of DNA contains nucleotides, which consist of a **nitrogenous base** (A, G, C, or T), **deoxyribose**, and **phosphate**.
   b. The bases are the **purines** adenine (A) and guanine (G) and the **pyrimidines** cytosine (C) and thymine (T).
   c. **Phosphodiester bonds** join the $3'$-carbon of one sugar to the $5'$-carbon of the next sugar (Figure 17-1).

2. **DNA double helix**
   a. Each DNA molecule is composed of two **polynucleotide chains** joined by hydrogen bonds between the bases (Figure 17-2).
      (1) **Adenine** on one chain forms a base pair with **thymine** on the other chain.
      (2) **Guanine** base pairs with **cytosine.**
      (3) The **base sequences** of the two strands are **complementary.** Adenine on one strand is matched by thymine on the other, and guanine is matched by cytosine.
   b. The **chains are antiparallel.** One chain runs in a **$5'$ to $3'$** direction; the other chain runs **$3'$ to $5'$** (Figure 17-3).
   c. The double-stranded molecule is twisted to form a **helix** with major and minor grooves (Figure 17-4).
      (1) The **base pairs** that join the two strands are **stacked** like a spiral staircase in the interior of the molecule.
      (2) The **phosphate groups** are on the outside of the double helix. Two hydroxyl groups of each phosphate are involved in phosphodiester bonds. The third is free and dissociates its proton at physiologic pH, giving the molecule a **negative charge** (Figure 17-1).
      (3) The **B form of DNA,** first described by Watson and Crick, is right-handed and contains **10 base pairs per turn.**
      (4) Other forms of DNA include the A form, which is similar to the B form but more compact, and the Z form, which is left-handed and has its bases positioned more toward the periphery of the helix.

3. **Denaturation, renaturation, and hybridization**
   a. **Denaturation: Alkali** or **heat** causes the **strands** of DNA to **separate** but does not break phosphodiester bonds.
   b. **Renaturation:** If strands of DNA are separated by heat and then the **temperature** is slowly **decreased** under the appropriate conditions, **base pairs reform,** and complementary strands of DNA come back together.
   c. **Hybridization:** A single strand of DNA or RNA pairs with complementary base sequences on another strand of DNA or RNA.

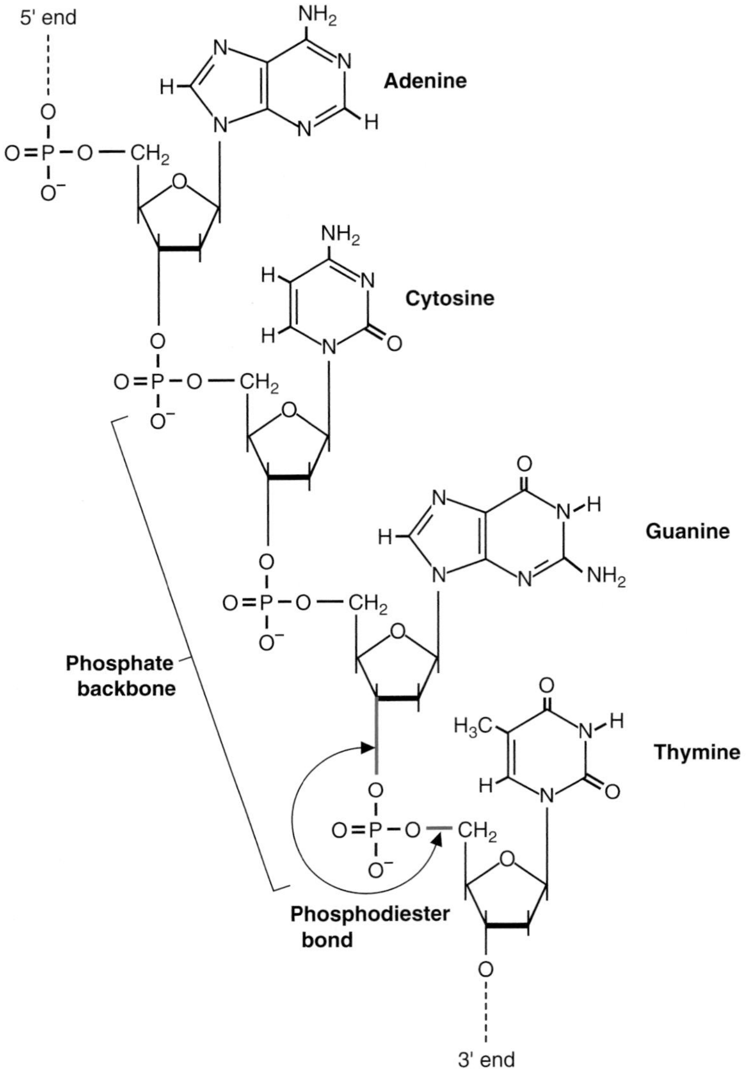

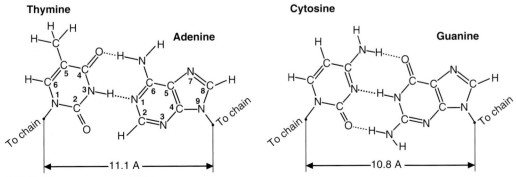

FIGURE 17-1 A segment of a polynucleotide strand. This strand contains thymine and deoxyribose, so it is a segment of DNA.

FIGURE 17-2 The base pairs of DNA.

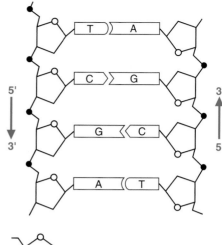

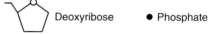

FIGURE 17-3 Antiparallel strands of DNA. Note that the strands run in opposite directions. A, adenine; C, cytosine; G, guanine; T, thymine.

4. **DNA molecules are extremely large**
   a. The entire chromosome of the bacterium *Escherichia coli* is circular and contains more than 4×10^6 base pairs.
   b. The DNA molecule in the longest human chromosome is linear and is over 7.2 cm long.
5. **Packing of DNA in the nucleus**
   a. The **chromatin** of eukaryotic cells consists of DNA complexed with histones in **nucleosomes** (Figure 17-5).
      (1) **Histones** are relatively small, basic proteins with a high content of **arginine** and **lysine**. (Prokaryotes do not have histones.)
      (2) Eight histone molecules form an octamer, around which about 140 base pairs of DNA are wound to form a nucleosome core.
      (3) The DNA that joins one nucleosome core to the next is complexed with histone H1.
   b. The "beads-on-a-string" nucleosomal structure of chromatin is further compacted to form solenoid structures (helical, tubular coils).
6. **Mitochondrial DNA**
   a. The mitochondrial genome is a **double-stranded circular DNA** molecule found within the **mitochondrial matrix.**
      (1) The genetic code for the mitochondria is slightly different than that of genomic DNA.
      (2) The genome codes for 13 **protein subunits of the electron transport chain,** a large and small **ribosomal RNA (rRNA),** and **22 transfer RNAs (tRNAs).**

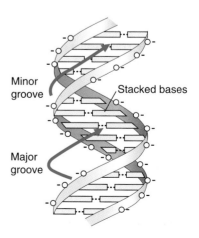

FIGURE 17-4 The DNA double helix.

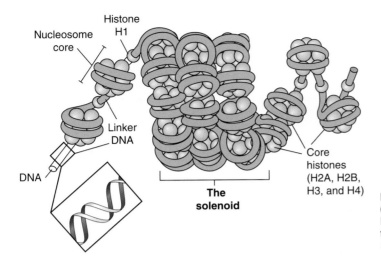

FIGURE 17-5 A polynucleosome. (Adapted from Olins DE, Olins AL: Nucleosomes: The structural quantum in chromosomes. *American Scientist* 66:708, 1978.)

   b. Mitochondrial DNA is maternally inherited.
     (1) Mitochondria from the egg contribute exclusively to the zygote.
     (2) The mitochondria autonomously reproduce, and therefore, all the mitochondria are of maternal origin.
   c. Mitochondrial DNA has a high mutation rate (about 5 to 10 times greater than the nuclear genome).

B. The structure of RNA
  1. RNA differs from DNA
   a. The polynucleotide structure of RNA is similar to DNA except that RNA contains the sugar **ribose** rather than deoxyribose and uracil (U) rather than thymine. (A small amount of thymine is present in tRNA.)
   b. RNA is generally **single stranded** (in contrast to DNA, which is double stranded).
     (1) When **strands loop back** on themselves, the bases on opposite sides can pair: adenine with uracil (A to U) and guanine with cytosine (G to C).
     (2) RNA molecules have extensive base pairing, which produces secondary and tertiary structures that are important for RNA function.
     (3) RNA molecules recognize DNA and other RNA molecules by base pairing.
   c. Some **RNA molecules** act as **catalysts** of reactions; thus, RNA, as well as protein, can have enzymatic activity.
     (1) Ribozymes, usually precursors of rRNA, remove internal segments of themselves, splicing the ends together.
     (2) RNAs also act as **ribonucleases,** cleaving other RNA molecules (e.g., RNase P cleaves tRNA precursors).
     (3) Peptidyl transferase, an enzyme in protein synthesis, consists of RNA.
  2. Messenger RNA (mRNA) contains a cap structure and a poly(A) tail.
   a. The **cap** consists of methylated guanine triphosphate (GTP) attached to the hydroxyl group on the ribose at the 5′ end of the mRNA.
     (1) The N7 in the guanine is methylated.
     (2) The 2′-hydroxyl groups of the first and second ribose moieties of the mRNA also may be methylated (Figure 17-6).

CLINICAL CORRELATES   Many viruses, such as the **influenza virus,** transfer the 7-methyl G cap from host cell mRNAs to viral mRNA, which functions to increase mRNA stability and increase translation of the mRNA.

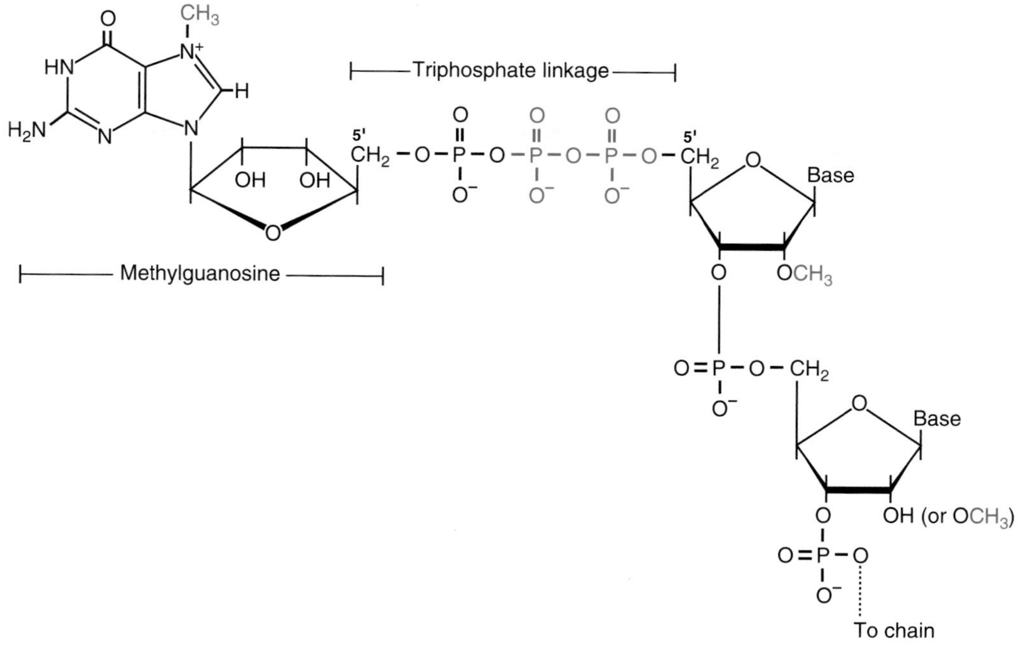

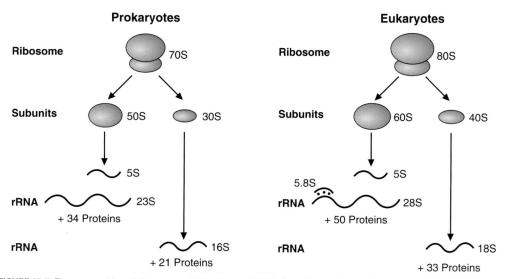

CH₃

HN

H₂N

Triphosphate linkage

Methylguanosine

FIGURE 17-6 The cap structure of messenger RNA.

b. The **poly(A) tail** contains up to 200 adenine (A) nucleotides attached to the hydroxyl group at the 3′ end of the mRNA.

3. **rRNA** contains many loops and extensive base pairing.
   a. rRNA molecules differ in their sedimentation coefficients (S). They associate with proteins to form **ribosomes** (Figure 17-7).
   b. **Prokaryotes** have three types of rRNA: 16S, 23S, and 5S rRNA.
   c. **Eukaryotes** have four types of cytosolic rRNA: 18S, 28S, 5S, and 5.8S rRNA. Mitochondrial ribosomes are similar to prokaryotic ribosomes.

4. **tRNA** has a cloverleaf structure and contains modified nucleotides. tRNA molecules are relatively small, containing about 80 nucleotides.

FIGURE 17-7 The composition of ribosomes. rRNA, ribosomal RNA; S, sedimentation coefficients.

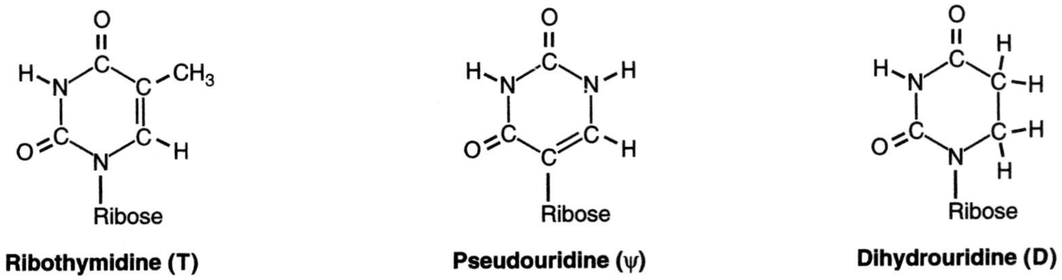

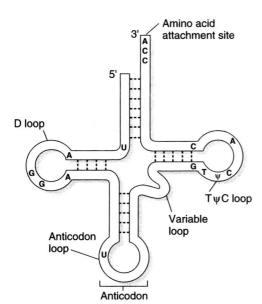

Ribothymidine (T)   Pseudouridine (ψ)   Dihydrouridine (D)

FIGURE 17-8 Three modified nucleosides found in most transfer RNAs.

   a. In eukaryotic cells, many nucleotides in tRNA are modified. Modified nucleotides con-
      taining **pseudouridine (Ψ), dihydrouridine (D),** and **ribothymidine (T)** are present in most
      tRNAs (Figure 17-8).
   b. All tRNA molecules have a similar **cloverleaf structure** even though their base sequen-
      ces differ (Figure 17-9).
      (1) The first loop from the 5′ end, the **D loop,** contains dihydrouridine.
      (2) The middle loop contains the **anticodon,** which base pairs with the codon in mRNA.
      (3) The third loop, the **TΨC loop,** contains both ribothymidine and pseudouridine.
      (4) The **CCA sequence** at the 3′ end carries the amino acid.

II. SYNTHESIS OF DNA (REPLICATION)

A. Mechanism of replication
   1. Replication is bidirectional and semiconservative (Figure 17-10).
      a. Bidirectional means that replication begins at a site of origin and simultaneously
         moves out in both directions from this point.
         (1) Prokaryotes have one site of origin on each chromosome.
         (2) Eukaryotes have multiple sites of origin on each chromosome.
      b. Semiconservative means that, following replication, each daughter molecule of DNA
         contains one intact parental strand and one newly synthesized strand joined by base
         pairs.

FIGURE 17-9 The cloverleaf structure of transfer RNA.
Bases that commonly occur in a particular position are indicated by *letters.* Base pairing in stem regions is indicated
by *dashed lines* between strands. Ψ, pseudouridine, T, ribothymidine; D, dihydrouridine.

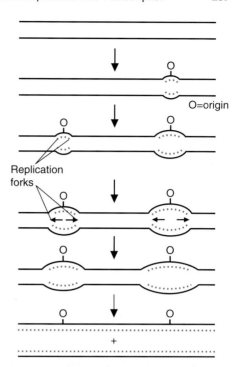

FIGURE 17-10 Replication of a eukaryotic chromosome. *Solid lines* are parental strands. *Dotted lines* are newly synthesized strands. Synthesis is bidirectional from each point of origin (O).

2. **Replication forks are the sites at which DNA synthesis is occurring.**
   a. The **parental strands** of DNA separate, and the helix unwinds ahead of a replication fork (Figure 17-11).
   b. **Helicases** unwind the helix, and single-strand binding proteins hold it in a single-stranded conformation.
   c. **Topoisomerases** act to prevent the extreme supercoiling of the parental helix that would result as a consequence of unwinding at a replication fork.
   d. Topoisomerases break and rejoin DNA chains.

CLINICAL CORRELATES The cancer drug **etoposide (VP-16)** inhibits **topoisomerase** and is widely used in the treatment of lung, ovarian, testicular, and prostate cancer.

---

   e. **DNA gyrase,** a topoisomerase, is found only in prokaryotes.

CLINICAL CORRELATES **Quinolone antibiotics,** such as **ciprofloxacin,** inhibit **DNA gyrase** and are used for numerous infections, including complicated **urinary tract infections** and lower respiratory tract infections.

---

3. **DNA polymerases catalyze the synthesis of DNA.**
   a. **Prokaryotes** have three DNA polymerases: **pol I, pol II,** and **pol III.** Pol III is the major replicative enzyme, and pol I is involved in both DNA replication and repair.
   b. **Eukaryotes** have at least five major species of DNA polymerase: α, β, γ, δ, and ε.
      (1) DNA polymerase α is involved in replication of nuclear DNA.
      (2) Polymerase δ acts in conjunction with α during replication.
      (3) Polymerases β and ε are involved in repair of nuclear DNA, and γ functions in mitochondria.
   c. **DNA polymerases** can only copy a DNA template in the 3′ to 5′ direction and produce the newly synthesized strand in the 5′ to 3′ direction.

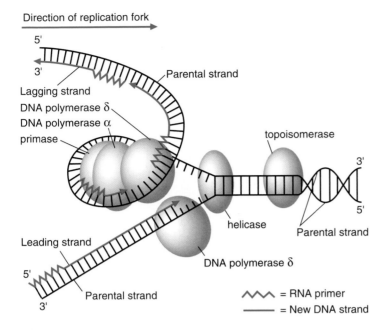

Direction of replication fork

5′
3′
Parental strand
Lagging strand
DNA polymerase δ
DNA polymerase α
primase
topoisomerase
3′
5′
helicase
Leading strand
Parental strand
5′
DNA polymerase δ
Parental strand
3′
〜〜〜 = RNA primer
——— = New DNA strand

FIGURE 17-11 The eukaryotic replication complex located at a replication fork. The lagging strand loops around the complex. Single-strand binding proteins (not shown) are attached to the regions of single-stranded DNA.

   d. Deoxyribonucleoside triphosphates (dATP, dGTP, dTTP, and dCTP) are the precursors for DNA synthesis.

     (1) Each precursor pairs with the corresponding base on the template strand and forms a phosphodiester bond with the hydroxyl group on the 3′-carbon of the sugar at the end of the growing chain (Figure 17-12).

CLINICAL CORRELATES Many of the antiviral drugs used in the treatment of human immunodeficiency virus (HIV) are **analogs of deoxyribonucleoside triphosphates.** For instance, the drug **zidovudine (AZT, ZDV)** is an analog of thymidine, which lacks the 3′-hydroxyl for the addition of the next nucleotide, thereby inhibiting the viral DNA polymerase. **Dideoxyinosine (ddI)** and **zalcitabine (ddC)** are similar agents used to treat HIV.

---

     (2) Pyrophosphate is produced and cleaved to two inorganic phosphates.

  4. DNA polymerase requires a **primer** (Figure 17-13).

   a. DNA polymerases **cannot initiate** synthesis of new strands.

   b. RNA serves as the primer for DNA polymerase in vivo. The RNA primer, which contains about 10 nucleotides, is formed by copying of the parental strand in a reaction catalyzed by **primase.**

   c. DNA polymerase adds deoxyribonucleotides to the 3′-hydroxyls of the RNA primers and subsequently to the ends of the growing DNA strands.

   d. DNA parental (template) strands are copied simultaneously at replication forks, although they run in opposite directions.

     (1) The **leading strand** is formed by continuous copying of the parental strand that runs 3′ to 5′ **toward** the replication fork.

     (2) The **lagging strand** is formed by discontinuous copying of the parental strand that runs 3′ to 5′ **away from** the replication fork.

       ● As more of the helix is unwound, synthesis of the lagging strand begins from another primer. The short fragments formed by this process are known as **Okazaki fragments.**

       ● The RNA **primers are removed by nucleases** (e.g., RNase H), and then the resulting **gaps are filled** with the appropriate deoxyribonucleotides by another DNA polymerase.

       ● Finally, the **Okazaki fragments are joined by DNA ligase,** an enzyme that catalyzes formation of phosphodiester bonds between two polynucleotide chains.

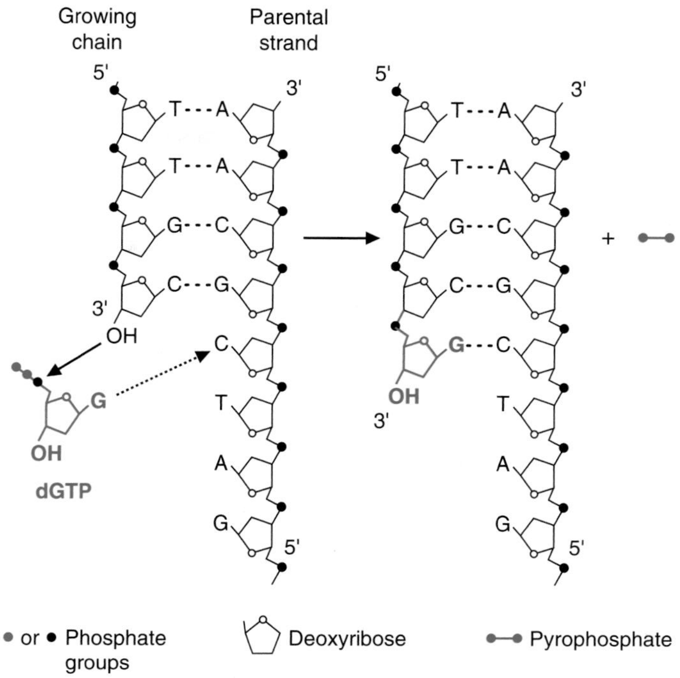

FIGURE 17-12 The action of DNA polymerase. dGTP, deoxyguanosine triphosphate.

● or ● Phosphate groups   ⬠ Deoxyribose   ●—● Pyrophosphate

    e. In eukaryotic cells, about 200 deoxyribonucleotides are added to the lagging strand in each round of synthesis, whereas in prokaryotes, 1000 to 2000 are added.

  5. The **fidelity of replication** is very high, with an overall error rate of 10^{-9} to 10^{-10}.

    a. Errors (insertion of an inappropriate nucleotide) that occur during replication can be corrected by editing during the replication process. This proofreading function is performed by a $3'$ to $5'$ exonuclease activity associated with the polymerase complex.

    b. Postreplication repair processes (e.g., mismatch repair) also increase the fidelity of replication.

B. Mutations

  1. Changes in DNA molecules cause mutations. After replication, these changes result in a permanent alteration of the base sequence in the daughter DNA.

  2. Changes causing mutations include:

    a. Uncorrected errors made during replication

    b. Damage that occurs to replicating or nonreplicating DNA caused by oxidative deamination, radiation, or chemicals, resulting in cleavage of DNA strands or chemical alteration or removal of bases

  3. Types of mutations include:

    a. Point mutations (substitution of one base for another)

    b. Insertions (addition of one or more nucleotides within a DNA sequence)

    c. Deletions (removal of one or more nucleotides from a DNA sequence)

C. DNA repair (Figure 17-14)

  1. In general, repair involves three steps:

    a. Removal of the segment of DNA that contains a damaged region or mismatched bases

    b. Filling in the gap by action of a DNA polymerase that uses the undamaged sister strand as a template

    c. Ligation of the newly synthesized segment to the remainder of the chain

  2. Endonucleases, exonucleases, a DNA **polymerase,** and a **ligase** are required for repair.

  3. Nucleotide excision repair involves the removal of a group of nucleotides (including the damaged nucleotide) from a DNA strand.

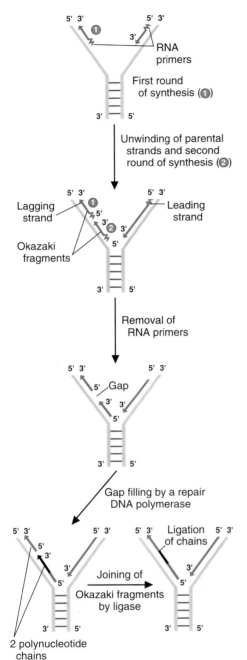

FIGURE 17-13 Mechanism of DNA synthesis at the replication fork. Two rounds of polymerase action are shown (❶ and ❷). The number of nucleotides added in each round is much larger than shown; in eukaryotes, about 10 ribonucleotides and 200 deoxyribonucleotides are polymerized on the lagging strand. Synthesis on the leading strand is continuous. The unshaded regions of the *arrows* indicate the nucleotides added by the repair action of a DNA polymerase.

4. **Base excision repair** involves a specific glycosylase that removes a damaged base by hydrolyz-ing an *N*-glycosidic bond, producing an apurinic or apyrimidinic site, which is cleaved and, subsequently, repaired.
5. **Mismatch repair** involves the removal of the portion of the **newly synthesized strand** of recently replicated DNA that contains a pair of mismatched bases.
   a. Bacteria recognize the newly synthesized strand because, in contrast to the parental strand, it has not yet been methylated.
   b. The recognition mechanism in eukaryotes is not known.

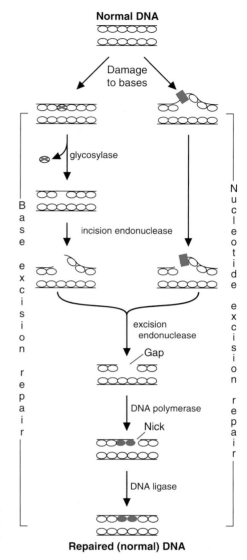

FIGURE 17-14 Base excision and nucleotide excision repair of DNA. Circles indicate normal bases; ⬡ and ◆ indicate damaged bases. The actual number of nucleotides removed (the size of the gap) is larger than that shown.

D. Rearrangements of genes
1. Several processes produce new combinations of genes, thus promoting genetic diversity.
2. **Recombination** occurs between homologous DNA segments, that is, those that have very similar sequences.
3. **Transposition** involves movement of a DNA segment from one site to a nonhomologous site. Transposons ("jumping genes") are mobile genetic elements that facilitate the movement of genes.

CLINICAL CORRELATES **Transposons** in bacteria are believed to mediate the **transfer of antibiotic resistance** between bacteria. The creation of **multidrug-resistant organisms** is a growing health concern worldwide.

E. Reverse transcription
1. Synthesis of DNA from an **RNA template** is catalyzed by reverse transcriptase.
2. **Retroviruses** contain RNA as their genetic material.
   a. The retroviral RNA serves as a template for synthesis of DNA by reverse transcriptase.
   b. The DNA that is generated can be inserted into the genome (chromosomes) of the host cell and be expressed.

HIV is **the retrovirus** that causes acquired immune deficiency syndrome (**AIDS**) in humans. **Hepatitis C**, a virus that causes **hepatitis, cirrhosis,** and hepatocellular carcinoma, is another human virus that encodes for a **reverse transcriptase.**

3. Reverse transcriptase also may play a role in normal development.

III. SYNTHESIS OF RNA (TRANSCRIPTION)

A. **RNA polymerase**
   1. RNA polymerase can **initiate** the synthesis of new chains. A primer is not required.
   2. The DNA template is copied in the 3' to 5' direction, and the RNA chain grows in the 5' to 3' direction.
   3. **Ribonucleoside triphosphates** (adenosine triphosphate [ATP], GTP, uridine triphosphate [UTP], and cytidine triphosphate [CTP]) serve as the precursors for the RNA chain. The process is similar to that for DNA synthesis (Figure 17-12).

B. **Synthesis of RNA in bacteria**
   1. The RNA polymerase of *E. coli* contains **four subunits:** $\alpha_2\beta\beta'$, which form the core enzyme; and a fifth subunit, the sigma factor (σ), which is required for initiation of RNA synthesis.

Rifampin is a bactericidal antibiotic that **inhibits the β subunit of bacterial DNA-dependent RNA polymerase.** It is used in the treatment of **tuberculosis** or as prophylaxis against some forms of bacterial meningitis.

   2. Genes contain a **promoter region** to which RNA polymerase binds.
      a. Promoters contain the consensus sequence **TATAAT** (called the *Pribnow* or *TATA box*) about 10 bases upstream from (before) the start point of transcription.
      b. A **consensus sequence** consists of the most commonly found sequence of bases in a given region of all DNAs tested.
      c. A **second consensus sequence (TTGACA)** is usually located upstream from the Pribnow box, about 35 nucleotides (-35) from the start point of transcription.
   3. When RNA polymerase binds to a **promoter,** local unwinding of the DNA helix occurs, so that the DNA strands partially separate. The polymerase then begins transcription, copying the template strand.
      a. As the polymerase moves along the DNA, the next region of the double helix unwinds, and the single-stranded region that has already been transcribed rejoins its partner.

Actinomycin D is an antibiotic-type compound that binds to DNA and **inhibits the elongation of RNA transcription by RNA polymerase.** Although highly toxic, it is used in the treatment of **some pediatric cancers** like neuroblastoma, Wilms tumor, and sarcomas.

      b. Termination occurs in a region in which the transcript forms a hairpin loop that precedes four U residues.
      c. The ρ (rho) factor aids in the termination of some transcripts.
   4. **mRNA** is often produced as a **polycistronic transcript** that is translated as it is being transcribed.
      a. A polycistronic mRNA produces several different proteins during translation, one from each cistron.
      b. *E. coli* mRNA has a short half-life. It is degraded in minutes.

5. rRNA is produced as a **large transcript** that is cleaved, producing the 16S rRNA that appears in the 30S ribosomal subunit.

   a. The 23S and 5S rRNAs appear in the 50S ribosomal subunit.

   b. The 30S and 50S ribosomal subunits combine to form the 70S ribosome.

6. tRNA usually is produced from **larger transcripts** that are cleaved. One of the cleavage enzymes, RNase P, contains an RNA molecule that acts as a catalyst.

C. Synthesis of RNA in nuclei of eukaryotes

1. mRNA synthesis (Figure 17-15)

   a. Eukaryotic genes that produce mRNA contain a **basal promoter** region. This region binds transcription factors, which are proteins that bind RNA polymerase II. Promoters contain a number of conserved sequences.

   (1) A **TATA** (Hogness) **box,** containing the consensus sequence TATATAA, is located about 25 base pairs upstream (−25) from the transcription start site.

   (2) A **CAAT box** is frequently found about 70 base pairs upstream from the start site.

   (3) GC-rich regions (GC boxes) often occur between −40 and −110 base pairs upstream from the start site.

   b. Enhancers are DNA sequences that function in the **stimulation** of the transcription rate.

   (1) Enhancers can be located thousands of base pairs upstream or downstream from the start site.

   (2) Other sequences called **silencers** function in the **inhibition** of transcription.

   c. RNA polymerase II initially produces a large primary transcript called **heterogeneous nuclear RNA (hnRNA),** which contains exons and introns.

CLINICAL CORRELATES α-Amanitin is a cellular toxin that binds and inhibits **RNA polymerase II,** thereby halting **mRNA synthesis** and ultimately protein synthesis. Ingestion of *Amanita phalloides* mushroom (death cap), which produces the toxin, results in severe gastrointestinal symptoms, **liver toxicity,** and, potentially, death.

   (1) Exons are sequences within a transcript that appear in the mature **mRNA.**

   (2) Introns are sequences within the primary transcript that are **removed** and do not appear in the mature mRNA.

   d. Processing of hnRNA yields mature mRNA, which enters the cytoplasm through nuclear pores (Figure 17-16).

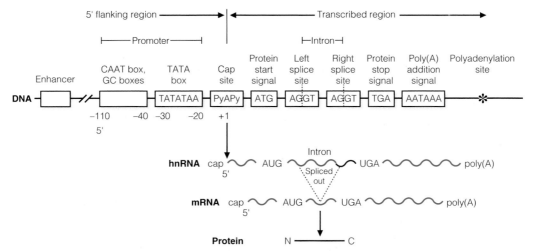

FIGURE 17-15 The structure of a eukaryotic gene and its products. As is customary, DNA sequences are given for the nontemplate strand. The DNA template strand, of course, is present. Its sequence is complementary and antiparallel to that of the nontemplate strand. The sequence of the RNA transcript is identical to that of the corresponding region of the nontemplate strand of the DNA, except that, in RNA, U replaces T. hnRNA, heterogeneous nuclear RNA; mRNA, messenger RNA; Py, pyrimidine.

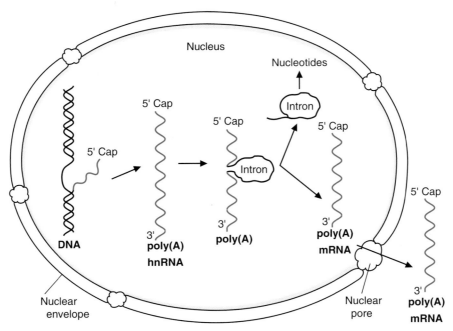

FIGURE 17-16 Synthesis of messenger RNA (mRNA) in eukaryotes. hnRNA, heterogeneous nuclear RNA.

(1) The **primary transcript** (hnRNA) is capped at its 5′ end as it is being transcribed.

(2) A **poly(A) tail,** 20 to 200 nucleotides in length, is added to the 3′ end of the transcript.

(3) The sequence AAUAAA in hnRNA serves as a signal for cleavage of the hnRNA and addition of the poly(A) tail by poly(A) polymerase. ATP serves as the precursor.

(4) **Splicing** reactions remove introns and connect the exons.

- The **splice point** at the **left** flank of an intron usually has the sequence AG followed by an **invariant GU.** At the **right** flank, an **invariant AG** is frequently followed by GU (Figure 17-15).
- Small nuclear RNAs complexed with protein (**snRNPs**) (e.g., U1 and U2) are involved in the cleavage and splicing process. A **lariat** structure is generated during the splicing reaction (Figure 17-16).

(5) Some hnRNAs contain 50 or more exons that must be spliced correctly to produce functional mRNA. Other hnRNAs have no introns.

2. **rRNA synthesis and assembly of ribosomes** (Figure 17-17)

a. A **45S precursor** is produced by RNA polymerase I from rRNA genes located in the fibrous region of the nucleolus. Many copies of the genes are present, linked together by spacer regions.

b. The **45S** precursor is modified by methylation and undergoes a number of cleavages that ultimately produce 18S rRNA and 28S rRNA; the latter is hydrogen-bonded to a 5.8S rRNA.

c. **18S rRNA** complexes with proteins and forms the 40S ribosomal subunit.

d. The **28S, 5.8S,** and **5S rRNAs** complex with proteins and form the 60S ribosomal subunit. 5S rRNA is produced by RNA polymerase III outside of the nucleolus.

e. The **ribosomal subunits** migrate through the nuclear pores into the cytoplasm where they complex with mRNA, forming 80S ribosomes. (Because sedimentation coefficients reflect both shape and particle weight, they are not additive.)

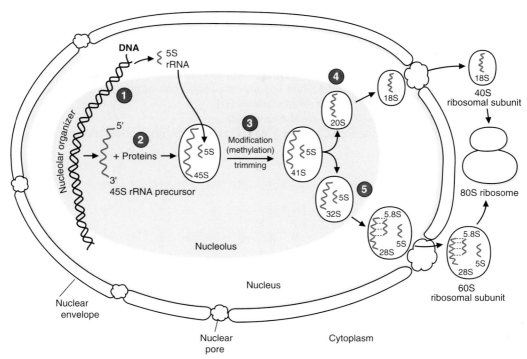

FIGURE 17-17 Synthesis of ribosomal RNA (rRNA) and assembly of ribosomes.

    f. rRNA precursors can contain introns that are removed during maturation. In some organisms, the enzymatic activity that removes rRNA introns resides in the rRNA precursor. No proteins are required. These autocatalytic RNAs are an example of **ribozymes,** RNA molecules that can catalyze reactions.

3. tRNA synthesis (Figure 17-18)

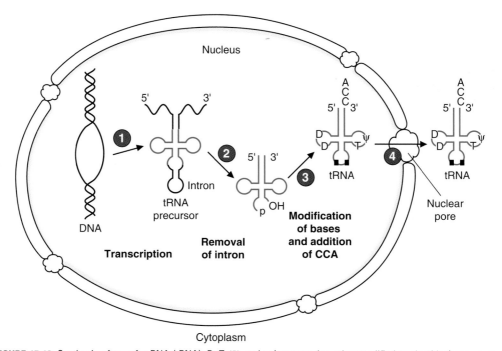

FIGURE 17-18 Synthesis of transfer RNA (tRNA). D, T, Ψ, and ■ (representing other modified nucleotides) are unusual nucleotides produced by post-transcriptional modifications.

    a. **RNA polymerase III** is the enzyme that produces tRNA. The promoter is located within the coding region of the gene.

    b. **Primary transcripts** for tRNA are cleaved at the 5′ and 3′ ends.

    c. Some precursors contain **introns** that are removed.

    d. During processing of tRNA precursors, **nucleotides are modified.**

        (1) Post-transcriptional modification includes the conversion of uridine to pseudouridine (Ψ), ribothymidine (T), and dihydrouridine (D).

        (2) Other unusual nucleotides are also produced.

    e. Addition of the sequence **CCA** to the **3′ end** is catalyzed by nucleotidyl transferase.

Review Test

Directions: Each of the numbered questions or incomplete statements in this section is followed by answers or by completions of the statement. Select the **one** lettered answer or completion that is **best** in each case.

1. A 23-year-old man presents to his family physician with a painless swelling of his testicles. An ultrasound is suspicious for a neoplasm, and a biopsy confirms the presence of cancer. He is referred to an oncologist, who begins treatment with the topoisomerase inhibitor etoposide. The normal function of this enzyme is to do which of the following?

(A) Repair nuclear DNA in the event of DNA damage
(B) Unwind the DNA helix during replication
(C) Break and rejoin the DNA helix during replication
(D) Prevent the single strands of DNA from reannealing during replication
(E) Synthesize RNA primers for DNA polymerase

2. A 33-year-old homosexual man is recently diagnosed with HIV. His CD4$^+$ T-cell count is dramatically decreased, and he has a high HIV viral load. He is referred to an infectious disease clinic where they begin him on a nucleoside analog. Certain nucleoside analogs inhibit DNA synthesis because they lack which of the following properties required for normal DNA polymerization?

(A) A 5′-phosphate
(B) A 3′-hydroxyl
(C) A 7-methyl G modification
(D) A poly(A) tail
(E) A consensus sequence

3. A 53-year-old man is referred to a neurologist because he is beginning to develop spastic-like movements in his lower limbs. Magnetic resonance imaging of the head shows loss of mass in the caudate nucleus, and a presumptive diagnosis of Huntington disease is made. The genetic basis of this disease is best described as which of the following?

(A) Triple repeat expansion
(B) Nucleotide deletion
(C) Point mutation

(D) Transposition of genetic material
(E) DNA methylation

4. A 37-year-old immigrant from Thailand develops fevers, night sweats, weight loss, and a blood-tinged cough. He present to the emergency room, where an infectious disease doctor is consulted and immediately prescribes a multidrug regimen that includes rifampin. Rifampin inhibits which one of the following types of enzymes?

(A) DNA-dependent DNA polymerase
(B) DNA-dependent RNA polymerase
(C) RNA-dependent DNA polymerase
(D) RNA-dependent RNA polymerase
(E) Reverse transcriptase

5. Two couples present to the emergency room with severe nausea, vomiting, and diarrhea. One of the patients admits that she had a dinner party and served a salad containing mushrooms she had picked during a hike in the forest earlier that day. Inhibition of which enzyme or process explains the clinical manifestations of α-amanitin poisoning seen in these patients?

(A) RNA polymerase II
(B) RNA polymerase I
(C) RNA splicing
(D) RNA polyadenylation
(E) RNA polymerase III

6. A 23-year-old diabetic woman reports having fevers and dysuria. Physical examination reveals costovertebral tenderness, and her urinary analysis shows the presence of bacteria in her urine. Her physician suspects a complicated urinary tract infection and begins a 5-day course of ciprofloxacin. Such quinolone antibiotics inhibit which one of the following enzymes?

(A) Eukaryotic topoisomerase
(B) Helicase
(C) Primase
(D) Gyrase
(E) Poly(A) polymerase

7. A 4-year-old child is referred by the pediatrician to a pediatric neurologist after presenting with myoclonic seizures and lactic acidosis. The neurologist orders a muscle biopsy, and the pathology returns with the appearance of "ragged red fibers." The parents are informed that the child has MERFF syndrome, a mitochondrial DNA (mtDNA) disorder. Which of the following statements best explains mtDNA?

(A) It is inherited equally from both parents.
(B) It is replicated with increased fidelity with respect to nuclear DNA.
(C) It shares the same genetic code as nuclear DNA.
(D) It is a double-stranded circular DNA.
(E) It encodes all the proteins necessary for the electron transport chain.

8. A 34-year-old man of Italian descent is seen for a yearly physical examination. He has no complaints and is in good health. However, he does relay a family history of anemia, and a complete blood count demonstrates a mild anemia; the physician suspects thalassemia minor in the patient. Thalassemia is often due to an alteration in RNA splicing, which is an essential part of mRNA processing in eukaryotes. Which of the following is a correct statement concerning mRNA processing?

(A) Poly(A) RNA is the initial transcript produced, which is subsequently spliced to mRNA.
(B) The coding region of the gene is found within introns.
(C) The coding regions of the gene are found within exons.
(D) All human genes require splicing of introns.

(E) The 5' end of the intron contains the nucleotides AG followed by an invariant GU.

9. A 4-year-old child, on a well-child checkup, is found to have a large flank mass. Computed tomography demonstrates a large mass arising from the kidney, and a subsequent biopsy reveals a diagnosis of Wilms tumor. A pediatric oncologist starts chemotherapy including the transcription inhibitor actinomycin D. Which of the following statements is correct regarding transcription regulation in bacteria?

(A) All mRNAs are monocistronic.
(B) RNA polymerase requires a primer.
(C) The RNA chain grows in the 3' to 5' direction.
(D) Rho factor is critical for initiation of RNA synthesis.
(E) The TATA box contains a consensus sequence for the binding of RNA polymerase.

10. A second-year medical student is working in a laboratory studying gene regulation in a mouse model of hepatocellular carcinoma. He isolates nucleic acids from the cells after exposure to a known carcinogen and has the sequences analyzed. He is surprised to find that some of the nucleotides are pseudouridine and ribothymidine. Which type of nucleic acid has the student likely isolated?

(A) tRNA
(B) rRNA
(C) hnRNA
(D) mRNA
(E) snRNP

Answers and Explanations

1. **The answer is C.** Topoisomerase creates double-stranded breaks ahead of the replication fork to relieve the supercoiling induced by the action of helicase, which unwinds the DNA helix during replication. DNA polymerase and ligase, along with specific endonucleases, are important in repairing DNA damage. Single-stranded binding proteins prevent the separated strands from reannealing during replication. Primase is required to synthesize primers for DNA replication by DNA polymerase.

2. **The answer is B.** DNA polymerase requires a free $3'$-hydroxyl group on the deoxyribonucleotide, which acts as a nucleophile to attack the $5'$-α-phosphate of the incoming nucleotide, which forms the phosphodiester bond. Nucleoside analogs inhibit polymerization because they lack the $3'$ OH for chain elongation. A 7-methyl G modification and a poly(A) tail are added to eukaryotic mRNA to stabilize the transcript, and are not found in nucleoside analogs. A consensus sequence is a DNA sequence that is found at the promoter region of genes and functions to bind various factors that regulate the transcription of the gene.

3. **The answer is A.** Huntington disease is a neurodegenerative disorder that results from a triplet repeat expansion (CAG) within the Huntington gene. The most common mutation leading to cystic fibrosis is an example of a deletion ($\Delta 508$, a loss of three nucleotides). Point mutations may cause disease when they occur either in coding or noncoding regions, such as the point mutation in the α_1-antitrypsin coding sequence or mutations in introns of certain types of β-thalassemia. Transposition is a phenomenon of transposons moving about the genome, but they are not responsible for Huntington disease. DNA methylation leads to the genetic phenomena of imprinting.

4. **The answer is B.** Rifampin is an important agent in a multidrug regimen for tuberculosis and works by inhibiting the β subunit of the bacterial DNA-dependent RNA polymerase (RNA polymerase). A DNA-dependent DNA polymerase, such as bacterial Pol III, directs DNA replication, whereas bacterial Pol I is involved with DNA repair and lagging strand DNA synthesis. An example of a RNA-dependent DNA polymerase is reverse transcriptase, found in retroviruses. Only certain RNA viruses, such as poliovirus, code for RNA-dependent RNA polymerases.

5. **The answer is A.** The cellular toxin α-amanitin from the *Amanita phalloides* mushroom (death cap mushroom) specifically inhibits RNA polymerase II, the enzyme required for mRNA synthesis. Loss of transcriptional activity results in severe gastrointestinal symptoms, liver toxicity, and sometimes death. Eukaryotic RNA polymerase I is responsible for the synthesis of rRNA, whereas RNA polymerase III produces tRNA. Small ribonucleoproteins are required for RNA splicing. RNA poly(A) polymerase normally adds stretches of adenine residues to the $3'$ end of mRNA. The only enzyme inhibited by α-amanitin is RNA polymerase II.

6. **The answer is D.** Quinolone antibiotics inhibit DNA gyrase, a prokaryotic topoisomerase, and are important drugs in the treatment of urinary tract infections. Ciprofloxacin in particular has high urinary excretion and is effective against urinary tract infections (although resistance to the drug is becoming more common). Eukaryotic topoisomerase inhibitors include etoposide, which is used in the treatment of some cancers. There are no current drugs regimens that target helicase, which unwinds DNA during replication, or primase, which creates the RNA primers during DNA replication, or poly(A) polymerase.

7. **The answer is D.** Mitochondrial DNA is a small double-stranded circular DNA. It is inherited exclusively from the mother because the ovum contributes the cytoplasm to the zygote, which contains all the mitochondria for the zygote. The mitochondrial DNA replication machinery is less evolved than nuclear DNA and replicates with an error rate that is 5 to 10 times greater than that of the nuclear genome. The genetic code within mitochondria is slightly different than that

of the nuclear genome. Finally, mitochondrial DNA encodes only 13 of the numerous subunits of the electron transport chain. The others are encoded by the nuclear genome.

8. **The answer is C.** The coding regions of genes are located within exons. Most, *but not all,* human genes contain introns, which are spliced out. The splice point at the 5′ end of an intron usually has the sequence GU (the 3′ end of the exon adjacent to this intron has an invariant AG). At the 3′ end, an invariant AG is frequently followed by GU, which are the first two nucleotides at the 5′ end of the next exon. Poly(A) RNA is added post-transcriptionally to a mRNA transcript, at the 3′ end, before export from the nucleus.

9. **The answer is E.** RNA polymerase binds to specific consensus sequences on DNA, with the TATA box being an example of such a sequence. The TATA box is also called the *Hogness box* in eukaryotic cells and the *Pribnow box* in prokaryotes. Prokaryotic cells produce both monocistronic and polycistronic mRNA, whereas eukaryotic cells only produce monocistronic mRNA. RNA polymerase, unlike DNA polymerase, does not require a primer. RNA polymerase synthesizes RNA in the 5′ to 3′ direction, reading the DNA template in the 3′ to 5′ direction. The rho factor (ρ) is critical for rho-dependent termination, whereas the sigma factor (σ) aids in bacterial transcriptional initiation.

10. **The answer is A.** tRNAs often contain post-transcriptionally modified bases, including the conversion of uridine to pseudouridine and ribothymidine. rRNAs are found within ribosomes and do not contain these modified bases. snRNPs (small nuclear RNAs complexed with protein) are involved in splicing and also lack ribothymidine and pseudouridine. hnRNA is processed to produce mRNA, which also lacks these modified bases.

18 RNA Translation and Protein Synthesis

I. PROTEIN SYNTHESIS (TRANSLATION OF MESSENGER RNA)

A. The genetic code (Table 18-1)

1. The **genetic code** is the collection of codons that specify all the amino acids found in proteins.

2. A **codon is a sequence of 3 bases** (triplet) in messenger RNA (mRNA) (5′ to 3′) that specifies (corresponds to) a particular amino acid. During translation, the successive codons in an mRNA determine the sequence in which amino acids add to the growing polypeptide chain.

3. The **genetic code is degenerate** (redundant). Each of the 20 common amino acids has at least one codon; many amino acids have numerous codons.

4. The genetic code is **non-overlapping** (i.e., each nucleotide is used only once).
   a. It begins with a start codon (**AUG**) near the 5′ end of the mRNA.
   b. It ends with a termination (stop) codon (**UGA, UAG,** or **UAA**) near the 3′ end.

5. The code is **commaless** (i.e., there are no breaks or markers to distinguish one codon from the next).

6. The code is **nearly universal**. The same codon specifies the same amino acid in almost all species studied; however, some differences have been found in the codons used in mitochondria.

7. The **start codon** (AUG) determines the **reading frame**. Subsequent nucleotides are read in sets of three, sequentially following this codon.

B. Effect of mutations on proteins

1. Mutations in DNA are transcribed into mRNA and thus can cause changes in the encoded protein.

2. The various types of mutations that occur in DNA have different effects on the encoded protein.

3. **Point mutations** occur when 1 base in DNA is replaced by another, altering the codon in mRNA.
   a. **Silent mutations** do not affect the amino acid sequence of a protein (e.g., CGA to CGG causes no change because both codons specify arginine).
   b. **Missense mutations** result in one amino acid being replaced by another (e.g., CGA to CCA causes arginine to be replaced by proline).

CLINICAL CORRELATES Hereditary hemochromatosis (HH) is one of the most common genetic diseases. It is associated with two well-known **missense mutations** in the *HFE* gene, namely the **C282Y** mutation, a substitution of tyrosine for cysteine at amino acid 282, and the **H63D** mutation, with a substitution of aspartic acid for histidine at position 63. These **mutations are used to screen** "at-risk populations" for this **disorder of iron metabolism**, which results in **cirrhosis, diabetes, skin pigmentation**, and **heart failure**.

---

   c. **Nonsense mutations** result in premature termination of the growing polypeptide chain (e.g., CGA to UGA causes arginine to be replaced by a stop codon).

t a b l e **18-1** The Genetic Code					
First Base	**Second Base**				**Third Base**
(5')	*U*	*C*	*A*	*G*	(3')
U	Phe	Ser	Tyr	Cys	U
	Phe	Ser	Tyr	Cys	C
	Leu	Ser	Term	Term	A
	Leu	Ser	Term	Trp	G
C	Leu	Pro	His	Arg	U
	Leu	Pro	His	Arg	C
	Leu	Pro	Gln	Arg	A
	Leu	Pro	Gln	Arg	G
A	Ile	Thr	Asn	Ser	U
	Ile	Thr	Asn	Ser	C
	Ile	Thr	Lys	Arg	A
	Met	Thr	Lys	Arg	G
G	Val	Ala	Asp	Gly	U
	Val	Ala	Asp	Gly	C
	Val	Ala	Glu	Gly	A
	Val	Ala	Glu	Gly	G

4. **Insertions** occur when a base or a number of bases are added to DNA. They can result in a protein with more or fewer amino acids than normal.
5. **Deletions** occur when a base or a number of bases are removed from DNA. They can result in a protein with fewer or more amino acids than normal.
6. **Frameshift mutations** occur when the number of bases added or deleted is not a multiple of three. The reading frame is shifted so that completely different sets of codons are read beyond the point at which the mutation starts.

C. **Formation of aminoacyl-transfer RNAs (tRNAs)** (Figure 18-1)
   1. **Amino acids are activated and attached to** their corresponding **tRNAs** by highly specific enzymes known as aminoacyl-tRNA synthetases.
   2. Each **aminoacyl-tRNA synthetase** recognizes a particular amino acid and the tRNAs specific for that amino acid.

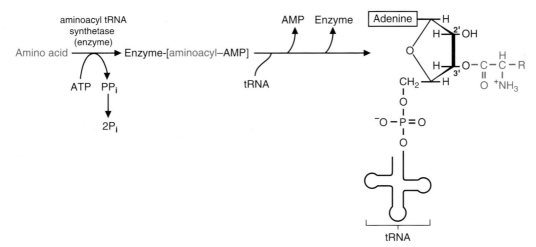

FIGURE 18-1 Formation of aminoacyl-transfer RNA (tRNA). AMP, adenosine monophosphate; ATP, adenosine triphosphate; PP_i, inorganic pyrophosphate.

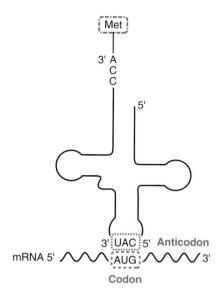

FIGURE 18-2 Antiparallel binding of aminoacyl-transfer RNA to messenger RNA (mRNA).

3. An **amino acid first** reacts with adenosine triphosphate (ATP), forming an activated amino acid (aminoacyl-adenosine monophosphate [AMP]) and pyrophosphate, which is cleaved to two inorganic phosphates (P_i).

4. The **aminoacyl-AMP** then **forms an ester** with the 2′- or 3′-hydroxyl of a tRNA specific for that amino acid, producing an aminoacyl-tRNA and AMP.

5. Once an amino acid is attached to a tRNA, insertion of the amino acid into a growing polypeptide chain depends on the codon–anticodon interaction (Figure 18-2).

D. **Initiation of translation** (Figure 18-3)

1. **In eukaryotes, methionyl-tRNA$_i$^{Met}** binds to the small **ribosomal subunit**.

a. The **5′ cap** of the mRNA binds to the small subunit, and the first AUG codon base pairs with the anticodon on the methionyl-tRNA$_i$^{Met}.

b. The methionine that initiates protein synthesis is subsequently removed from the N terminus of the polypeptide.

c. **In bacteria**, the methionine that initiates protein synthesis is **formylated** and is carried by tRNA$_f$^{Met}.

CLINICAL CORRELATES   Tetracyclines are a class of antibiotics that bind to the **30S ribosomal subunit**, thereby blocking the access of the aminoacyl-tRNA to the mRNA–ribosomal complex.

CLINICAL CORRELATES   Aminoglycosides, such as gentamicin, are a class of antibiotics that bind to the 30S ribosomal subunit, thus interfering with the assembly of the functional ribosomal apparatus.

---

d. **Prokaryotes do not contain a 5′ cap** on their mRNA. An mRNA sequence upstream from the translation start site (the Shine-Dalgarno sequence) binds to the 3′ end of 16S ribosomal RNA (rRNA) to position the small ribosomal subunit on the mRNA.

2. The **large ribosomal subunit binds**, completing the initiation complex.

a. The methionyl-tRNA$_i$^{Met} is bound at the **P (peptidyl) site** of the complex.

b. The **A (acceptor or aminoacyl) site** of the complex is unoccupied.

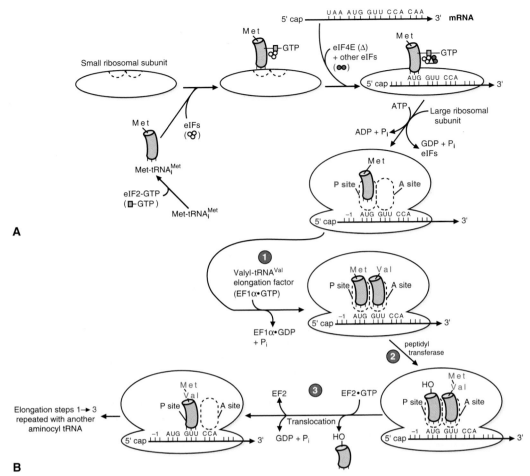

FIGURE 18-3 The initiation **(A)** and elongation **(B)** reactions of protein synthesis. eIFs are initiation factors in eukaryotes (IFs in prokaryotes). EF-1 and EF-2 are eukaryotic elongation factors corresponding with EF-Tu and EF-G in prokaryotes. A site, aminoacyl site; P site, peptidyl site. ADP, adenosine diphosphate; ATP, adenosine triphosphate; GDP, guanosine diphosphate; GTP, guanosine triphosphate; P_i, inorganic phosphate; tRNA, transfer RNA.

CLINICAL CORRELATES   Both **erythromycin** and **clindamycin** are antibiotics that inhibit protein synthesis as they **bind the 50S ribosomal subunit** of bacteria. This results in inhibition of translocation of the growing peptide.

---

   3. Initiation factors (IFs), ATP, and guanosine triphosphate (GTP) are required for formation of the initiation complex.
      a. The **initiation factors** are designated IF-1, IF-2, and IF-3 in prokaryotes. In eukaryotes, they are designated eIF-1, eIF-2, and so on. Seven or more may be present.
      b. Release of the initiation factors involves hydrolysis of GTP to guanosine diphosphate (GDP) and P_i.

E. Elongation of polypeptide chains (Figure 18-3B)
   1. The addition of each amino acid to the growing polypeptide chain involves binding of an aminoacyl-tRNA at the A site, formation of a peptide bond, and translocation of the peptidyl-tRNA to the P site.

2. **Binding of aminoacyl-tRNA to the A site** (Step 1, Figure 18-3B)
   a. The **mRNA codon** at the A site determines which aminoacyl-tRNA will bind.

CLINICAL CORRELATES   The antibiotic **puromycin** is an analog of **aminoacyl-tRNA**. It inhibits both prokaryotic as well as eukaryotic **translation** as it acts as a chain terminator in protein synthesis.

---

   (1) The codon and the anticodon bind by base pairing that is antiparallel (Figure 18-2).
   (2) Internal methionine residues in the polypeptide chain are added in response to AUG codons. They are carried by $tRNA_m^{Met}$, a second tRNA specific for methionine.
   b. An **elongation factor** (EF) (EF-Tu in prokaryotes and EF-1 in eukaryotes) and hydrolysis of GTP are required for binding.
3. **Formation of a peptide bond** (Step 2, Figure 18-3B)
   a. A peptide bond forms between the amino group of the aminoacyl-tRNA at the **A site** and the carbonyl of the aminoacyl group attached to the tRNA at the **P site**. Formation of the peptide bond is catalyzed by **peptidyl transferase**, which is rRNA.

CLINICAL CORRELATES   **Chloramphenicol**, an antibiotic rarely used because of the potential to develop decreased white blood cells, **inhibits peptidyltransferase**, thus halting protein synthesis.

---

   b. The tRNA at the P site now does not contain an amino acid. It is "uncharged."
   c. The growing polypeptide chain is attached to the tRNA in the A site.
4. **Translocation of peptidyl-tRNA** (Step 3, Figure 18-3B)
   a. The peptidyl-tRNA (along with the attached mRNA) moves from the A site to the P site, and the uncharged tRNA is released from the ribosome. An **elongation factor** (EF-2 in eukaryotes or EF-G in prokaryotes) and the hydrolysis of **GTP** are required for translocation.

CLINICAL CORRELATES   **Diphtheria toxin** is produced from phage genes incorporated into the bacterium *Corynebacterium diphtheriae*. The toxin causes diphtheria, a lethal disease of the respiratory tract. The A fragment of the toxin catalyzes the adenosine diphosphate **(ADP)-ribosylation** of **EF-2**, thus inhibiting translocation in eukaryotes.

---

   b. The next codon in the mRNA is now in the A site.
   c. The elongation and translocation steps are repeated until a termination codon moves into the A site.

F. **Termination of translation**
   1. When a termination codon (UGA, UAG, or UAA) occupies the A site, release factors cause the newly synthesized polypeptide to be released from the ribosome.
   2. The ribosomal subunits dissociate from the mRNA.

G. **Polysomes** (Figure 18-4)
   1. More than one ribosome can be attached to a single mRNA at any given time. The complex of mRNA with multiple ribosomes is known as a **polysome**.
   2. Each ribosome carries a nascent polypeptide chain that grows longer as the ribosome approaches the 3′ end of the mRNA.

H. **Post-translational processing**
   ● After synthesis is completed, **proteins can be modified** by phosphorylation, glycosylation, ADP-ribosylation, hydroxylation, and addition of other groups.

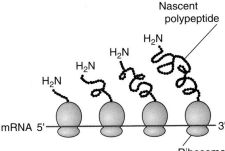

FIGURE 18-4 A polysome. mRNA, messenger RNA.

I. **Synthesis and release of secretory proteins**
  1. **Secretory proteins**, destined for release from the cell, are synthesized on ribosomes attached to the **rough endoplasmic reticulum (RER)** in eukaryotic cells.
  2. A **hydrophobic signal sequence** at the N terminus of a secretory protein causes the nascent protein to pass into the lumen of the RER. The signal sequence is cleaved from the N terminus, and the protein may be glycosylated within the RER.
  3. The protein travels in vesicles to the **Golgi**, where it may be glycosylated further and is packaged in secretory vesicles.
  4. **Secretory vesicles** containing the protein travel from the Golgi to the cell membrane. The protein is released from the cell by **exocytosis**.

II. REGULATION OF PROTEIN SYNTHESIS

A. **Regulation of protein synthesis in prokaryotes**
  1. **Relationship of protein synthesis to nutrient supply**
     a. **Prokaryotes** respond to changes in their supply of nutrients in a way that allows them to obtain or conserve energy most efficiently.
        (1) Prokaryotes, such as *Escherichia coli*, require a source of **carbon**, which is usually a sugar that is oxidized for energy.
        (2) A source of **nitrogen** is also required for the synthesis of amino acids from which structural proteins and enzymes are produced.
     b. *E. coli* uses **glucose** preferentially whenever it is available. The enzymes in the pathways for glucose utilization are made **constitutively** (i.e., they are constantly being produced).
     c. **If glucose is not present** in the medium but another sugar is available, *E. coli* produces the enzymes and other proteins that allow the cell to derive energy from that sugar. The process by which synthesis of the enzymes is regulated is called **induction**.
     d. **If an amino acid is present in the medium**, *E. coli* does not need to synthesize that amino acid and conserves energy by ceasing to produce the enzymes required for its synthesis. The process by which synthesis of these enzymes is regulated is called **repression**.
  2. **Operons**
     a. An operon is a **set of genes** that are **adjacent** to one another in the genome and are coordinately controlled; that is, the genes are either all turned on or all turned off (Figure 18-5).
     b. The **structural genes** of an operon **code** for a series of different proteins.
        (1) A single **polycistronic mRNA** is transcribed from an operon. This single mRNA codes for all the proteins of the operon.
        (2) A series of **start** and **stop codons** on the polycistronic mRNA allows a number of different proteins to be produced at the translational level from the single mRNA.
     c. Transcription begins near a **promoter region**, which is located upstream from the group of structural genes.

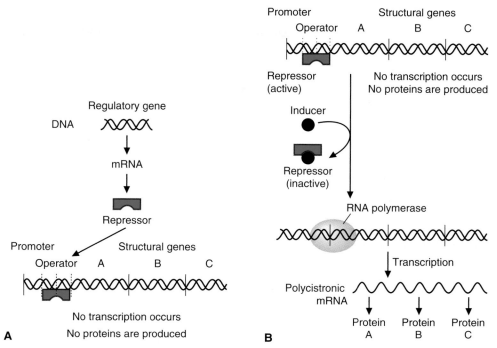

FIGURE 18-5 An inducible operon (e.g., the *lac* operon). **(A)** If the inducer is absent, the repressor is active and binds to the operator, preventing RNA polymerase from binding. Thus, transcription does not occur. **(B)** If the inducer is present, it binds to and inactivates the repressor, which then does not bind to the operator. Therefore, RNA polymerase can bind and transcribe the structural genes. mRNA, messenger RNA.

    d. Associated with the promoter is a short sequence, the **operator**, which determines whether or not the genes are expressed.

    e. **Binding of a repressor protein** to the operator region prevents binding of RNA polymerase to the promoter and **inhibits transcription** of the structural genes of the operon.

    f. Repressor proteins are encoded by regulatory genes, which may be located anywhere in the genome.

3. Induction (Figure 18-5B)

    a. Induction is the process whereby an **inducer** (a small molecule) stimulates transcription of an operon.

    b. The inducer is frequently a sugar (or a metabolite of the sugar), and the proteins produced from the inducible operon allow the sugar to be metabolized.

        (1) The inducer binds to the **repressor**, inactivating it.

        (2) The inactive repressor does not bind to the operator.

        (3) **RNA polymerase**, therefore, can **bind** to the promoter and **transcribe** the operon.

        (4) The structural **proteins** encoded by the operon are **produced**.

    c. The **lactose (*lac*) operon** is **inducible**.

        (1) A metabolite of lactose, **allolactose**, is the inducer.

        (2) Proteins produced by the genes of the *lac* operon allow the cell to oxidize lactose as a source of energy. Gene Z produces a **β-galactosidase;** gene Y, a lactose permease; and gene A, a transacetylase.

        (3) The *lac* operon is induced only in the **absence of glucose**. It exhibits **catabolite repression** (see section II.A.6 below).

4. Repression

    a. Repression is the process whereby a **co-repressor** (a small molecule) **inhibits transcription** of an operon.

    b. The **co-repressor** is usually an amino acid, and the proteins produced from the repressible operon are involved in the synthesis of the amino acid.

    (1) The co-repressor binds to the repressor, activating it.

    (2) The active repressor binds to the operator.

    (3) **RNA polymerase**, therefore, cannot bind to the promoter, and the operon is not transcribed.

    (4) The cell stops producing the structural proteins encoded by the operon.

  c. The **tryptophan (*trp*) operon** is **repressible**.

    (1) **Tryptophan** is the corepressor.

    (2) The proteins encoded by the *trp* operon are involved in the synthesis of tryptophan.

    (3) The *trp* operon is repressed in the presence of tryptophan because cells do not need to make the amino acid if it is present in the growth medium.

5. Positive control

  a. Some operons are turned on by mechanisms that **activate transcription**.

  b. When the repressor of the arabinose (*ara*) operon binds arabinose, it changes conformation and becomes an activator that stimulates binding of RNA polymerase to the promoter. The operon is then transcribed, and the proteins required for oxidation of arabinose are produced.

6. Catabolite repression (Figure 18-6)

  a. Cells preferentially use **glucose** when it is available.

A. In the presence of lactose and glucose

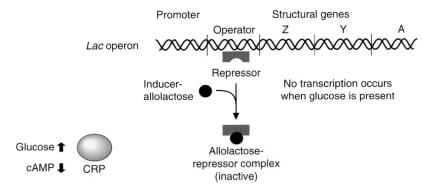

B. In the presence of lactose and absence of glucose

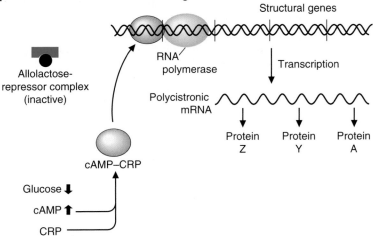

FIGURE 18-6 Catabolite repression. The operon is transcribed only when glucose is low. Cyclic adenosine monophosphate (cAMP) is elevated, and the inducer binds to the repressor, inactivating it. Under these conditions, the cAMP–cyclic receptor protein (CRP) complex forms and binds to the DNA, facilitating the initiation of transcription by RNA polymerase. The *lac* operon exhibits catabolite repression. mRNA, messenger RNA.

b. Some operons (e.g., *lac* and *ara*) are not expressed when glucose is present in the medium. These operons require **cyclic adenosine monophosphate (cAMP)** for their expression
   (1) Glucose causes cAMP levels in the cells to decrease.
   (2) When glucose decreases, cAMP levels rise.
   (3) **cAMP** binds to the catabolite-activator protein (**CAP or CRP**).
   (4) The **cAMP–CAP complex** binds to a site near the **promoter** of the operon and facilitates binding of RNA polymerase to the promoter.

c. The *lac* **operon** exhibits **catabolite repression**.
   (1) In the **presence of lactose** and the **absence of glucose**, the *lac* repressor is inactivated, and the high levels of cAMP facilitate binding of RNA polymerase to the promoter.
   (2) The **operon is transcribed**, and the proteins that allow the cells to utilize lactose are produced.

7. Attenuation
   a. In bacterial cells, **transcription and translation occur simultaneously**.
   b. Attenuation occurs by a mechanism by which **rapid translation** of the nascent transcript causes **termination of transcription**.
   c. As the transcript is being produced, if ribosomes attach and **rapidly translate** the transcript, a secondary structure is generated in the mRNA that is a **termination signal** for RNA polymerase.
   d. If **translation is slow**, this termination structure does not form, and **transcription continues**.
      (1) Within operons that code for amino acid biosynthetic enzymes, multiple codons for the amino acid are located near the translation start site of the mRNA.
      (2) When cells contain low levels of the amino acid (which is produced by the enzymes encoded by the operon), less aminoacyl-tRNA is available to bind to these codons, and translation slows.
   e. The *trp* operon is regulated by attenuation.

8. Factors, such as sigma, affect RNA polymerase activity. These factors bind to the core RNA polymerase and increase its ability to bind to specific promoters.

B. Differences between eukaryotes and prokaryotes
   1. Eukaryotic cells undergo differentiation, and the organisms go through various developmental stages.
   2. Eukaryotes contain nuclei. Therefore, transcription is separated from translation. In prokaryotes, transcription and translation occur simultaneously.
   3. DNA is complexed with histones in eukaryotes, but not in prokaryotes.
   4. The **mammalian genome** contains about **1000 times more DNA** than *E. coli* (10^9 versus 10^6 base pairs).
   5. Most **mammalian** cells are **diploid**.
   6. The **major part of the genome** of mammalian cells **does not code for proteins**.
   7. Some eukaryotic genes, like most bacterial genes, **are unique** (i.e., they exist in one or a small number of copies per genome).
   8. Other eukaryotic genes, unlike bacterial genes, **have many copies** in the genome (e.g., genes for tRNA, rRNA, histones).
   9. Relatively **short, repetitive DNA sequences** are dispersed throughout the eukaryotic genome. They do not code for proteins (e.g., Alu sequences).
   10. Eukaryotic genes contain introns. Bacterial genes do not.
   11. Bacterial genes are organized in **operons** (sets that are under the control of a single promoter). **Each eukaryotic gene has its own promoter.**

C. Regulation of protein synthesis in eukaryotes
   1. Regulation can result from changes in genes or from mechanisms that affect transcription, processing, and transport of mRNA, mRNA translation, or mRNA stability.
   2. Changes in genes
      a. Genes can be lost (or partially lost) from cells, so that functional proteins can no longer be produced (e.g., during differentiation of red blood cells).

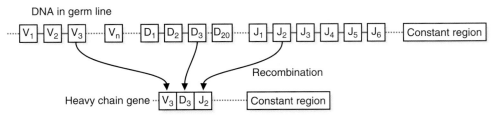

DNA in germ line

FIGURE 18-7 Rearrangement of DNA. Specific V, D, and J segments from among a large number of potential sequences in the DNA of precursor cells combine to form the heavy-chain gene from which lymphocytes produce immunoglobulins (antibodies).

b. Genes can be amplified.

> **CLINICAL CORRELATES**   Gene amplification is common in tumor cells. For instance, in one of the most common childhood solid tumors, **neuroblastoma**, patients have up to **300 copies** of the growth-promoting **N-*myc* gene**.

c. Segments of DNA can move from one location to another on the genome, associating with each other in various ways so that different proteins are produced.

> **CLINICAL CORRELATES**   Both **T and B lymphocytes undergo DNA rearrangements**, with loss of intervening DNA (Figure 18-7). Such rearrangements create a **single transcriptional unit** for the formation of a diverse repertoire of **antibodies and T-cell receptors** for a competent immune system.

    d. Modification of the **bases in DNA** affects the **transcriptional activity** of a gene.
        (1) Cytosine can be methylated at its 5 position.
        (2) The greater the extent of methylation, the less readily a gene is transcribed.
3. Regulation of the level of transcription
    a. Histones, which are small, basic proteins associated with the DNA of eukaryotes, act as nonspecific repressors.
    b. The **expression** of specific genes is stimulated by **positive** mechanisms.
    c. Inducers (e.g., steroid hormones) enter cells, bind to protein receptors, interact with chromatin in the nucleus, and **activate specific genes**.
    d. Some genes have **more than one promoter**. Thus, the promoter that is used can differ under different physiologic conditions or in different cell types.
4. Regulation during processing and transport of mRNA
    a. Regulatory mechanisms that occur during capping, polyadenylation, and splicing can alter the amino acid sequence or the quantity of the protein produced from the mRNA. Editing of mRNA also occurs, and the rate of degradation of mRNA is also regulated.
    b. Alternative splice sites can be used to produce different mRNAs.

> **CLINICAL CORRELATES**   The use of different splice sites results in the production of **calcitonin in the C cells of the thyroid** or, alternatively, in the brain, the neuropeptide **calcitonin gene–related peptide** (CGRP) (Figure 18-8).

    c. Alternative polyadenylation sites can be used to generate different mRNAs.

> **CLINICAL CORRELATES**   **Immunoglobulin M (IgM)** genes contain **two distinct polyadenylation sites**. One poly(A) site is at the 3′ end of the hydrophobic transmembrane region, found in IgM that is anchored to the cell surface. The second poly(A) site is at the 5′ end of the transmembrane region. Alternative splicing at this second poly(A) site results in a soluble **secreted IgM molecule**.

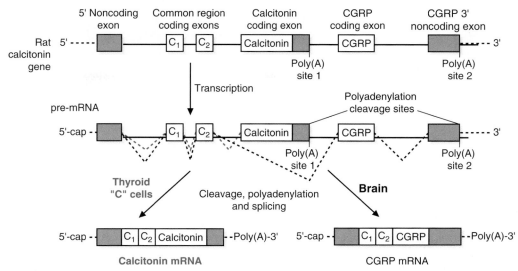

FIGURE 18-8 Alternative splicing of the calcitonin gene. In thyroid cells, heterogeneous nuclear RNA (hnRNA) transcribed from the calcitonin gene is processed to form the messenger RNA (mRNA) that produces calcitonin. In the brain, the same transcript of this gene is spliced differently. The first polyadenylation site is cleaved out, and a second polyadenylation site is used. The protein product is the calcitonin gene–related protein (CGRP).

    d. mRNAs can be degraded by nucleases after their synthesis in the nucleus and before their translation in the cytoplasm. Some mRNAs are degraded more rapidly than others.

    e. RNA editing involves the alteration ("editing") of bases in mRNA after transcription (Figure 18-9).

  5. Protein synthesis can be **regulated at the translational level**, during the initiation or elongation reactions.

CLINICAL CORRELATES Interferon-α, an antiviral cytokine, has several important functions to prevent the spread of viral infection. It stimulates the **synthesis of 2′,5′-oligo(A)**, which activates a nuclease that **degrades mRNA**. Additionally, it stimulates the **phosphorylation of eIF-2**, causing **inhibition of initiation**.

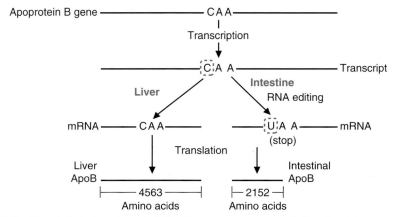

FIGURE 18-9 RNA editing. In liver, the apoprotein B (ApoB) gene produces a protein (Apo B100) that contains more than 4000 amino acids. It is the major apoprotein of very-low-density lipoprotein (VLDL). In intestinal cells, the same gene produces a protein that contains only 48% of this number of amino acids. This protein (Apo B48) is the major apoprotein of chylomicrons. "Editing" of mRNA (conversion of a C to a U) generates a stop codon in the intestinal messenger RNA (mRNA).

Review Test

Directions: Each of the numbered questions or incomplete statements in this section is followed by answers or by completions of the statement. Select the **one** lettered answer or completion that is **best** in each case.

1. A 14-year-old African American girl with sickle cell anemia presents with extreme pain in her chest and legs. A peripheral smear shows sickling of her red blood cells, and her reticulocyte count is 6.7%. She is diagnosed with an acute pain crisis secondary to microvascular occlusion from sickled erythrocytes. Sickle cell anemia is caused by a mutation that results in one amino acid being replaced by another, which results from which of the following?

(A) A missense point mutation
(B) A nonsense point mutation
(C) An insertion
(D) A deletion
(E) A frameshift mutation

2. A 53-year-old man sees his family physician with concerns that his skin is "bronzing." He is found to have diabetes as well as an elevated ferritin level (a sign of iron overload). The physician suspects hemochromatosis and confirms the diagnosis with genetic testing. It is found that the patient's DNA carries a mutation in which tyrosine is substituted for cysteine at position 282 (C282Y) within the *HFE* gene. What word below best describes this type of mutation?

(A) Silent
(B) Missense
(C) Nonsense
(D) Frameshift
(E) Deletion

3. A 43-year-old woman, who has recently had difficulty getting up and out of a chair and finds going up stairs to be troublesome, is referred to a rheumatologist for her progressive weakness. A full rheumatologic workup reveals anti–Jo-1 antibodies, indicating that the patient likely has polymyositis. The physician explains to the patient that she has autoantibodies directed against histidinyl-tRNA synthetase (the Jo-1 antigen). Which of the following best describes a property of this protein?

(A) To form an aminoacyl-tRNA synthetase complex in the absence of energy
(B) To initiate transcription by interacting with the 30S subunit of the ribosome
(C) To recognize and covalently link a particular amino acid and a particular tRNA for that amino acid
(D) To bind puromycin, which terminates protein synthesis
(E) To covalently link amino acids to the 5′ end of a corresponding tRNA

4. A 54-year-old man presents to his family physician with a 3- to 4-week history of a nonproductive cough and a low-grade fever. The physician suspects an atypical pneumonia from *Mycoplasma pneumoniae*, and decides to treat the patient empirically with erythromycin. Which of the following best describes the mechanism of action of erythromycin?

(A) Binds to the 5′ cap of mRNA and prevents translation
(B) Binds to the 30S ribosomal subunit and blocks peptidyl transferase activity
(C) Binds to the Shine-Dalgarno sequence of mRNA and prevents translation
(D) Binds to and inhibits initiation factor IF-1 from binding to the initiation complex
(E) Binds to the 50S ribosomal subunit and blocks translocation during translation

5. A 27-year-old man is seen by his physician for a week-long cough, sore throat, and difficulty swallowing. He is diagnosed with diphtheria, which has reactivated because of waning immunity. One way in which diphtheria toxin leads to cell death is through the inhibition of eEF-2. Which statement best explains the function of eEF-2?

(A) It is required for the translocation of peptidyl-tRNA during translation.
(B) It is required for the initiation of protein synthesis.

(C) It is the agent that binds to, and is inactivated by, chloramphenicol.
(D) It functions as a peptidyl transferase.
(E) It is analogous to the prokaryotic factor eIF-1.

6. A third-year medical student joins a laboratory that studies gene regulation. The laboratory uses bacteria to study gene expression and metabolic regulation after exposure to toxic compounds. The goal is to generalize the observations seen in prokaryotic cells in response to the toxins and to compare the response to eukaryotic cells. Which of the following statements is true regarding prokaryotic and eukaryotic genomes?

(A) They are both diploid.
(B) They both organize and compact their DNA with histones.
(C) They both have short repetitive DNA sequences throughout their genome.
(D) They both organize their genes into operons.
(E) They both use the same genetic code to convert codons to amino acids.

7. A 23-year-old man is seen in the gastroenterologist's office for a referral concerning a family history of α_1-antitrypsin deficiency. The physician arranges for the interventional radiologist to perform a liver biopsy, which will allow a determination of the extent of accumulation of nonsecreted protein in the hepatocyte. Which of the following statements is true concerning proteins like α_1-antitrypsin that are normally secreted from the cell?

(A) They are synthesized on ribosomes attached to the smooth endoplasmic reticulum.
(B) They contain a hydrophilic signal sequence.

(C) The signal sequence is found on the C terminus of the protein.
(D) Glycosylation takes place only in the endoplasmic reticulum.
(E) Proteins travel from the endoplasmic reticulum to the Golgi apparatus and are ultimately secreted by exocytosis.

8. One colony of bacteria is split into two Petri plates: one plate with growth medium containing glucose and all 20 amino acids and one medium with one sugar (lactose) and one nitrogen source (NH_4^+). Which of the following statements is correct concerning the cells growing in the second medium?

(A) cAMP levels will be lower than cells growing in the presence of glucose.
(B) CAP protein (cAMP-binding protein) will be bound to the *lac* promoter.
(C) The *lac* repressor will be bound to the *lac* operator.
(D) RNA polymerase will not bind to the *trp* promoter.
(E) Attenuation of transcription of the *trp* operon will increase.

9. Gene transcription rates and mRNA levels were determined for an enzyme that is induced by glucocorticoids. Compared with untreated levels, glucocorticoid treatment caused a 10-fold increase in the gene transcription rate and a 20-fold increase in both mRNA levels and enzyme activity. These data indicate that a primary effect of glucocorticoid in this assay is to decrease which of the following?

(A) The activity of RNA polymerase II
(B) The rate of mRNA translation
(C) The ability of nucleases to act on mRNA
(D) The rate of binding of ribosomes to mRNA
(E) The activity of RNA polymerase III

Answers and Explanations

1. **The answer is A.** A missense point mutation is the change of 1 base in the DNA that changes the "meaning" of a codon. In this case, the 1 base change is in an exon and leads to a glutamate codon (GAG) being changed to a valine codon (GTG). This change in primary structure of the β-globin protein alters its properties, which leads to the sickling observed under low-oxygen conditions. A nonsense point mutation is due to a change in a single base in DNA that converts a codon into a stop codon. This will result in premature termination of the growing polypeptide chain. Insertions occur when 1 base or more are added to DNA. Deletions occur when 1 base or more are removed from DNA, such as the Δ508 mutation, which leads to cystic fibrosis. Frameshift mutations occur when the number of bases added or deleted is not in a multiple of three, and the reading frame of the mRNA is altered.

2. **The answer is B.** A missense mutation results from a nucleotide change within the DNA, which results in a change in the meaning of the codon, such that a different amino acid is placed within the protein. This is the case of the C282Y mutation in hereditary hemochromatosis. A silent mutation does not result in an amino acid change, by definition, owing to the degenerate nature of the genetic code, even though there has been a base change in the DNA (e.g., UUU and UUC both code for phenylalanine). A frameshift mutation, as in Duchenne muscular dystrophy, can result in premature termination of protein synthesis with a dysfunctional protein and requires either the insertion or deletion of 1 base or more. Deletion mutations, as in the most common mutation leading to cystic fibrosis, are due to the loss of one or more amino acids. A nonsense mutation is a single base change that converts a codon to a stop codon, leading to premature termination of protein synthesis.

3. **The answer is C.** Each aminoacyl-tRNA synthetase recognizes a single amino acid and a particular tRNA specific for that amino acid. The enzyme then covalently links the two, forming an aminoacyl-tRNA, in a reaction requiring the hydrolysis of ATP. The amino acid is added to the 3′ end of the tRNA. The initiation of transcription requires the interaction of the small ribosomal subunit and an initiator methionyl-tRNA, not an aminoacyl tRNA synthetase. Puromycin inhibits translation by binding to the ribosome, not to the aminoacyl tRNA synthetase.

4. **The answer is E.** Erythromycin, as well as clindamycin, binds to the 50S ribosomal subunit of bacteria and blocks translocation, thereby inhibiting translation. Aminoglycosides, like gentamicin, tetracycline, and streptomycin, bind to the 30S ribosomal subunit to elicit their effects. The ribosomes bind to the 5′ cap of the eukaryotic mRNA (prokaryotic mRNA lacks a cap). The Shine-Dalgarno sequence in prokaryotic mRNA allows proper binding of the mRNA to the 30S ribosomal subunit; erythromycin does not bind to this sequence. IF-1, IF-2, and IF-3 are bacterial initiation factors required for the formation of the initiation complex, although they are not the targets of any antibiotic.

5. **The answer is A.** Eukaryotic elongation factor 2 (eEF-2) is required for eukaryotic translation in that it facilitates the translocation of peptidyl-tRNA along the mRNA. The elongation reaction requires GTP hydrolysis. The corresponding elongation factor in bacteria is EF-G. Diphtheria toxin ADP-ribosylates eEF-2, leading to its inactivation. Initiation of eukaryotic protein synthesis requires several initiation factors, designated eIF-1, eIF-2, etc. Peptidyl transferase is an rRNA (within the large ribosomal subunit) involved in formation of the peptide bond between the amino acid groups within the A and P sites of the ribosome. This activity is not affected by the toxin. Chloramphenicol inhibits prokaryotic peptidyl transferase. Prokaryotes are not affected by diphtheria toxin because they do not contain eEF-2.

6. **The answer is E.** Although there are some differences in mitochondria, the genetic code is nearly universal. Only eukaryotes have a diploid genome, which is organized into chromatin with the aid of highly positively charged histones. Only eukaryotes have numerous short repetitive DNA

sequences throughout their genome, like Alu sequences, which are found in primates and humans. Lastly, prokaryotes, but not eukaryotes, organize transcriptional units as operons, multiple gene products obtained from a single mRNA.

7. **The answer is E.** Proteins destined to be secreted from the cell travel to the cell membrane via the endoplasmic reticulum and the Golgi apparatus. Such proteins are synthesized on ribosomes attached to the RER. The proteins enter the endoplasmic reticulum lumen with the aid of a hydrophobic signal sequence at the N terminus of the protein. Glycosylation takes place in both the endoplasmic reticulum and the Golgi before sorting and sending the protein to its final destination.

8. **The answer is B.** In the absence of glucose and the presence of lactose (growth medium #2), the *lac* repressor will be inactive, cAMP levels will rise, and the cAMP–CAP complex will bind to the *lac* promoter, stimulating transcription of the operon. Tryptophan levels in the cell will be low; thus, the repressor for the *trp* operon will be inactive, and the operon will be transcribed by RNA polymerase. Attenuation of transcription of this operon will decrease.

9. **The answer is C.** If the rate of degradation of mRNA is not altered by glucocorticoids, the increase in mRNA levels should reflect the increase in transcription rate (10-fold in this case). Because the increase in mRNA level (20-fold) is greater than the increase in transcription rates (10-fold), the glucocorticoids must also be increasing mRNA stability (i.e., decreasing the rate of degradation by nucleases). The activity of RNA polymerase II is increased (transcription is increased), and the rate of translation (the binding of ribosomes to mRNA) is increased (the enzyme activity is increased).

I. CHROMOSOMES

A. DNA within the human nucleus is organized into chromosomes. Normal human somatic cells are diploid with **46 chromosomes**: 22 pairs of **autosomes** and 1 pair of **sex chromosomes**, either XY (male) or XX (female). Mature gametes have a **haploid** number of chromosomes (22 autosomes and either an X or Y sex chromosome). There are more than 3 billion base pairs in the human haploid chromosome.

B. Composition of chromosomes
   1. **Chromatin:** The combination of DNA and protein on a chromosome. The DNA is tightly packed around histones and other DNA binding proteins.
   2. **Telomere:** Repetitive DNA sequences **(TTAGGG)** at the ends of chromosomes
      a. Protects the ends of chromosomes from shortening with each successive semiconservative replication of the DNA
      b. Maintained by the activity of a ribonucleoprotein enzyme complex, **telomerase**, an RNA-dependent DNA polymerase (**reverse transcriptase**)
      c. Cell senescence is thought to be a function of the downregulation of telomerase. Cancer cells frequently have upregulated telomerase.
   3. **Centromere:** Highly repetitive sequences where two sister chromatids attach and proteins assemble to form the **kinetochore**. The positioning of the centromere forms the "arms" of the chromosome: labeled **p** (the **shorter** of the two) and **q** (the **longer**) (Figure 19-1).
      a. Metacentric: Both arms are the same length.
      b. Submetacentric: The arms are different lengths.
      c. Acrocentric: The p (short) arm is so short that is hard to observe, but is still present.
      d. Telocentric: The chromosome's centromere is located at the terminal end of the chromosome (as in the Y chromosome).

II. CELL CYCLE

A. Cells destined to **divide** into two identical daughter cells normally progress through a sequence of duplicating the cell contents (**interphase**), nuclear division (**mitosis**), and cytoplasmic division (**cytokinesis**).

B. G_0 is the **quiescent state** in which cells, which are not in the process of cellular division, are maintained.
   1. At this point, the cells contain the **diploid amount of genetic material (2n)**, where n represents the number of individual chromosomes, which number **23 in humans** (the haploid number).
   2. These cells **express proteins** required for cellular housekeeping as well as proteins required to perform the specialized function of that cell type.

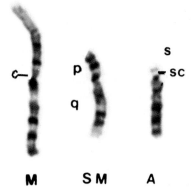

FIGURE 19-1 Chromosomes are numbered according to size and centromere (C) position, and the bands are numbered from centromere toward telomere. Examples of a metacentric (M), submetacentric (SM), and acrocentric (A) chromosome are shown. The letters p and q refer to the short and long arms of the chromosome, respectively. For the acrocentric chromosome, the S refers to the stalk (the very short p arm), and SC refers to the location of the centromere on this acrocentric chromosome.

C. Interphase

1. **Interphase is the period between cell divisions,** which is further divided into the following distinct periods: gap 1, synthesis of DNA, and gap 2 (Figure 19-2).

2. **G_1 (gap 1):** Point of entry for cells to divide and enter the cell cycle. A time of intense messenger RNA **(mRNA) transcription** for the production of proteins required to produce a full complement of proteins for the **resultant two daughter cells** as well as producing all the proteins required for the **duplication of the genome**

3. **S (synthesis of DNA):** Results in the **semiconservative replication** of cellular DNA with the production of two copies of the cellular DNA (**4n**)

4. **G_2 (gap 2):** The cell prepares for cell division with further protein and organelle synthesis. Also, the integrity of the **replicated DNA is assessed** before proceeding to mitosis.

D. Mitosis (Figure 19-2)

1. The process of nuclear division is further broken into the following microscopically discernible stages: prophase, metaphase, anaphase, and telophase.

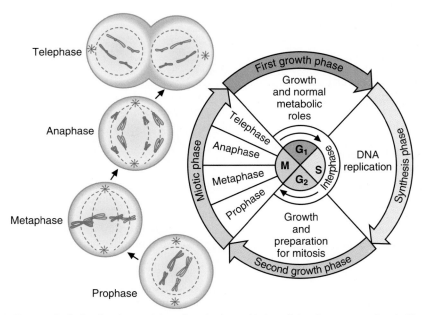

FIGURE 19-2 Diagram displaying the phases of the cell cycle along with the cellular changes associated with each stage of mitosis.

2. **Prophase** is the initial stage of mitosis encompassing the following changes:
   a. **Chromosomes** can be identified due to the condensation of the newly replicated chromatin. The condensation is promoted by the phosphorylation of histone.
   b. The organization network of structural proteins, known as the **centrioles**, begins moving to opposite poles of the cell.
   c. Breakdown of proteins known as **lamins** results in the dissolution of the nuclear membrane because the genetic material will be segregated to opposite sides of the cell during the division process.
3. **Metaphase** is the most distinctively visualized stage (Figure 19-2) of mitosis.
   a. Duplicated genetic material, **sister chromatids**, line up along the **equatorial plane** of the cell.
   b. Cytoskeletal elements **radiating from the polar centrioles** connect to the junction between the two sister chromatids, the **kinetochore**.
4. **Anaphase** is the "action" stage of mitosis.
   a. Separation of the two sister chromatids occurs by movement of the separate chromatids toward the polar centrioles on the network of cytoskeletal elements.

CLINICAL CORRELATES   The chemotherapy agent paclitaxel **(Taxol)** prevents the **cytoskeletal** remodeling required to complete the migration of the replicated chromatids to the cell poles for the formation of replicated daughter cells. It is an important agent in the treatment of many cancers, including breast cancer.

---

   b. The separation of sister chromatids is simultaneous for all chromosomes, ensuring the **segregation of equal genetic material** (2n) to the daughter cells.
5. **Telophase**
   a. **Chromosomes decondense**, with the return of less highly organized chromatin.
   b. A new nuclear membrane is formed, encapsulating the newly divided daughter genomes.
   c. **Cytokinesis**, the final step in telophase as well as cell division, requires **the pinching off of the plasma membrane** and the formation of two separate membrane-bound daughter cells.

III. CONTROL OF THE CELL CYCLE

A. Progression of the cell cycle
   1. Progression is orchestrated through an elaborate series of check points.
   2. The check points are mediated by interactions between proteins such as cyclins, cyclin-dependent kinases (CDKs), and CDK inhibitors.

B. Entry into the cell cycle
   1. **The $G_0 \rightarrow G_1$ transition** (Figure 19-3)
      a. Cells in the G_0 phase may remain so **indefinitely** as in the case of **neuronal or cardiac muscle cells** or, under certain circumstances, may enter into the cell cycle (as is often the case with epithelial **cells of the gastrointestinal tract**).
      b. The transition of cells from $G_0 \rightarrow G_1$ is contingent on the presence of one or more **growth factors**, which are produced in a regulated manner when a particular cell type needs to be increased in number.
   2. **The $G_1 \rightarrow S$ transition** (Figure 19-3)
      a. The boundary between the G_1 and S phase is often referred to as the **restriction point**. Once cells traverse this boundary, the cell is committed to completion of the S phase.
      b. **Cyclin D** levels begin to rise late in G_1 and bind to constitutively expressed **CDK4** and **CDK6**.

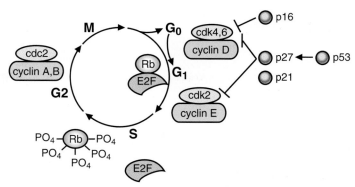

FIGURE 19-3 Diagram displaying some of the many proteins involved in the transitions between various points in the cell cycle.

  c. CDK4 and CDK6 **phosphorylate cyclin D**, which, together as cyclin D–CDK4 or cyclin D–CDK6 complexes, **phosphorylate** the nuclear **retinoblastoma (Rb) protein**.
  d. **Rb** protein is normally bound to and **inhibits transcription factor E2F**, which is **released when Rb is phosphorylated** by the cyclin–CDK complexes.
  e. E2F, when free of its Rb-mediated repression, initiates the transcription of **genes** required for **cell cycle progression**.
  f. The cyclin–CDK complexes can be inhibited by a family of proteins known as the **CDK inhibitors, which include p21, p27, and p16**. These inhibitors block progression through the cell cycle.
  3. **The $G_2 \rightarrow$ M transition** (Figure 19-3)
  a. As the G_2 phase progresses, a group of cyclins, predominantly **cyclin A and cyclin B**, begin to accumulate.
  b. Cyclin A associates with **CDK1** and **CDK2**, which form activated complexes required for further progression through the cell cycle.
  c. Targets of the G_2 phase CDKs include **topoisomerase**, which, when phosphorylated, results in **condensation of chromosomes** and phosphorylation of **lamins and** leads to the fragmentation of the nuclear membrane.

C. Progression through the various phases of mitosis requires the phosphorylation of numerous proteins, primarily by the cyclin B–CDK1 complex.

IV. MEIOSIS (FIGURE 19-4)

A. The process of **reductive division** of the diploid chromosomes to the haploid number occurs within the gametes.

B. The production of haploid gametes allows for the restoration of the diploid number with the union of male and female gametes during the process of **fertilization**.

C. **Meiosis is composed of two successive nuclear divisions following DNA replication.**
  1. **Meiosis I:** separation of **homologous** chromosome pairs in a tetraploid cell producing two diploid cells.
  a. **Prophase 1:** Duplicated chromatin condenses. Each chromosome consists of two, closely associated **sister chromatids**.
  (1) **Synapsis** brings together paired chromosomes to form **tetrads**, two chromosomes and four chromatids, with one chromosome coming from each parent.
  (2) The process of **crossing over** is an exchange of genetic material from one chromatid of a chromosome with the corresponding region of its homologous chromatid of the other chromosome in the tetrad.

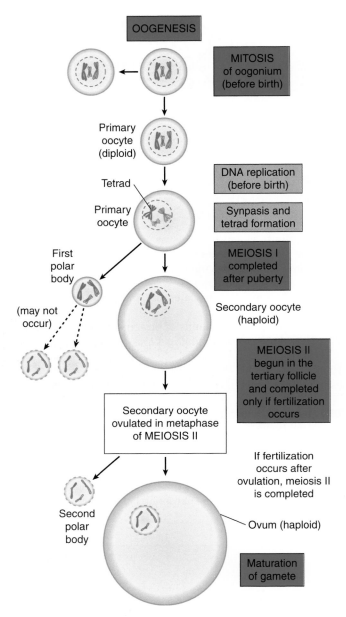

FIGURE 19-4 Diagram displaying the process of meiosis in the female gamete.

    (3) The homologous chromosomes appear to repel each other and remain held together only at **chiasmata** (until anaphase I), **the points at which crossing over has occurred**, and at the centromere.

  b. Metaphase I: The tetrads attach to the meiotic spindle and align.

  c. Anaphase I: Each tetrad divides so that one chromosome moves to one pole and the second chromosome moves to the other. (**Note: each chromosome is still composed of two chromatids**.)

  d. Telophase I: The nuclear membranes form, and the cell completes division.

    (1) In the case of spermatogenesis, the cell division is equal.

    (2) During **oogenesis**, the division is **unequal** with the formation of the larger primary oocyte and the smaller **first polar body** (which may not continue into meiosis II).

2. Meiosis II

  a. Meiosis II proceeds, without DNA synthesis, through prophase II, metaphase II, and anaphase II with the events similar to the respective stages of mitosis, except in this case, the diploid number of chromosomes will yield progeny with only a haploid number of chromosomes.

   b. The **second meiotic division** in the egg is **not completed until fertilization by a sperm** and again is unequal, giving rise to the mature egg and a small **second polar body**.

3. Errors occurring during meiosis

   a. Variations in the normal diploid number of chromosomes

     (1) Aneuploid: A number of chromosomes that is not a multiple of the haploid number (23) usually resulting from a **non-disjunction** event during meiosis.

     (2) Polyploid: A number of chromosomes more than 2 times the haploid number; this is incompatible with life.

   b. Non-disjunctions

     (1) Failure of the homologous chromosomes to separate during meiosis.

     (2) Results in partial or total **aneuploidy** in gametes.

     (3) Most often occurs in **female gametes** and correlates with advanced **maternal age**. (Table 19-1 lists some clinically relevant disorders that result from non-disjunctions.)

   c. Deletions

     (1) Loss of a **portion of a chromosome**.

     (2) The nomenclature is such that a ($-$) follows specific deletion (i.e., 46,XY, 5p$-$, denotes the lost genetic material on the short arm (p) of chromosome 5 in an otherwise karyotypically normal male).

CLINICAL CORRELATES   **Cri du chat syndrome** (deletion 5p syndrome): A rare genetic disorder caused by loss of genetic material on the **short arm of chromosome 5**. Affected individuals have delayed growth and development, neurocognitive delay, wide-set eyes (hypertelorism), and a distinctive **catlike cry**.

   d. Inversions: Occur when a chromosome experiences two internal breaks, with a subsequent rejoining of the internal fragment in the reverse orientation

   e. Translocations

     (1) An exchange of chromosome segments **between two nonhomologous chromosomes**

     (2) The nomenclature for a translocation includes a "t" followed in parentheses by the involved chromosomes in numeric order. For example, 46, XY t(14;21)(q6;p11) denotes the translocation of genetic material on the long arm of chromosome 14 with material from the short arm of chromosome 21.

     (3) Types of Translocations

       (a) Reciprocal (balanced) translocation: A translocation occurring without any loss of genetic information and therefore typically "clinically" **silent**.

       (b) Robertsonian translocation: A variant translocation between two acrocentric chromosomes, whereby two long arms are joined at the centromere with the loss of the two short arms.

table 19-1 Clinically Relevant Disorders that Result from Non-disjunctions

Syndrome	Karyotype	Clinical Manifestations
Down syndrome	Trisomy 21	Flat nasal bridge, low-set ears, and epicanthal folds; congenital heart disease at birth. Main problems: mild mental retardation with IQ of 30 to 60; increased risk for leukemia, Alzheimer disease (premature senility)
Patau syndrome	Trisomy 13	Growth and mental retardation, central nervous system malformations, microcephaly, microphthalmia, malformed ears, often cleft lip and palate, hand abnormalities
Edwards syndrome	Trisomy 18	Mental retardation, failure to thrive, hypertonia, prominent occiput, receding jaw, low-set ears, rocker-bottomed feet, severe heart malformations

CLINICAL CORRELATES   Heterozygous carriers of the **robertsonian translocation** are **phenotypically normal** because there are two copies of all major chromosome arms. However, **children of this carrier** may inherit an unbalanced **trisomy 21**, causing **Down syndrome**. (47,XX, +21) or (47,XY, +21).

f. **Isochromosomes:** Formed during meiosis as a result of the transverse, rather than the longitudinal, division of chromosomes. The result is two new chromosomes containing the two short arms and the two long arms.

g. **Ring chromosomes:** occur during development when the ends of a chromosome are lost and the two arms of the chromosome fuse to form a closed circle.

V. GENE DOSAGE

● Not all genetic material is equivalent during development. The developing human may or may not accommodate additional genetic information. Examples are:

A. **Sex chromosomes:** Females inherit two X chromosomes (one from each parent); however, during development, one of the X chromosome within the cell randomly inactivates (a process called **lyonization**) (Table 19-2 list some disorders involving sex chromosomes).

1. The **randomly inactivated X chromosome** (see later) becomes heterochromatin and can be seen microscopically within the nucleus as a **Barr body**.

   a. Normal females have one Barr body, and normal males have none.

   b. As the X inactivation is random, females express the genes on the X chromosome from both parents in different cells and therefore are **mosaic**.

2. The inactivation of the X chromosome requires the expression of a large untranslated RNA known as the **X-inactive–specific transcript (XIST)** from the second X, which binds DNA sequences on the X chromosome to inactivate genes.

B. **Genetic imprinting and uniparental disomy**

1. Some genes are expressed in a **parent-specific manner** defying normal rules of mendelian inheritance. At least one mechanism involves **methylation of DNA** on chromosomes. This is **epigenetic**, referring to **factors affecting phenotype without a change in genotype. X inactivation** is also epigenetic.

2. An example occurs in humans with del(15)(q11q13).

   a. **Paternal transmission** of this deletion results in **Prader-Willi syndrome**.

table **19-2**   Disorders Involving Sex Chromosomes

Syndrome	Karyotype	No. of Barr Bodies	Clinical Manifestations
Turner Syndrome	45XO	0	Short stature, characteristic facies, neck webbing, broad chest, widely spaced nipples, gonadal dysgenesis (infertility).
Klinefelter Syndrome	47XXY	1	At puberty: hypogonadism, failed 2nd sex characteristics to develop, often female body habitus. Infertile germ cells fail to develop during embryogenesis.
XYY Syndrome	47XYY	0	Normal phenotype, no dysmorphology. When diagnosed, $1/2$ have language delays in reading and spelling. Increased risk of ADHD, impulsiveness.

CLINICAL CORRELATES Patients with **Prader-Willi syndrome** present with developmental delay, an insatiable appetite (**hyperphagia**), and **hypogonadism**.

    b. **Maternal transmission** of this deletion results in **Angelman syndrome**.

CLINICAL CORRELATES Patients with **Angelman syndrome** present with developmental delay, epilepsy, neurocognitive defects, abnormal gait, and **frequent inappropriate laugh** (leading to the term **happy puppet syndrome**).

C. Trinucleotide repeats
   1. The expansion of the number of trinucleotide (three base repeats of CG-rich units) within a gene is sometimes associated with deleterious consequences.
   2. The number of repeats may **increase** from generation to generation as they are transmitted, leading to **earlier and more severe manifestations**, a phenomenon known as **anticipation**.
   3. Sometimes, the number of repeats is so large that visible changes in the appearance of the chromosome occur, as in the case of **fragile X syndrome**.

CLINICAL CORRELATES Fragile X syndrome is the **second leading inherited cause of mental retardation**. The trinucleotide repeat CGG can be expanded over 200-fold within the *FMR1* gene on the X chromosome. Males present with retardation, elongated faces, large ears, and large testicles (**macro-orchidism**).

VI. FUNDAMENTALS OF MENDELIAN GENETICS

● Tenets for the transmission of heritable characteristics from parent to offspring developed by Gregor Mendel.

A. Law of segregation
   1. Phenotypic variation observed for various traits is the result of **alternative versions of genes at specific genetic loci** known as alleles.
   2. The offspring inherit one allele at each locus from each of the parents.
      a. **Dominant alleles** (denoted by an **uppercase letter** as in A) are those that when co-inherited with another allele **dictate the phenotype** of the offspring.
      b. **Recessive alleles** (denoted by a **lower case letter** as in a) are those that when co-inherited with another allele have **no tangible effect** on the phenotype.
      c. The offspring may inherit the same allele from each of the parents (AA or aa), in which case they are **homozygous**, or different alleles from each parent (Aa or aA), in which case they are **heterozygous**.
   3. The two alleles for each gene segregate during gamete production.

B. Law of independent assortment
   1. The inheritance pattern of one trait is **independent** and does not influence the inheritance of another trait.
   2. Independent assortment occurs during **anaphase I of meiosis** after crossover has occurred.
   3. Genes may be linked together because of their physical proximity on the chromosomes and therefore may segregate together to affect phenotype.

VII. THE PUNNETT SQUARE

A. A diagram predicting the outcome of a mating between individuals with different genotypes.

B. Provides a graphic representation of all **possible genotypes of the offspring** of the cross.

C. The interpretation of such data leads to the determination of the **frequency** of offspring affected by the various modes of transmission (as described further later).

D. The simplest example is the mating of two individuals who are heterozygous at a single genetic locus (Figure 19-5).

    1. By convention, the two maternal alleles are written over the columns, and the paternal alleles are written in the side rows.
    2. The genotypes and the phenotypes of the offspring are determined by the combination of the maternal and paternal alleles.
        a. In the mating of heterozygotes, the probability of an individual offspring having the genotype **AA** is 25%, **Aa** is 50%, and **aa** is 25%.
        b. **Seventy-five percent** of the offspring will have the dominant phenotype (**AA** or **Aa**), whereas only 25% will have the recessive phenotype (**aa**).

VIII. MODES OF INHERITANCE (FIGURE 19-6)

A. Autosomal dominant inheritance
    1. One affected parent (likely a heterozygote) mates with a normal individual, resulting in the transmission of the trait to the offspring.
    2. The likelihood of **affected offspring is 50%**, regardless of sex.
    3. Every generation of the pedigree is likely to be affected.

B. Autosomal recessive inheritance
    1. The effects of the trait only manifest **when two copies of the allele are present** (homozygous).
    2. Most of the time, transmission of the trait occurs when two carriers (individuals heterozygous for the allele) mate.

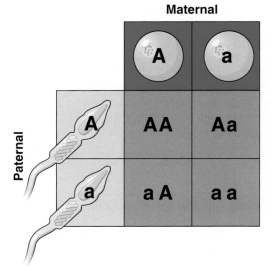

FIGURE 19-5 A Punnett square demonstrating the mating between two individuals who are heterozygote (A, a) at a particular allele.

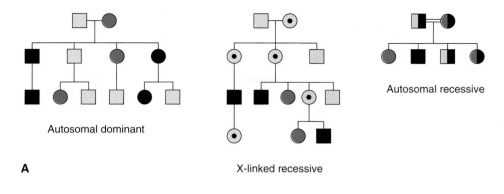

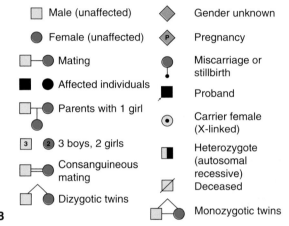

FIGURE 19-6 **(A)** The genetic pedigree for autosomal dominant, X-linked recessive and autosomal recessive inheritance. **(B)** Common symbols used in a pedigree.

    a. Twenty-five percent of offspring will be homozygous for the allele and will **manifest the trait.**
    b. Fifty percent of offspring will be heterozygous carriers.
    c. Twenty-five percent of offspring will be neither affected nor carriers.
  3. The transmission is equally distributed between males and females.
  4. Affected individuals may not be seen in every generation; however, matings between familial descendants in the pedigree (**consanguinity**) may increase the occurrence within the pedigree.

C. X-linked recessive inheritance
  1. Occurs when an allele for a particular trait is located on the **X chromosome**.
  2. Most often occurs when a **heterozygous female** mates with an unaffected male.
    a. Fifty percent of male children will be affected.
    b. Fifty percent of female children will be carriers.

CLINICAL CORRELATES   Hemophilia A is an **X-linked recessive disease** caused by a deficiency of the clotting **factor VIII**. Patients are at risk for **life-threatening bleeds** from minor trauma. They often experience bleeding into joint spaces (**hemarthrosis**) and serious **gastrointestinal bleeds**.

D. Other modes of inheritance
  1. X-linked dominant: Rather rare and observed when a gene on the X chromosome leads to expression of a disease or trait in both hemizygous males and heterozygous females. All the daughters and none of the sons of affected males will be affected.

2. **Mitochondrial inheritance:** Because all the mitochondria in the developing zygote originate from the ovum, defects in the mitochondrial genome are exclusively maternally transmitted. The mutation rate in mitochondrial DNA is much higher than in genomic DNA.

CLINICAL CORRELATES   **Leber hereditary optic neuropathy (LHON)** is due to mutations in the complex I genes in the mitochondrial DNA (mtDNA). The disorder results in **degeneration of the retinal ganglion cells and optic nerve** resulting **in progressive, bilateral loss of vision** in young adults.

3. **Multifactorial inheritance:** Disorders due to the interplay of multiple genes as well as environmental influences.

IX. MODERATORS OF INHERITANCE

- Sometimes, the observed characteristics of a person (phenotypes) do not agree with the predicted genetic constitution of the individual (genotype).

1. **Variable penetrance:** Although an individual may harbor the genotype, he or she fails to express the phenotype.
2. **Variable expressivity:** Refers to the range of signs and symptoms that can occur in different people with the same genetic condition.
3. **Mosaicism:** The presence of two populations of cells with **different genotypes in one individual,** who has developed from a single fertilized egg.

X. HARDY-WEINBERG PRINCIPLE

- Just as the frequency of genotypes between individual mating can be predicted using the Punnett square, the Hardy-Weinberg principle can be used to calculate the frequency of particular alleles based on frequency of a phenotype within a population.

A. **The Hardy-Weinberg principle is based on the binomial theorem: $p^2 + 2pq + q^2 = 1$.**
   1. For normal allele (A), the frequency in the population is p.
   2. For the mutant allele (a), the frequency in the population is q.
   3. Because there are assumed to be only 2 alleles, $p + q = 1$.
   4. The frequency of the homozygote A $= p^2$, the heterozygote Aa $= 2pq$, and the frequency of the mutant homozygote a $= q^2$.

B. **Application in the cases of modes of inheritance.**
   1. **Autosomal recessive inheritance**
      a. For a disorder with an incidence of 1/10000 persons, $q^2 = 1/10000$ and $q = 1/100$.
      b. $p = 1 - 1/100$ or 99/100, and the frequency of AA is $p^2 = 98/100$.
      c. The frequency of the heterozygote is $2pq \sim 1/50$.
   2. **Autosomal dominant inheritance**
      a. The incidence of the disorder in the population $= 2pq$.
      b. The frequency of the mutant allele $=$ half the incidence.
      c. For simplicity, the homozygous affected individuals are ignored because such diseases are typically lethal.
   3. **X-linked inheritance**
      a. The frequency is equal to the incidence of the trait in males.
      b. The carrier frequency in females is 2pq.

C. **Exceptions:** For a population to be in Hardy-Weinberg equilibrium, the following conditions must be met in the population:
1. **Random mating:** None of the matings can result from inbreeding, from selection for traits, or from assertion of traits.
2. **Constant mutation rates**
3. **Absence of selection**
4. **Large population sizes** to avoid random fluctuations by chance
5. **Absence of migration**

XI. GENETIC TESTING

A. **Fetal testing for screening abnormalities in the fetus**
1. **Amniocentesis**
   a. Performed between 14 and 20 weeks' gestation and advised for women older than 35 years for **detecting chromosomal abnormalities, genetic defects, and neural tube defects**.
   b. Amniotic fluid can be used to measure enzymes and hormones from cells within the fluid (shed from amnion, fetal skin, fetal lungs, and urinary tract epithelium). The cells that are collected can be cultured for genetic analysis (chromosomal analysis by karyotyping or polymerase chain reaction (PCR) analysis of specific markers).
   c. Amniocentesis also provides access to **DNA for paternity testing** before delivery. DNA is collected from the potential father and compared with fetal DNA.
   d. **Miscarriage is the primary risk** related to amniocentesis (about 1 in 200).
2. **Chorionic villus sampling (CVS)**
   a. Performed between 9 and 12 weeks' gestation with a sample of chorionic villus surrounding the sac obtained. Villi are dissected from decidual tissue in a small placental sample. **Chromosomal analysis on these cells determines the karyotype of the fetus**.
   b. **DNA may be extracted** from these cells for molecular analysis **and amplified** by **PCR**.
   c. A major **advantage of CVS** is that abnormalities may be identified in early pregnancy.
   d. The major **disadvantage is a 2% to 3% risk for miscarriage** and higher rate of maternal cell contamination.
3. **Karyotyping: visualizing chromosomes for abnormalities in number and size** (Figure 19-7)
   a. **Giemsa staining**
      (1) A light microscopy procedure for **visualizing chromosomes** yielding **banding patterns** on each chromosome in addition to morphology.
      (2) A band is a chromosomal area, lighter or darker than its neighboring region. **Heterochromatin stains darker than euchromatin**, indicating tighter chromatin packing and consisting of genetically inactive DNA sequences.
   b. **Fluorescent in situ hybridization (FISH) analysis**
      (1) FISH uses different **fluorescent-labeled probes** (single-stranded DNA conjugated to fluorescent dyes) **specific to regions of individual chromosomes** to detect chromosomal abnormalities.
      (2) Whole chromosome probes are applied to metaphase spreads for the identification of translocations or aneuploidy within the genome. Repetitive probes, such as α-satellite sequences located in the centromere, are also used in the identification of marker chromosomes and aneuploidy.

B. **Maternal blood testing**
1. **Triple screen**
   a. Provides a **statistical risk assessment** but is not a definitive answer regarding chromosomal composition. **Requires accurate fetal number (single versus multiples) and maternal age**. Performed at 15 to 20 weeks' gestation **and is most accurate with samples obtained from between 16 and 18 weeks' gestation** (Table 19-3).

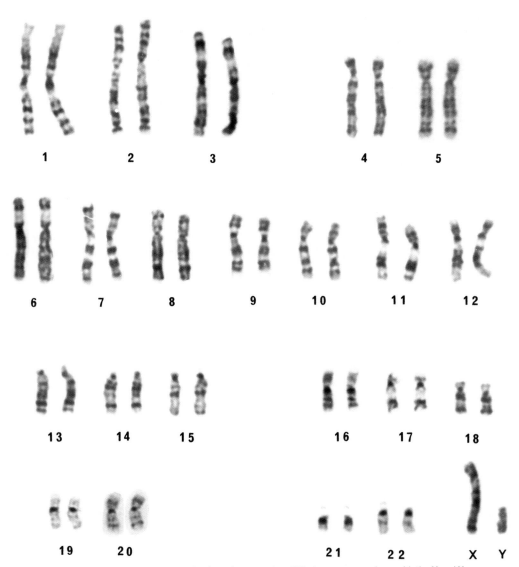

FIGURE 19-7 A human karyotype demonstrating homologous pairs of 22 chromosomes along with the X and Y.

table 19-3		Interpretations of Results from Maternal Blood Screening with the Triple Screen[*]
Test Results	**Clinical Findings**	**Other Interpretations**
AFP diffusing and rising rapidly	**Open neural tube defect** (anencephaly or spina bifida) or abdominal wall defects	Gestational age, gestational diabetes, intrauterine growth retardation, bleeding.
Falling AFP and low estriol	Down syndrome, other chromosomal aneuploidy	Failing pregnancies.
Rise in hCG with decreased AFP mid-/late-second trimester	Down syndrome.	Beta-hCG produced by trophoblasts indicate pregnancy
Rising inhibin A	Down syndrome, other chromosomal aneuploidy	Smoking may increase. Obesity may decrease.

*Adding inhibin A yields the quad screen.

   b. Assays for three specific substances:

   (1) AFP: α-fetoprotein: produced by yolk sac, later by liver, enters amniotic fluid then maternal serum.

   (2) hCG: human chorionic gonadotropin: a protein hormone produced in the placenta.

   (3) Estriol: an estrogen produced by both the fetus and the placenta.

2. **Quad screen:** Triple screen (see earlier) **adding inhibin A**, a protein produced by the placenta and ovaries.

Review Test

Directions: Each of the numbered questions or incomplete statements in this section is followed by answers or by completions of the statement. Select the **one** lettered answer or completion that is **best** in each case.

1. An 8-year-old boy of Ashkenazi Jewish descent presents with bone pain and easy bruising. His parents have no known history of serious medical ailments. He is found to have hepatosplenomegaly (enlarged liver and spleen), anemia, and an Erlenmeyer flask deformity of his distal femur. Which of the following is true for this patient?

(A) The likelihood of another, to be born, sibling being affected with the disease is 50%.

(B) At least one person in every generation of his pedigree is likely to be affected.

(C) His disease will only affect males.

(D) The probability that the patient's unaffected siblings will be heterozygous carriers is 67%.

(E) His parents will become affected with the disease.

2. A 2-year-old boy with Down syndrome requires intubation in the intensive care unit due to difficulty breathing. He is afflicted with congenital heart disease associated with the disease, and he dies shortly after admission. What is the most common genetic cause of Down syndrome?

(A) Meiotic nondisjunction
(B) Autosomal dominant inheritance
(C) X-linked recessive inheritance
(D) Decreased maternal age
(E) Monosomy 21

3. A 30-year-old woman presents to her obstetrician for her 6-month pregnancy examination. The patient has already had one son born with Edwards syndrome, who died after 1 week of life. She is concerned about the fate of the current pregnancy because after her first child was born she was seen by a clinical geneticist who told her that she is a mosaic for trisomy 18. Which of the following statements is true for this patient?

(A) She will develop severe trisomy 18 later in her life.

(B) Her baby will definitely have Edwards syndrome if the child is a boy.

(C) Her baby will not have trisomy if the child is a girl.

(D) Trisomy 18 in her son was likely due to some of her primary oocytes being 45,XX, −18

(E) Some of her primary oocytes are 47,XX, +18.

4. A 50-year-old woman presents with spleen enlargement and a decreased red blood cell count. She is diagnosed with chronic myelogenous leukemia (CML), a blood cell cancer in which a portion of chromosome 9 is aberrantly attached to chromosome 22. CML thus serves as a paradigm for other blood cell cancers, as an example of which of the following?

(A) Transgenic expression
(B) Reciprocal gene translocation
(C) Robertsonian translocation
(D) Gene knockout
(E) Single gene defect disease

5. A 10-year-old boy with Lesch-Nyhan syndrome presents with kidney stones from high levels of uric acid. This X-linked recessive syndrome is due to a genetic defect, which leads to deficiency of hypoxanthine-guanine phosphoribosyl transferase (HGPRT), an enzyme crucial in the purine salvage pathway. Which of the following is most indicative of this patient's family pedigree?

(A)

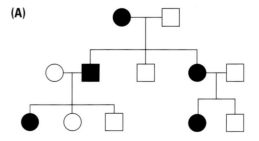

300

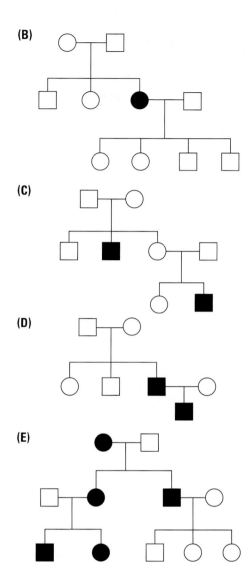

(B)

(C)

(D)

(E)

on amniotic fluid reveals 47,XY, +21. Which of the following statements is true of amniocentesis?

(A) The procedure can be performed at 4 to 10 weeks
(B) The procedure is unlikely to reveal a cyto-genetic abnormality
(C) Risk includes miscarriage and spontaneous abortion
(D) A biopsy of chorionic villus undergoes DNA analysis
(E) The procedure is offered to women younger than 35 years.

8. A 17-year-old boy receives a pediatric consult for an upper respiratory infection with jaundice. History reveals he frequently becomes jaundiced when he has minor infections. The patient's history contains no evidence of consanguinity. His father had a few mild cases of hyperbilirubinemia, and his paternal grandmother had episodic fatigue with mild scleral icterus. Based on the family history, what is the most plausible inheritance pattern of this hyperbilirubinemia?

(A) X-linked dominant
(B) X-linked recessive
(C) Autosomal dominant
(D) Autosomal recessive
(E) Mitochondrial

9. A 50-year-old man undergoes genetic testing for hemochromatosis, an autosomal recessive disease characterized by abnormally elevated serum iron levels leading to organ toxicity. He is positive for a genetic mutation and is diagnosed with the disease. However, he never develops signs of elevated serum iron levels or organ toxicity. Which of the following terms best describes this patient's disease?

(A) Low penetrance
(B) Low expressivity
(C) Low mosaicism
(D) Low lyonization
(E) Low mendelian inheritance

6. A 50-year-old man presents with personality changes and an uncontrolled choreic (dancing) movement of one arm. His mother has Huntington disease, which is an autosomal dominant disease characterized by an abnormally long trinucleotide repeat sequence in a specific area on one chromosome. He would like to know if he also has Huntington disease. Which of the following techniques would be most precise in detecting this genetic abnormality?

(A) Karyotyping
(B) Phenotype characterization
(C) DNA sequencing
(D) Amniocentesis
(E) Chorionic villus sampling

7. A woman is pregnant with her fourth child. She has had an uneventful pregnancy and is offered amniocentesis. Cytogenetic analysis performed

10. A 30-year-old man is a heterozygote for a disease that is prevalent in the population. If the population is in Hardy-Weinberg equilibrium, then $p^2 + 2pq + q^2 = 1$ and $p + q = 1$. Which of the following in this equation indicates the prevalence of heterozygotes?

(A) p^2
(B) q^2
(C) $2pq$
(D) p
(E) q

Answers and Explanations

1. **The answer is D.** The patient is exhibiting the signs of Gaucher disease, an autosomal recessive disorder. This means that each of the child's parents are carriers of Gaucher, and they have a 25% chance of having an affected offspring (not 50%, so answer A is incorrect). In an autosomal recessive pedigree, the probability of an unaffected sibling of an affected child being a carrier is 67% (of the four genetic possibilities for a child, the one chance of being affected is eliminated, leaving three possibilities; two of those three are carrier status, and the other is noncarrier, non-affected status). Because Gaucher is an autosomal recessive disorder, generations can be skipped in terms of an individual expressing the disease. In autosomal dominant disorders, it is likely that at least one person in every generation of the pedigree is affected (answer B is incorrect). Autosomal recessive disorders are not X-linked (the term autosomal refers to chromosomes 1 to 22, not the X and Y chromosomes, which are the sex chromosomes), so there is an equal probability of males and females being affected (answer C is incorrect). Carriers of autosomal recessive disorders do not develop the disease later in life (answer E is incorrect).

2. **The answer is A.** Meiotic nondisjunction is the failure of chromosomes to separate and move to opposite poles of the dividing cell. This results in two copies of the same chromosome (chromosome 21 in this case) in one gamete, and nullisomy (no chromosome 21) in the other gamete. If the gamete with two copies of chromosome 21 is fertilized by a gamete with another chromosome 21, trisomy 21 will result. This is the most common cause of Down syndrome (monosomy 21 is incompatible with life). Down syndrome does not occur due to autosomal dominant inheritance. There is no dominant gene that offspring can inherit that would lead to this disorder. Because Down syndrome is due to trisomy 21, it is clearly not X-linked. The incidence of Down syndrome is essentially equal between boys and girls. Increased (not decreased) maternal age is associated with increased incidence of meiotic nondisjunction.

3. **The answer is E.** A mosaic individual originated from a single cell line within the zygote, but because of a mitotic event during development, two separate cell lines are created. In this case, the patient originated as 46,XX cells, but a mitotic disjunction (mosaicism) event resulted in 45,XX, −18 cells (monosomy 18 cells typically do not survive) and 47,XX, +18 cells. She would therefore be a mosaic of 46,XX cells and 47,XX, +18 cells. Severity of disease in a mosaic depends on how many of her cells are 47,XX, +18, but because this patient is healthy, she will not develop symptoms later in life. Transmission of trisomy 18 from a female mosaic to her child occurs from a 47,XX, +18 primary oocyte from the mosaic, which generates an egg with two copies of chromosome 18. Transmission will not likely occur from a mosaic to her child if all of her primary oocytes are 46,XX (normal). Trisomy 18 is not determined by gender and can occur in both males and females. One cannot predict the occurrence of trisomy based on the X and Y chromosomes. Trisomy 18 in her son was likely due to at least some of her primary oocytes being 47,XX, +18, not 45,XX, −18. If the latter were correct, there would be a chance of monosomy 18, which is incompatible with life.

4. **The answer is B.** Gene translocation in CML refers to the reciprocal gene translocation between chromosomes 9 and 22. Gene translocation occurs in other blood cell cancers as well. Transgenic expression refers to intentional expression of a gene, as opposed to expression of that gene due to spontaneous mutation as occurs in CML. Creation of the Philadelphia chromosome is not due to transgenic expression. Robertsonian translocation is a type of nonreciprocal chromosomal translocation that only occurs with the 5 acrocentric chromosomes (chromosomes with centromeres near their ends, which includes chromosomes 13, 14, 15, 21, and 22). Nonhomologous acrocentric chromosomes can break at their centromeres, and their long arms can join at a single centromere. For example, the long q arm of 21 can fuse to a q arm of chromosome 14 at a single centromere. The short p arm of 21 and the short p arm of chromosome 14 fuse and are lost after a few cell divisions. Gene knockout refers to intentional genetic engineering in which a

gene is eliminated or "knocked out" of a genome. This does not occur in CML. A single gene defect disease refers to a disease in which a mutation or deficiency of a single gene determines disease diagnosis and manifestation. It does not apply to creation of a new gene by translocation of genetic material between chromosomes.

5. **The answer is C.** Pedigree C is indicative of X-linked recessive inheritance. Disease can be present in multiple generations, but there is no male-to-male transmission. Essentially, only males are affected. Pedigree A is indicative of autosomal dominant inheritance. Many generations, and multiple individuals per generation, are affected. Both males and females can be affected. Pedigree B is indicative of autosomal recessive inheritance. Disease is usually present in only one generation in a pedigree. Both males and females can be affected. Pedigree D is close to X-linked recessive inheritance, but there is no male-to-male transmission in X-linked recessive diseases. Pedigree E is indicative of mitochondrial inheritance. Many generations can be affected, but transmission can only be through a mother. Both males and females can be affected.

6. **The answer is C.** DNA sequencing is the most precise way of detecting small genetic changes in a specific area on one chromosome. Karyotyping enables visualization of chromosomes under light microscopy. Chromosomes are arrested in metaphase and are differentiated according to size and centromere location. This technique is useful for chromosomal abnormalities such as gene translocations but usually is not precise enough to detect small genetic changes on the scale of several to tens of nucleotides, as would occur with an expansion of a trinucleotide repeat. Characterizing the patient's phenotype or clinical manifestation is helpful for diagnosis, but it will not detect a patient's genetic abnormality. Amniocentesis and chorionic villus sampling are helpful for detecting fetal genetic abnormalities but are not useful for detecting genetic abnormalities in adults.

7. **The answer is C.** The primary risk for amniocentesis is miscarriage. Spontaneous abortion can occur if the procedure is done earlier than the recommended time period, which is typically between 14 and 20 weeks's gestation, not as early as 4 to 10 weeks. Amniocentesis is a reliable and accurate procedure for obtaining fetal cells for the detection of cytogenetic abnormalities in the fetus. A biopsy of the chorionic villus is taken for chorionic villus sampling, which is usually performed earlier (at 9 to 12 weeks) than amniocentesis. This is a different procedure than amniocentesis. Amniocentesis is routinely offered to women older than 35 years because advanced maternal age increases the risk for incidence of cytogenetic fetal abnormalities. It is not routinely offered to women younger than 35 years.

8. **The answer is C.** Inheritance of an autosomal dominant trait exhibits the following characteristics: transmission from father to son, variable expressivity, a recurrence rate risk of 50%, potential of reduced penetrance, and a significant spontaneous mutation rate. X-linked dominant transmission is excluded on the basis of male-to-male inheritance, as is a mitochondrial inheritance pattern. X-linked recessive transmission is excluded because females as well as males are affected in this family. Assuming no consanguinity, autosomal recessive transmission is unlikely because there is transmission of the disorder through three generations of the family.

9. **The answer is A.** Low penetrance indicates that a patient carrying the disease allele does not manifest the traits that are typical for that disease, whereas low expressivity indicates that a patient carrying the disease allele shows a decreased degree of expression of the traits typical for that disease, but traits or signs are still detectable (and none are detectable in our patient). Mosaicism indicates that some of the patient's cells are positive for a specific genetic abnormality, and some of the patient's cells are negative for the same genetic abnormality. This is not the case for our patient. Lyonization refers to X-inactivation in females, which could manifest as expression of an X-linked recessive disease in heterozygous females. This is a rare occurrence, and our patient is a male. Mendelian inheritance refers to inheritance of genes from parents to their offspring, but this term does not describe clinical manifestations of a genetically inherited disease.

10. **The answer is C.** The Hardy-Weinberg equilibrium espouses genetic equilibrium—that genotype frequencies in a population remain constant or in equilibrium from generation to generation—assuming there is random mating, constant mutation rates, absence of selection, a large

population size avoiding random, chance fluctuations, and no significant migration in or out of a population. A single locus has two alleles, p and q. The p allele can represent one allele A, and q can represent the other allele a. The p^2 allele would then represent the frequency of AA homozygotes in the population, whereas q^2 would represent the frequency of aa homozygotes in the population. The 2pq allele represents the frequency of Aa heterozygotes in the population.

chapter 20

Biochemistry of Cancer

I. ONCOGENES

A. **Proto-oncogenes** are normal cellular proteins that work to regulate normal growth and development. If mutated or misexpressed, the proto-oncogenes become **oncogenes** and lead to aberrant cell cycle control.

1. The aberrant expression of oncogenes results in entry of the cell into the cell cycle with **abnormal cell growth**, suggesting a **gain of function**.
2. There are several classes of such genes, which perturb cell growth through a variety of mechanisms.

B. **Growth factors**

1. **Aberrant production of these proteins** or response to the signals they elicit (in cells normally in the G_0 phase) **can result in aberrant transition from $G_0 \to G_1$, with subsequent uncontrolled growth**.
2. **Growth factors**
   a. Overexpression of a member of these **polypeptide growth hormones** stimulates the proliferation of restricted cell types, leading to their aberrant growth.
   b. **Fibroblast growth factors** (FGFs) are a family of proteins that are normally expressed during the proliferation of cells required for **normal wound healing**, but overexpression can lead to tumor formation.
   c. **Platelet-derived growth factor** (PDGF) is a polypeptide that is normally important for **extracellular matrix production**, but overexpression may result in proliferation as a result of **autocrine stimulation**.
3. **Growth factor receptors**
   a. The normal binding of growth factors to their receptors results in signal transduction in response to receptor dimerization.
   b. Several growth factor receptors have been identified that are capable of **activation, even in the absence of specific ligand**. Many of these receptors have intracellular domains that function as **tyrosine kinases**.
   c. **Epidermal growth factor receptors (EGFRs):** There are at least three members of this family of tyrosine kinase receptors, *erb* b-1, *erb* b-2, and *erb* b-3, which, when mutated, lead to aberrant signaling and growth in the absence of the cognate ligand (epidermal growth factor [EGF]).

CLINICAL CORRELATES Overexpression of the growth factor receptor *erb* b-1, also known as *HER2/neu*, is associated with the development of breast cancers. Patients who overexpress **HER2** (human epidermal growth factor receptor 2) in their breast tumors can be treated with a monoclonal antibody to HER2, trastuzumab (**Herceptin**), which blocks signaling through this oncogenic pathway.

   d. Rearranged during transfection (RET): Although this tyrosine kinase receptor does not directly bind growth factors, it is important in the transduction of a signal upon binding of glial cell line–derived neurotrophic factor (GDNF), with mutations resulting in autonomous growth-promoting signals in the absence of ligand binding.

CLINICAL CORRELATES   **Mutations in RET** are commonly associated with **multiple endocrine neoplasia (MEN) syndromes**, including **MEN I**, which is characterized by pancreatic, pituitary, and parathyroid tumors, and **MEN II**, which is characterized by adrenal, thyroid, and parathyroid tumors.

C. Signal transducing proteins
   1. The next level at which defects in cell growth and development can occur is at the level of **downstream signal transduction** proteins. Two such examples are given: the *ras* gene and non-receptor tyrosine kinase proteins.
   2. The *ras* gene (Figure 20-1)
      a. A guanine triphosphate **(GTP)-binding protein** anchored to the **inner cell membrane** via a covalently attached **farnesyl moiety**
         (1) In the **inactive state**, Ras binds guanosine diphosphate **(GDP)**.
         (2) In stimulation of the cell by growth factor–ligand interactions, Ras **exchanges GTP for GDP**, leading to activation of downstream signaling events.
      b. The ras protein has **intrinsic GTPase activity**, terminating the signal transduction events when **GTP is hydrolyzed back to GDP**, returning *ras* to its **inactive** state.

CLINICAL CORRELATES   The *ras* gene is the **most commonly mutated oncogene in cancer**, with 10% to 20% of tumors harboring mutations in *ras*. Mutations in *ras* are found in a large number of tumors of the colon, pancreas, and thyroid.

   3. Another important grouping of signaling molecules is the **nonreceptor tyrosine kinase proteins**.
      a. These proteins include molecules such as the proto-oncogenes *abl* and *src*.
      b. These proteins function as **intermediaries** in signal transduction pathways resulting in the promotion of cellular growth.

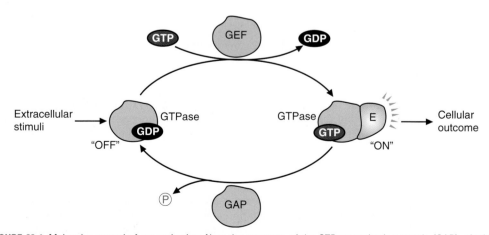

FIGURE 20-1 Molecular control of *ras* activation. Note the presence of the GTPase-activating protein (GAP), of which neurofibromatosis-1 is an example. GDP, guanosine diphosphate; GTP, guanosine triphosphate; GEF, guanine nucleotide exchange factor.

D. **Nuclear transcription proteins**
1. These transcription proteins, such as the proto-oncogene *myc*, integrate divergent growth-promoting pathways and ultimately lead to the production of proteins that allow the cell to advance through the cell cycle.
2. Nuclear transcription factors contain amino acid sequences dictating three-dimensional motifs such as **helix-loop-helix, leucine zipper,** and **zinc finger domains**, which allow them **to bind to DNA**.

> **CLINICAL CORRELATES** The nuclear transcription protein **WT-1**, coded for on chromosome **11p13**, is mutated in **Wilms tumors**. Wilms tumors are the most common **tumors of the kidney** in children.

3. Such genes are **rapidly induced** when quiescent cells receive signals to divide and are rapidly translocated to the nucleus to mediate **gene transcription**.

E. **Cell cycle regulators**
1. Alterations in the normal function of cyclins, cyclin-dependent kinases (CDKs), and CDK inhibitors, often result in unchecked cell growth.
2. **Cyclin D:** Increased expression of this regulator of the $G_1 \to S$ **transition** is commonly found in tumors.
3. **CDK4:** This regulator is among the most commonly altered genes in this class of genes.

II. TUMOR-SUPPRESSOR GENES

A. **Tumor-suppressor genes are cellular proteins,** which when their activity is reduced, result in uncontrolled cell growth.

B. **Cell surface molecules**
1. **There are numerous cell surface molecules that antagonize normal cell growth and development**.
2. **Transforming growth factor-β (TGF-β) receptor** mediates its inhibitory effects by stimulating the production of CDK inhibitors.
3. The protein product of the deleted in colon carcinoma (*DCC*) gene regulates cell growth through the integration of signals from the cellular environment.

C. **Molecules that regulate signal transduction**
1. These molecules possess an antagonistic role to the actions of intracellular proto-oncogenes.
2. **Neurofibromatosis-1 (*NF-1*) gene product** and **GTPase-activating protein** (GAP) activate **the GTPase function of *ras***, converting GTP to GDP and **suppressing** the growth-promoting function of *ras* (Figure 20-1).

> **CLINICAL CORRELATES** **Von Recklinghausen disease**, which is also known as **neurofibromatosis-1**, results from **mutations of *NF-1***. This **autosomal recessive** disorder results in the development of **café-au-lait spots** as well as multiple tumors of the peripheral nerve sheath (**schwannomas**) and tumors of cranial nerve 7 (**acoustic neuromas**).

3. The **adenomatous polyposis coli (*APC*)** gene product promotes the **degradation of β-catenin**, which otherwise normally translocates to the nucleus to induce cellular proliferation.

> **CLINICAL CORRELATES** **Familial adenomatous polyposis (FAP)** syndromes result from mutations of the *APC* gene located on **chromosome 5**. Such patients have a **100% chance** of developing **colon cancer**.

D. **Molecules that regulate nuclear transcription**
1. Several tumor-suppressor genes residing in the nucleus encode proteins that play an important role in the integration of growth-promoting and growth-inhibiting signals.
2. The **retinoblastoma (*Rb*)** gene, as discussed, is an important negative regulator of cell growth.

> **CLINICAL CORRELATES** Patients with ***Rb* loss of function** are prone to the development of **tumors of the retina** early in life and **osteosarcomas** of the bone later in life.

3. The *p53* gene has an important gate-keeper role in cellular proliferation.
   a. The *p53* gene is **induced when DNA is damaged** by irradiation, ultraviolet (UV) light, or chemical mutagenesis.
   b. The *p53* gene then exerts its growth-inhibitory function in one of two ways to ensure adequate **repair of the damaged DNA before proceeding through the cell cycle**.
      (1) The *p53* gene induces the transcription of the **CDK inhibitor *p21***, which **inhibits** the CDK- and cyclin-mediated **phosphorylation of *Rb*** required for the cell to transition to the S phase.
      (2) If DNA damage inflicted on the cell cannot be successfully repaired, ***p53* mediates the transcription of genes implicated in the process of programmed cell death, or apoptosis**.

> **CLINICAL CORRELATES** Mutations in the tumor-suppressor gene, ***p53***, are the **most common molecular alterations in cancer**, with more than 50% of human tumors harboring mutations in *p53*. **Germline mutations in *p53*** result in **Li-Fraumeni syndrome**. Patients in families with a history of Li-Fraumeni syndrome inherit one mutant copy of *p53* in their cells, thereby requiring only one sporadic mutation in their other allele to develop cancer. These patients develop **sarcomas, breast cancers, tumors of the central nervous system**, and leukemias at an increased frequency and decreased age compared with normal individuals.

III. APOPTOSIS

A. **Apoptosis is defined as the programmed destruction of the cell.**
1. It is characterized by a decrease in cell volume, mitochondrial destabilization, chromatin condensation with nuclear fragmentation, and cellular dispersion into fragmented apoptotic bodies without the release of cellular material.
2. Apoptosis is the **endpoint of a cascade** of converging events that **results in cell death**.
   a. **Growth factor withdrawal** occurs with the activation of the proto-oncogene *myc* in conditions of sparse nutrients in the cellular milieu.
   b. Signals are provided by the **proapoptotic cytokines**, tumor necrosis factor (**TNF**), and **Fas ligand**, whose receptors stimulate the activation of proapoptotic enzymes, called **caspases**.

> **CLINICAL CORRELATES** Agents such as **infliximab (Remicade)** and **etanercept (Enbrel)** are biologic agents that are used in the treatment of **autoimmune diseases**. These drugs trigger TNF receptors on autoreactive immune cells, inducing these cells to undergo apoptosis.

   c. Activation of the **proapoptotic gene *Bax*** by the tumor-suppressor gene *p53* occurs if DNA mutations detected during the G_1/S **checkpoint** cannot be repaired with adequate fidelity.

B. Terminal events in the process of apoptosis
  1. The release of the electron transport chain protein **cytochrome c** located on the outer mitochondrial membrane is a **critical regulator** in the process of apoptosis.
   a. Cytochrome c is normally prevented from translocating out of the mitochondria by the **antiapoptotic gene, *bcl-2*** (Figure 20-2).
   b. The exiting of cytochrome c occurs via the mitochondrial channel protein **Bax**.
   c. The **relative abundance of *bcl*-2 and *Bax*** determines the ultimate fate of the cell.
   d. If ***Bax* predominates**, cytochrome c is liberated through the channel and associates with the cytoplasmic molecule, proapoptotic protease activating factor (**Apaf-1**).
   e. Apaf-1 then activates a **cascade of proteolytic events** via the activation of **caspases**.
  2. Caspases contain both "**C**" (**cysteine**) and "**aspase**" (**aspartic acid**) **protease activity**, and once activated, they begin the apoptotic cascade.
   a. Caspases normally exist in the cytoplasm as inactive **zymogens** until stimulated through any of the major pathways triggering apoptosis.
   b. Caspases degrade intracellular proteins and **activate DNases**, with resultant DNA fragmentation, or **DNA laddering**, which is characteristic of apoptosis.

C. The normal programmed cell death pathway, when perturbed, can also result in the **accumulation of cells and uncontrolled cell growth.**

IV. MECHANISM OF ONCOGENESIS

A. Numerous mechanisms exist to create the genetic changes that result in uncontrolled cell growth.

B. Point mutations
  1. Point mutations are changes in the individual nucleotides in the gene encoding either proto-oncogenes or tumor-suppressor genes that can result in cancer.
  2. *ras*: Mutations in codon 12 of the *ras* proto-oncogene results in the **loss of GTPase activity**. This results in continuous activation and the conversion to an oncogene.
  3. *p53*: A wide spectrum of point mutations have been reported, and most **compromise the ability to survey the integrity of the replicate genome** during the cell cycle, with gradual increase in **additional mutations** in other critical regulators of cell growth.

C. Chromosomal translocations (Table 20-1)
  1. Such translocations occur during chromosomal replication, with whole segments of different chromosomes becoming aberrantly attached and fused, resulting in two distinct mechanisms of aberrant growth factor production.
  2. Insertional inactivation
   a. Insertional activation results when normally tightly **regulated growth-promoting genes** come under the control of the regulatory elements of **constitutively expressed** genes

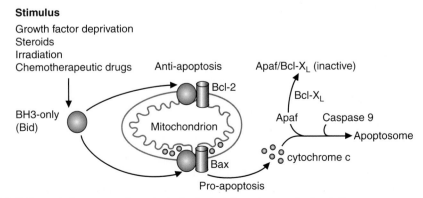

FIGURE 20-2 Pathways in the process of apoptosis. Apaf, apoptotic protease activating factor.

table **20-1** Examples of Chromosomal Translocations Underlying the Development of Cancer

Chromosomal Translocation	Malignancy	Mechanism of Oncogenesis
t(8;14)	Burkitt lymphoma	Expression of the **myc** oncogene (normally **on chromosome 8**), under the control of the immunoglobulin (**Ig**) **gene** promoter (normally on **chromosome 14**)
t(14;18)	Follicular lymphoma	Control of the antiapoptotic gene **bcl-2** (normally on **chromosome 18**) by the regulators of the **Ig** gene (**chromosome 14**)
t(11;14)	Mantle cell lymphoma	Aberrant expression of **cyclin D**
t(9;22)	Chronic myelogenous leukemia	The **bcr-abl** fusion protein results from the translocation between **chromosomes 9 and 22.**
t(15;17)	Acute myelogenous leukemia	Results in a mutant form of **the retinoic acid receptor** that blocks white blood cell differentiation

because of the close proximity resulting from the **repositioning of chromosomal elements** not normally in juxtaposition.

b. Insertional activation is illustrated by the **t(8;14)** translocation with the expression of the **myc** oncogene (normally **on chromosome 8**), under the control of the immunoglobulin (**Ig**) **gene** promoter (normally on **chromosome 14**). **This results in Burkitt lymphoma and acute lymphoblastic leukemia.**

c. Similarly, the **t(14;18)** translocation results in the control of the antiapoptotic gene, **bcl-2** (normally on **chromosome 18**) by the regulators of the **Ig** gene (**chromosome 14**). Such translocations result in malignant lymphomas.

3. **Chimeric protein formation**

a. This results when the reading frame of a protein becomes fused, in-frame, with that of another protein by virtue of a genetic rearrangement between chromosomes.

b. The **bcr-abl** fusion protein results from the translocation between **chromosomes 9 and 22**, with the formation of the **Philadelphia chromosome**.

(1) The resultant protein, **p210**, is derived from the fusion of the proto-oncogene **c-abl** (from **chromosome 9**) and the **bcr** gene (from **chromosome 22**).

(2) The **p210 abl** gene is a potent tyrosine kinase with **50-fold greater activity than the normal gene**, resulting in dramatic cell cycle progression.

CLINICAL CORRELATES **Imatinib (Gleevec)** is a recently developed **tyrosine kinase inhibitor** that inhibits the active site of the **p210** gene and is used in the treatment of **chronic myelogenous leukemia**. It also has been found to inhibit the receptor tyrosine kinase c-*Kit*, which is overexpressed in some gastrointestinal stromal tumors. It is one of the first drugs developed solely based on rational drug design.

c. Other such translocations are known to occur between multiple transcription factors, resulting in inappropriate protein production and subsequent cell growth.

4. **Gene amplification**

a. Defined as overexpression of proto-oncogenes, gene amplification can result from aberrant duplication of their DNA sequences, often resulting in several hundred copies of the proto-oncogene and abnormal growth.

b. These duplicated regions can be seen on the chromosome as **homogeneous staining regions (HSRs)**.

CLINICAL CORRELATES **Breast cancers** are routinely screened for the presence of an **amplified *HER2/ neu*** oncogene. *HER2/neu* expression has been associated with a **poor prognosis**. However, patients with *HER2/neu* overexpression are candidates for **Herceptin therapy**.

c. In the event that the HSRs cause genetic instability, these amplified regions form **double-minute (dm) chromosomes**.

N-*myc*, which is normally found on **chromosome 2**, is often **grossly amplified** in one of the most common pediatric solid tumors, **neuroblastoma**. Up to 300 copies of the N-*myc* gene have been found both as HSRs and dm chromosomes. **N-*myc* amplifications carry a poor prognosis in neuroblastoma**.

V. MOLECULAR CARCINOGENESIS

A. As cells proceed through the multiple rounds of division during the growth and maintenance of the organism, mistakes in the replication of the genome are inevitable. As the cell is subjected to insults, such as chemicals, radiant energy, or viruses, the normal DNA repair mechanisms may become overwhelmed, leading to the chemical changes that result in mutations.

B. Chemical carcinogenesis
   1. Both natural and synthetic compounds are capable of damaging cells either directly, after being acted on by the cell, or in synergy with other chemicals (Table 20-2).
   2. Initiators
      a. These compounds cause direct damage to cellular macromolecules, but their effects are not sufficient, in and of themselves, for tumor formation.
      b. Direct acting compounds are usually **highly reactive electrophiles**, such as **alkylating agents** that **form adducts** with various cellular components (DNA, RNA, proteins, or lipids).

Aflatoxin B$_1$ is associated with the development of the most common cancer worldwide, **liver cancer**. This substance is produced by molds that grow on desperately needed grains that are consumed by developing nations.

   c. Indirect acting compounds (procarcinogens)
      (1) This larger group requires enzymatic activation to produce an **ultimate carcinogen**.
      (2) This enzymatic conversion is often the product of the **P-450 mono-oxygenase system**.
      (3) Such enzyme systems are capable of transforming **polyaromatic hydrocarbons**, such as **benzopyrene (found in cigarette smoke)**, into a reactive species that binds to GC base pairs in DNA, creating **distortions in the helical structure** of DNA.

table **20-2** Association of Environmental and Industrial Exposures with Various Cancers

Substance	Cancer
Aniline dyes	Bladder cancer
Asbestos	Mesotheliomas
Radon	Lung cancer
Arsenic	Skin cancer
Chromium and nickel	Lung cancer
Vinyl chloride	Angiosarcoma of the liver
Diethylstilbestrol (DES)	Vaginal cancer
Nitrosamines (food preservatives)	Stomach cancer

3. **Promoters**
   a. These compounds are noncarcinogenic but facilitate the abnormal growth of cells that have been exposed to initiators.
   b. These compounds facilitate tumor formation by **stimulating proliferation of the cell mutated by the initiator**.

C. **Radiation carcinogenesis**
   1. DNA and other macromolecules are capable of being damaged by different wavelengths of electromagnetic radiation including both UV and ionizing radiation.
   2. **UV radiation** from the sun is responsible for causing mutations in DNA by the formation of **dimers between two adjacent pyrimidines (thymine dimers)**, which must be removed for normal replication to proceed.
   3. **Ionizing radiation:** High-energy radiation (**x-rays and gamma rays**) causes direct damage **to DNA** and **creates highly reactive hydroxyl and hydrogen radicals** that further interact with various cellular macromolecules.

D. **Viral carcinogenesis**
   1. Viruses, both DNA and RNA, have evolved numerous strategies for promoting the aberrant growth of their host cell types.
   2. **DNA viruses**
      a. **Human papilloma virus (HPV):** Members of this family are capable of causing **abnormal cell cycle progression** as the HPV **viral E6 protein binds** to and facilitates the degradation of **cellular *p53***, whereas another viral protein **E7 perturbs** the normal function of the protein **Rb**.

CLINICAL CORRELATES   HPVs, particularly the more aggressive subtypes **HPV-16 and HPV-18**, are closely associated with the development of **cervical cancers**. The development of the **Papanicolaou (Pap) smear** to detect abnormal cervical cells has expedited the screening for cervical cancer, dramatically improving the early detection and treatment of this gynecologic malignancy.

   b. **Epstein-Barr virus (EBV)** causes abnormal accumulation of cells through the production of the protein **LMP-1** (latent membrane protein-1), which promotes the expression of ***bcl-2***, leading to protection from the normal **apoptotic pathways** that trigger cell death.

CLINICAL CORRELATES   EBV is associated with several malignant conditions including Burkitt lymphoma, Hodgkin lymphoma, and nasopharyngeal carcinoma (especially in Southeast Asia).

   c. **Hepatitis B virus (HBV):** Although this virus does not encode any known oncoproteins, its association with human liver cancer has been clearly demonstrated as most likely multifactorial.

CLINICAL CORRELATES   HBV is the leading cause of **hepatocellular carcinoma** worldwide. It is believed that the repeated viral damage to liver cells followed by regeneration leads to increased accumulation of mutations, which culminates in the development of liver cancer. As mentioned before, **aflatoxin B_1** also promotes hepatocellular pathology and, along with HBV, works as a **cocarcinogen**, synergistically increasing the development of liver cancer.

3. **RNA viruses**
   a. RNA **retroviruses** have clearly demonstrated a link to carcinogenesis through two distinct mechanisms.

b. Insertional activation occurs when viral regulatory elements come **in juxtaposition with cellular proto-oncogenes** on **retroviral integration**, resulting in aberrant expression of host cell genes and leading to uncontrolled growth.

Human T-cell lymphotrophic virus type 1 (HTLV-1) is an oncogenic RNA virus. HTLV-1 plays a causative role in the development of a rare set of human T-cell **leukemias and lymphomas**.

c. Viral oncogenes: Some animal retroviruses contain **viral homologues (v-oncs)** of normal **cellular proto-oncogenes (c-oncs)**, which, when expressed in high levels, lead to cellular transformation.

VI. DNA REPAIR AND CARCINOGENESIS

A. The cell has evolved several mechanisms for the **repair of DNA** damaged by the multitudes of insults encountered in the environment. Multiple proteins exist to correct such errors in two major DNA repair pathways (Table 20-3; also see Figure 17-14).

B. **Nucleotide excision repair**
   1. This repair mechanism is responsible for **surveying the topology of the DNA double helix** and **removing such local distortions**.
   2. This occurs through endonuclease cleavage of the damaged bases and restoration of the original segment through the concerted actions of a DNA polymerase **using the intact strand as a template**, to correct the complementary strand.

C. **Mismatch repair**
   1. Sometimes during replication, DNA polymerases insert nucleotides that defy the normal **Watson-Crick base pairing** (i.e., a G may pair with a T instead of the normal A to T pairing.)
   2. Such "misspellings" need to be recognized and corrected before perpetuation of the error to the next round of division.

t a b l e 20-3 Hereditary DNA Repair Defect Syndromes

Genetic Syndrome	Defective Repair System	Associated Malignancies
Ataxia telangiectasia	DNA damage as a result of **ionizing radiation**	T-cell leukemias and lymphomas
Bloom syndrome	DNA damage as a result of **UV exposure**	Skin cancers
Fanconi anemia	DNA cross-linking repair with sensitivity to **nitrogen mustards**	Nonlymphoid hematopoietic malignancies
Li-Fraumeni syndrome	Germline mutations in *p53*	Multiple cancers, especially neoplasms of breast, soft tissue, and central nervous system
Hereditary nonpolyposis colon carcinoma (HNPCC)	Defect in **DNA mismatch repair**	Colon cancer as well as other gastrointestinal malignancies
Xeroderma pigmentosum	DNA damage due to **UV-induced thymidine dimers**	Skin and ocular cancers

UV, ultraviolet.

> **CLINICAL CORRELATES** The genes **BRCA-1** and **BRCA-2**, located on **chromosomes 17 and 13**, respectively, are DNA repair genes implicated in human cancers. **Mutations** in these genes underlie 5% to 10% of **familial cases of breast cancer**. Both genes also are implicated in the development of **ovarian cancer**.

VII. MOLECULAR PROGRESSION OF CANCER

A. Many genetic alterations are required for the about **10^9 tumor cells required to form 1 g of tissue mass**, which corresponds to the smallest clinically detectable mass.
   1. Every human cancer reveals the **activation of several oncogenes and the loss of two or more tumor-suppressor genes**.
   2. This is evidenced in the molecular model of colon carcinogenesis known as the *adenoma-carcinoma sequence* (Figure 20-3).

B. **Tumor growth**
   1. Numerous variables contribute to the growth of transformed cells.
   2. **Growth factors**
      a. Many tumors require the presence of various **hormones or other growth factors** to fuel the growth of the tumor mass.
      b. The lack of such factors retards the growth of the developing mass.

> **CLINICAL CORRELATES** **Breast cancers** are often responsive to estrogen. Therefore, once breast cancers have been shown to express **estrogen receptors**, the estrogen antagonist **tamoxifen** is often used as antihormonal therapy in such patients.

   3. **Angiogenesis**
      a. Tumor cell growth requires the presence of nutrients and oxygen, and because of normal diffusion limits, tumors can only grow to a thickness of **about 2 mm without a nutrient supply**.
      b. As such, **hypoxic conditions** elicit the production of **angiogenic molecules**, such as **vascular endothelial growth factor (VEGF)**, which promotes vascularization of the growing tumor mass.

> **CLINICAL CORRELATES** **Avastin** is a monoclonal antibody that **inhibits VEGFs**, thus inhibiting new blood vessel formation. Avastin is used in the treatment of **colon cancer**.

C. **Invasion**
   1. To disseminate throughout the body, the cancer must gain access to the circulation. This requires **breaking through the basement membrane**, the thick extracellular matrix that separates tissue layers.
   2. Such steps are facilitated by the rendering of various proteases, such as **matrix metalloproteinases (MMPs)**, **cathepsin D** (a cysteine protease), and **urokinase-type plasminogen activator** (a serine protease).

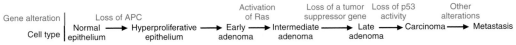

FIGURE 20-3 The adenoma-carcinoma sequence of colon carcinogenesis. APC, adenomatous polyposis coli.

D. Metastasis. Once in the circulation, tumor cells alter the expression of adhesion molecules, allowing them to deposit as "**seeds**" to distant sites, which serve as the "**soil**" for continued growth of the transformed cells.

VIII. MOLECULAR MARKERS IN CANCER BIOLOGY

A. There are **numerous proteins** that are **overexpressed in cancer cells**. Some are actually capable of being detected in the serum of patients with specific cancers. Many of these proteins are simple markers and have no special significance with respect to the pathology of the disease.

B. Many of these proteins lack either the specificity or sensitivity needed for their use as screening tests. Their true utility is in monitoring the progression of the disease once confirmed or in monitoring therapy or recurrence (Table 20-4).

t a b l e **20-4** Molecular Markers in Cancer Biology

Marker	Cancer
Carcinoembryonic antigen (CEA)	Colon cancer
Human chorionic gonadotropin (hCG)	Trophoblastic tumors; testicular tumors
Calcitonin	Medullary carcinoma of the thyroid
Catecholamines	Tumors of the adrenal cortex
Prostate-specific antigen (PSA)	Prostate cancer
Cancer antigen (CA) 125	Ovarian cancer
CA 19-9	Pancreatic cancer
α-Fetoprotein (AFP)	Liver cancer; testicular tumors

Review Test

Directions: Each of the numbered questions or incomplete statements in this section is followed by answers or by completions of the statement. Select the **one** lettered answer or completion that is **best** in each case.

1. A 56-year-old woman is recently diagnosed with breast cancer. She undergoes a lumpectomy and a lymph node dissection. The biopsy results indicate that tumor cells have migrated to the lymph nodes. Her oncologist recommends chemotherapy including the agent paclitaxel (Taxol), which blocks microtubule depolymerization, thereby interfering with the cells' ability to traverse the cell cycle. During which phase of mitosis and the cell cycle would this drug be most active?

(A) Cytokinesis
(B) Metaphase
(C) Anaphase
(D) Telophase
(E) Interphase

2. A 7-year-old child presents to the pediatrician for the development of numerous pigmented lesions on his body (café-au-late spots), difficulty hearing, and tinnitus. Magnetic resonance imaging confirms the presence of cerebellopontine angle acoustic neuromas, and the patient is diagnosed with neurofibromatosis-1. The defective protein in this disease normally has which of the following functions?

(A) Activates the GTPase function of *ras*
(B) Integrates signals from the extracellular environment
(C) Mediates proliferation of cells during normal wound healing
(D) Acts as a transcription factor
(E) Is the primary regulator for the G_1 to S transition of the cell cycle

3. A 23-year-old woman develops a tumor of the soft tissue of her arm (sarcoma) and is being evaluated by an oncologist. The physician learns that her older brother had leukemia when he was 12 years old, her grandmother died of a brain tumor, and her aunt has breast cancer. With this clustering of tumors, the oncologist suspects Li-Fraumeni syndrome and orders molecular studies on the patient's tumor for which of the following genes?

(A) TNF
(B) *p53*

(C) WT-1
(D) *Rb*
(E) RET

4. A 35-year-old woman is found to have breast cancer. A core biopsy is sent for molecular studies to guide treatment, and the pathology report indicates that the tumor is *HER2/neu* positive. Which of the following correctly describes *HER2*?

(A) A tumor-suppressor gene
(B) An anti-apoptotic gene
(C) A growth factor receptor
(D) A steroid hormone
(E) A cell cycle regulator

5. While on an aid mission to central Africa with Doctors Without Borders, a physician encounters a 23-year-old man who appears to have metastatic liver cancer. The grain storage facility outside his village was found to be contaminated with aflatoxin B_1. In addition to this carcinogen, which of the following might act as a cocarcinogen in the development of this patient's cancer?

(A) HTLV-1
(B) HBV
(C) Asbestos
(D) Vinyl chloride
(E) Aniline dyes

6. A 23-year-old woman has come to your clinic because of a lump in her breast that she palpated on breast self-examination. Family history reveals that her mother and her aunt both had breast and ovarian cancer. Given this presentation, you suspect the patient may have a hereditary mutation. Which one of the following genes, when mutated, is implicated in breast and ovarian cancer?

(A) *BRCA-1*
(B) *MLH-1*
(C) Ataxia telangiectasia (*AT*)
(D) *p53*
(E) *Rb*

Answers and Explanations

1. **The answer is C.** The ability of paclitaxel (Taxol) to inhibit microtubule depolymerization results in the cells being unable to complete anaphase. The cells complete metaphase, but the spindle fibers cannot shorten to allow anaphase to initiate. The replicated chromatids are unable to move to opposite ends of the cell for daughter cell formation. Metaphase occurs when the sister chromatids align on the equatorial plane. Telophase and cytokinesis are not completed if anaphase does not occur. Very few chemotherapy agents work during interphase (the portion of the cell cycle when the cell is preparing to divide).

2. **The answer is A.** The protein defective in neurofibromatosis-1 is neurofibrin, which is a GAP. GAPs function to activate the GTPase activity of *ras*. As the bound GTP is converted to guanosine diphosphate, *ras* signaling will be terminated. *DCC* is an example of a gene that integrates signals from the extracellular environment. *DCC* acts as a membrane-bound receptor, binding ligands and initiating signal transduction pathways. FGF is an example of a growth factor involved in wound healing, and aberrant expression of FGF is sometimes found in tumors. WT-1, the protein mutated in Wilms tumor, is a nuclear transcription factor. Cyclin D, which is mutated in some tumors, is the primary regulator of the G_1 to S transition of the cell cycle

3. **The answer is B.** Li-Fraumeni syndrome is a familial DNA repair syndrome caused by mutation in the tumor-suppressor gene *p53*. The *p53* gene is the most common genetic alteration in cancer, and patients who inherit a mutated copy of the *p53* gene have an increased predisposition to soft tissue neoplasms, leukemias, central nervous system tumors, and breast cancer. TNF is a proapoptotic molecule. Mutations in TNF do not lead to Li-Fraumeni syndrome. WT-1 is mutated in Wilms tumor, the most common malignancy of the kidney in children. The function of WT-1 is still controversial. Patients with hereditary *Rb* mutations develop retinoblastoma or osteosarcoma. *Rb* is important in regulating the E2F family of transcription factors. RET is mutated in patients, some with thyroid tumors and some with MEN. RET is a receptor tyrosine kinase.

4. **The answer is C.** *HER2/neu* is a growth factor receptor that is sometimes overexpressed in breast cancer, in which case it is considered to be a marker of poor prognosis. Patients who overexpress this protein can be treated with trastuzumab (Herceptin), which is a monoclonal antibody that blocks growth-promoting signals via the HER2 receptor. The *p53* gene is a tumor-suppressor gene, whereas *bcl-2* is an antiapoptotic gene. Estrogen is an example of a steroid hormone. Estrogen acts as a growth factor for breast tumors that overexpress the estrogen receptor. Cyclin D is an example of a cell cycle regulator that is aberrantly expressed in mantle cell lymphoma and other tumors.

5. **The answer is B.** Hepatocellular carcinoma is the most common cancer worldwide. HBV is a major contributor to the development of this cancer, by acting as a cocarcinogen with aflatoxin B_1. HTLV-1, a retrovirus related to HIV, is associated with a form of leukemia and lymphoma. Asbestos, used as an insulator, is closely associated with a tumor of the pleural linings of the lung, a mesothelioma. Vinyl chloride is associated with a rare form of liver cancer, angiosarcoma. Finally, aniline dyes, used in the clothing industry, have been associated with bladder cancer. There is no evidence to suggest that HTLV-1, asbestos, vinyl chloride, or aniline dyes contribute to aflatoxin B_1–induced liver cancer.

6. **The answer is A.** *BRCA-1* is a gene implicated in breast and ovarian cancer (as is *BRCA-2*). About 5% of breast cancers are due to mutations in this gene, and a strong family history of both breast and ovarian cancer is highly suspicious, especially in such a young patient. Mutations in *MLH-1*,

a gene involved in DNA repair, are correlated with hereditary nonpolyposis colon cancer (HNPCC). Patients with *AT* mutations demonstrate an increase in leukemias and lymphomas. Loss of *p53* function is found in many tumor types (not just breast and ovarian cancers). Mutations in *p53*, associated with breast cancer, signal an aggressive cancer type, with a poor prognosis for recovery. Mutations in *Rb* lead to retinoblastoma and lung tumors, but not to tumors of the breast and ovary.

chapter 21

Techniques in Biochemistry, Molecular Biology, and Genetics

I. BIOTECHNOLOGY INVOLVING RECOMBINANT DNA

A. Strategies for obtaining copies of genes or fragments of DNA
1. Short sequences of DNA (**oligonucleotides**) can be synthesized in vitro and used as **primers** for DNA synthesis or as **probes** for detection of DNA or RNA sequences.
2. Restriction endonucleases **cleave DNA into fragments.**
   a. Restriction endonucleases recognize short sequences in DNA and cleave both strands within this region (Figure 21-1).
   b. Most DNA sequences recognized by these enzymes are **palindromes** (i.e., both DNA strands have the same base sequence in the 5′ to 3′ direction).
      (1) The enzymes cleave a sequence-specific region on each strand, generating two products and allowing them to reanneal or to recombine with other DNA that has been cleaved by the same restriction endonuclease.
   c. A **DNA fragment,** which contains a **specific gene,** can be isolated from the genome with restriction enzymes. Genes isolated from eukaryotic cells usually contain **introns,** whereas those from bacteria do not.
   d. The messenger RNA (**mRNA**) for a gene can be isolated, and a DNA copy (**cDNA**) can be produced by reverse transcriptase. cDNA does not contain introns.

B. Techniques for identifying DNA sequences
1. **Use of probes to detect specific DNA or RNA sequences**
   a. A **probe** is a single strand of DNA that can **hybridize (base pair)** with a **complementary sequence** on another single-stranded polynucleotide composed of DNA or RNA.
   b. The probe must contain a **label,** so that it can detect complementary DNA or RNA. The label may be radioactive (detected by autoradiography) or fluorescent.
2. **Gel electrophoresis of DNA**
   a. Gel electrophoresis **separates** DNA **chains** of varying length. Polyacrylamide gels separate short DNA chains that differ in length by only one nucleotide. Agarose gels separate chains of larger size.
   b. Because DNA contains negatively charged phosphate groups, it will **migrate** in an electric field **toward the positive electrode.**
   c. Shorter chains migrate more rapidly through the pores of the gel, so **separation depends on length.**
   d. DNA **bands** in a gel can be **visualized** by various techniques; staining with dyes (e.g., ethidium bromide) and autoradiography (DNA is labeled radioactively). **Labeled probes** detect **specific DNA sequences.**
   e. **Blots** of gels can be made using nitrocellulose paper (Figure 21-2).
      (1) **Southern blots** are produced when a radioactive **DNA** probe hybridizes with **DNA** on a nitrocellulose blot of a gel. It is often used to detect DNA mutations.
      (2) **Northern blots** are produced when a radioactive **DNA** probe hybridizes with **RNA** on a nitrocellulose blot of a gel.

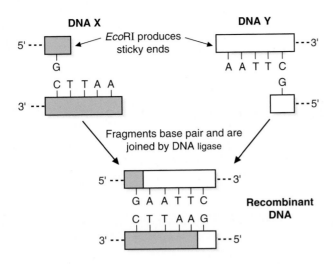

Recombinant DNA

FIGURE 21-1 Action of restriction enzymes. *Eco*RI cleaves a palindrome (5′-GAATTC-3′). Two fragments are produced containing complementary single-stranded regions (sticky ends). If two different DNAs (e.g., X and Y) are cleaved by *Eco*RI, the sticky ends can pair to form a recombinant DNA.

   (3) A **Western blot** is a related technique in which **proteins** are separated by gel electrophoresis and probed with **antibodies** that bind a specific protein.
3. DNA sequencing by the Sanger dideoxynucleotide method (Figure 21-3)
   a. Dideoxynucleotides are added where DNA polymerase is catalyzing polymerization of a DNA chain.
   b. A dideoxynucleotide lacks a 3′-hydroxyl group, so **polymerization of the chain is terminated** wherever a dideoxynucleotide is incorporated into the growing chain.

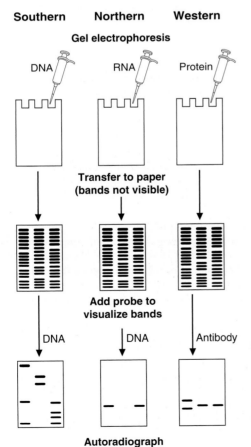

FIGURE 21-2 Southern, Northern, and Western blots. In Southern blots, DNA is electrophoresed, denatured with alkali, transferred to nitrocellulose paper ("blotted"), and hybridized with a DNA probe. In Northern blots, RNA is electrophoresed and hybridized with a DNA probe. (In this case, alkali is not used because RNA is already single stranded, and alkali would hydrolyze the RNA.) Western blots involve electrophoresis of proteins that are visualized by binding to antibodies. The nucleic acids and proteins can only be seen on the gel after the gel is treated with a labeled probe (i.e., labeled DNA or antibodies).

A. Terminates with ddATP

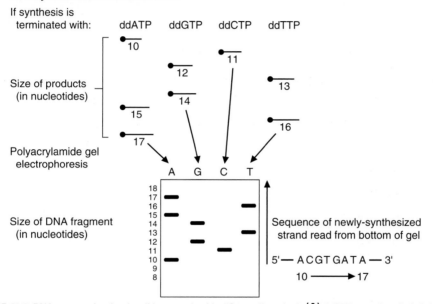

B. If synthesis is terminated with:

FIGURE 21-3 DNA sequencing by the dideoxynucleotide "Sanger" method. **(A)** A DNA template is hybridized with a primer. **(B)** DNA polymerase is added plus dATP, dGTP, dCTP, and dTTP. Either the primer or the nucleotides must have a radioactive label, so bands can be visualized on the gel by autoradiography. Samples are placed in each of four tubes, and one of the four dideoxyribonucleotides (ddNTPs) is added to each tube to cause random termination of DNA synthesis. Strands of different sizes are produced in each tube, electrophoresed, and visualized. The sequence of the newly synthesized strand is read from the bottom to the top of the gel.

    c. Because the dideoxynucleotide competes with the normal nucleotide for incorporation into the growing chain, **DNA chains of varying lengths are produced.** The shortest chains are nearest the 5′ end of the DNA chain (which grows 5′ to 3′).

    d. The sequence of the growing chain can be read (5′ to 3′) from the bottom to the top of the gel on which the DNA chains are separated.

  4. DNA microarrays or DNA chips produce a "genetic portrait" by screening for thousands of genes simultaneously. cDNAs or oligonucleotide probes for different genes are spotted or arrayed individually in high density on a glass slide or on nitrocellulose paper (as blots, described previously). Probes are hybridized to the microarray, and binding is quantified.

    a. Genotyping of **genomic DNA** can commence to detect mutations or polymorphisms.

    b. Gene expression uses **mRNA from two different sources** for a comparative analysis (e.g., normal versus cancerous tissue). mRNA is converted to cDNA, and each population of cDNA is labeled with a different fluorescent dye, mixed together, and hybridized to examine the relative abundance of genes.

CLINICAL		
CORRELATES		

CLINICAL CORRELATES   **DNA microarrays** can predict response to cancer treatment. Analysis of **chronic lymphocytic leukemia (CLL)** identifies genes associated with pathogenesis, and sensitivity or resistance to fludarabine or rituximab, two current treatments.

C. Techniques for amplifying DNA sequences

1. Polymerase chain reaction (PCR)
  a. PCR is a technique for rapidly producing large amounts of DNA (Figure 21-4).
  b. It is suitable for clinical or forensic testing because only small quantities of DNA are required as the starting material.

CLINICAL CORRELATES   **PCR** is used to detect **very-low-abundance nucleic acid transcripts. Human immunodeficiency virus (HIV),** with its long latency of infection, is difficult to test early after infection but can be detected with PCR. The 3–base pair deletion, the most common mutation in **cystic fibrosis,** is also easily detected.

2. Cloning of DNA (Figure 21-5)
  a. DNA from one organism ("foreign" DNA, obtained as described earlier) can be inserted into a DNA vector and used to transform cells from another organism, usually a bacterium, that grows rapidly, replicating the foreign DNA as well as its own.
  b. Large quantities of the foreign DNA can be isolated, or the DNA expressed, and its protein product can be obtained in large quantities.

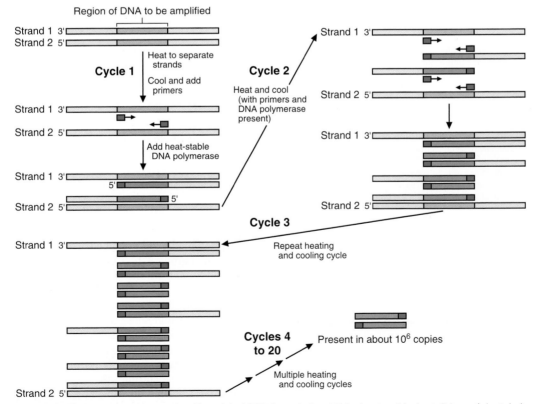

FIGURE 21-4 Polymerase chain reaction. The original DNA (strands 1 and 2) is denatured by heat. Primers (*short dark-green rectangles*) are added that bind to each DNA strand when the solution is cooled. A heat-stable DNA polymerase (Taq) is added, and polymerization is allowed to proceed. The *green areas* represent the regions that are replicated by extension of the primers. Heating and cooling cycles are repeated until the DNA is amplified many times.

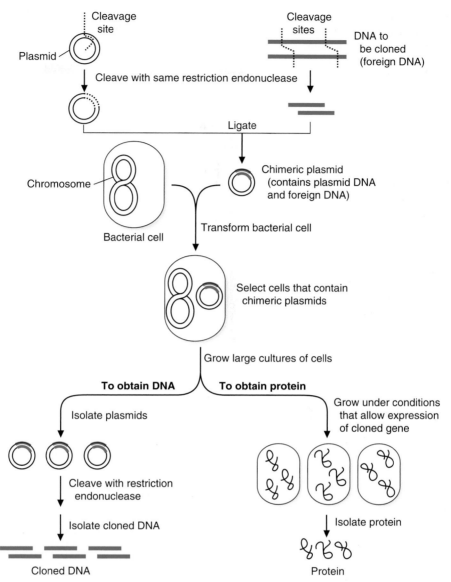

FIGURE 21-5 Cloning foreign DNA in bacteria. A vector for transferring foreign DNA into a bacterium, such as a plasmid, is cleaved with the same restriction endonuclease as the foreign DNA. The plasmid and foreign DNA, both cleaved by the same restriction enzyme, are mixed together and treated with DNA ligase. Some interactions produce chimeric plasmids, containing the foreign DNA integrated into the plasmid DNA. The plasmids are introduced into bacterial host cells (by transformation). Clones containing chimeric plasmid are selected and cultured. To obtain large quantities of the foreign DNA, the plasmids are isolated from cells and treated with the restriction enzyme to release the foreign DNA, which is then isolated. To obtain large quantities of the protein product of the foreign DNA, the cells are grown to promote synthesis of the protein, and the protein is isolated from the cells. The DNA used to express foreign proteins in bacterial cells must not contain introns because bacteria cannot remove them. Bacterial promoters must be inserted into the DNA so that the gene can be expressed.

D. Use of recombinant DNA techniques to detect polymorphisms

1. Humans differ in their genetic composition. **Polymorphisms** (variations in DNA sequence) occur frequently in the genome both in coding and in noncoding regions. Point mutations are simple polymorphisms, but insertions and deletions also occur.

CLINICAL CORRELATES Individual variations in DNA sequences among people occur at a frequency of about 1 per 1500 nucleotides. **Polymorphisms** are harmless, whereas **mutations** can be detrimental and are associated with a clinical disorder.

2. Restriction fragment length polymorphism (RFLP)

    a. Occasionally, a **mutation** occurs **in a restriction enzyme cleavage site** that is within or tightly linked to a gene.

        (1) The enzyme can cleave the normal DNA at this site, but not the mutant DNA.

        (2) Thus, two smaller restriction fragments will be obtained from this region of the normal DNA, compared with only one larger fragment from the mutant DNA.

CLINICAL CORRELATES   The classic **RFLP in prenatal disease screening** involves **sickle cell anemia.** A single nucleotide change (A → T) at codon 6 of β-globin results in a **Glu → Val** amino acid substitution, abolishing an *Mst*II restriction endonuclease site. A β-globin gene probe detects different *Mst*II restriction fragments. RFLP analysis detects both the affected and unaffected alleles.

---

    b. Sometimes, **a mutation creates a restriction site** not present in or near the normal gene. In this case, the mutant yields two smaller restriction fragments, and only one larger fragment will be obtained from the normal gene (Figure 21-6).

CLINICAL CORRELATES   RFLPs are considered alleles because they are heritable in a mendelian manner. **Huntington disease (HD)** is a progressive neurodegenerative disease with onset in the 40s. Before the human genome was sequenced, RFLP analyses identified an HD marker with appearance of two *Hind*III restriction sites.

---

    c. Normal human DNA has many regions that contain a highly **variable number of tandem repeats (VNTR).** The number of repeats differs from one individual to another (and from one allele to another).

        (1) Restriction enzymes that cleave on the flanks of VNTRs produce **DNA fragments of variable length.** The length depends on the number of repeats (Figure 21-7).

        (2) Fragments produced by various restriction enzymes from a number of different loci can be used to identify individuals; this is called **"DNA fingerprinting."**

CLINICAL CORRELATES   **DNA fingerprinting** is used legally to determine parentage or genealogy, or to implicate or free suspects in law enforcement investigations involving violent crimes. The combination of more than eight markers can exclude false suspects and can narrow positive suspects to a probability of a few billion to 1.

---

3. Single nucleotide polymorphisms (SNPs)

    a. SNPs are single bases in DNA differing in at least 1% of the population, occurring about once per gene, mostly in introns (noncoding).

    b. More than 99% do not change the amino acid sequence.

CLINICAL CORRELATES   An SNP in the ***APO-E* (apolipoprotein E)** gene is associated with an earlier onset of Alzheimer disease. Another SNP within the **chemokine-receptor gene *CCR-5*** leads to resistance to HIV and acquired immunodeficiency syndrome (AIDS).

---

4. Detection of mutations by allele-specific oligonucleotide probes

    a. An **oligonucleotide probe** is synthesized **complementary** to a region of DNA that contains a **mutation.** A different probe is made for the normal DNA (Figure 21-8).

    b. If a *mutant* probe binds to a DNA, the sample contains DNA from a *mutant* allele.

        (1) If the *normal* probe binds, the sample contains DNA from a *normal* allele.

        (2) If *both probes* bind, the sample contains DNA from both a mutant and a normal allele (i.e., the person providing the DNA sample is a carrier of the mutation).

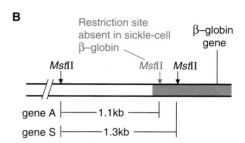

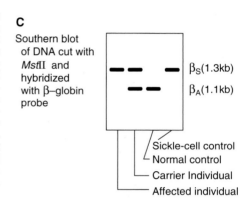

FIGURE 21-6 Restriction fragment length polymorphism is caused by loss of a restriction site. If a mutation occurs in a cleavage site for a restriction enzyme, the pattern of restriction fragments differs from normal. **(A)** The mutation that causes sickle cell anemia results in the loss of an MstII site in the β-globin gene. **(B)** Samples of DNA from individuals are treated with restriction endonucleases and then subjected to electrophoresis on gels. **(C)** With the Southern blot technique, the restriction fragments on the gel are hybridized with a radioactive cDNA probe for the β-globin gene. The sickle cell allele produces a fragment of 1.3 kilobases (kb) when treated with MstII. A normal allele produces a fragment of 1.1 kb (plus a fragment of 0.2 kb that is not seen on the gel). For a person with sickle cell disease, both alleles produce 1.3-kb restriction fragments. In a normal person, both alleles produce 1.1-kb fragments. For a carrier, both the 1.3- and 1.1-kb fragments are observed.

5. Testing for mutations by PCR
   a. An oligonucleotide complementary to a mutant region is used as a **primer for PCR.**
   b. If the primer binds to a DNA sample (i.e., if the sample contains the mutation), amplification of the DNA occurs (i.e., the primer is extended).
   c. If the primer does not bind, extension does not occur (i.e., the DNA is normal).

E. Alterations in the genetic composition of animals
   1. If a **gene** from another organism is **inserted into a blastocyst** (very early embryo) contributing to the germline (eggs or sperm), a **transgenic animal** can be produced with extra genetic material in every cell. The nucleus of the fertilized egg is then transplanted into the uterus of a foster female for development.

CLINICAL CORRELATES Apolipoprotein(a) [Apo(a)], when added to low-density lipoprotein (LDL), increases atherosclerosis risk associated with myocardial infarction, stroke, and restenosis. When fed an atherogenic diet, **Apo(a) transgenic mice developed lesions 15 times faster** than nontransgenic littermates. Mice with high levels of Apo(a) are a good model of atherosclerosis in humans.

   2. A special case of transgenesis, termed a **"knockout,"** inactivates a given gene in all cells, creating strains of animals that lack the protein product of the gene.

CLINICAL CORRELATES Knockout mice are models for human diseases. A **defective leptin or leptin receptor** gene yields animals with prodigious weight gain. Defects in metabolic pathways aid discovery of **causes of obesity** and testing possible drugs as treatments.

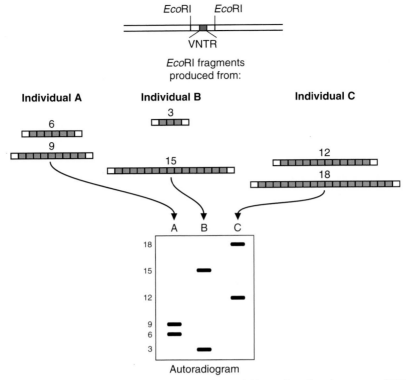

FIGURE 21-7 Restriction fragments produced from a gene with a variable number of tandem repeats (VNTR). DNA from three individuals, each with two alleles for this gene and a different number of repeats in each allele, was cleaved, electrophoresed, and treated with a probe for this gene. The length of the fragments depends on the number of repeats that they contain.

3. **RNA interference (RNAi)** is a precise process of mRNA degradation to **silence expression of a specific gene**.
   a. RNAi is mediated by a short 21- to 25–base pair, **double-stranded RNA** (dsRNA) recognizing an exact sequence functioning as a silencing complex. In evolution, this mechanism protects the host and its genome against viruses and rogue dsRNAs.
   b. RNA silencing has been adapted for roles in regulation of cell growth, death, differentiation, and oncogenesis using other small RNAs called **micro RNAs (miRNAs)**.

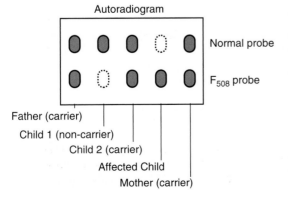

FIGURE 21-8 The use of oligonucleotide probes to test for cystic fibrosis (CF). Oligonucleotide probes complementary to the 3-base deletion located in the CF gene were synthesized. One probe binds only to the mutant (ΔF_{508}), and the other probe binds only to the normal region. DNA was isolated from individuals and amplified by polymerase chain reaction. Two spots were placed on nitrocellulose paper for each person. One spot was treated with the probe for the mutant region of the gene, and the other spot was treated with the probe for the normal region. *Dark spots* indicate binding of a probe. Only the normal probe binds to the DNA from a normal person, and only the mutant probe binds to the DNA from a person with CF. Both probes bind to DNA from a carrier. In carriers, one allele is normal and the other has the CF mutation.

    c. Silencing RNAs are being developed as therapeutics with clinical trials targeting the VEGF pathway involved in age-related macular degeneration, characterized by retinal neovascularization, fluid leakage, and scar tissue leading to central vision impairment.

F. Mapping of the human genome

    1. A massive effort was mounted to **sequence the entire** 3 billion base pairs of the **human genome,** culminating in 2001 with results expected to provide a better understanding of normal function and to elucidate specific defects resulting in inherited disease.

    2. There are only about **30,000 genes in the human genome,** less than the number in rice. Current drugs only target about 3% of the known genes.

G. Gene therapy (Figure 21-9)

    1. Transgenesis with humans could eliminate disease genes, but technical and ethical issues prevail regarding using human eggs.

    2. Some diseases have responded to efforts to introduce normal functioning genes into individuals with defective genes by introduction of the normal gene (**gene replacement**) in a viral vector to infect patient cells into production of the required protein.

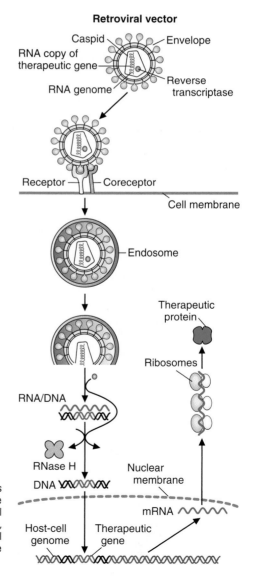

FIGURE 21-9 Use of retroviruses for gene therapy. The retrovirus carries an RNA copy of the therapeutic gene into the cell. The endosome that carries the virus dissolves, and the RNA and viral reverse transcriptase are released. This enzyme copies the RNA, making a double-stranded DNA that integrates into the host cell genome. Transcription and translation of this therapeutic gene produces the therapeutic protein. mRNA, messenger RNA.

CLINICAL CORRELATES An early success targets the X-linked autoimmune disease **severe combined immunodeficiency disease (SCID)**. The defective gene is corrected by retroviral delivery into hematopoietic cells by an interleukin receptor subunit and adenosine deaminase (ADA) in ADA-SCID. Other vectors for gene delivery have been developed.

H. Stem cells

1. These pluripotent cells can develop into many different cell types.
2. **Embryonic** stem cells are undifferentiated cells from an embryo with potential to become a variety of specialized cell types, whereas **adult** stem cells can differentiate to specialized cell types of the tissue from which it originated.

CLINICAL CORRELATES The potential for human stem cells is in **regenerative cell-based therapy**. The need for transplantable tissue outstrips supply. Stem cells are targeted to treat Parkinson disease, Alzheimer disease, spinal cord injury, diabetes, and heart disease.

I. Organismal cloning (Figure 21-10)

1. Organismal cloning produces **genetically identical offspring** to the animal being cloned.
2. This process removes the nucleus of an egg, replacing it with a diploid nucleus from the organism to be cloned. The egg is induced to divide and is placed in the uterus of a foster mother, where gestation occurs.

J. Pharmacogenomics or Personalized Medicine

1. Characterizing genetic variations in individuals to drug response, efficacy and side effects.
2. The major drug metabolizing enzymes are products of the cytochrome P-450 pathway, encoded by the *CYP* genes. People are characterized as extensive (normal) metabolizers, poor–intermediate metabolizers with reduced ability to clear or activate drugs, or ultra metabolizers who exhibit accelerated clearance or enhanced activation of drugs.

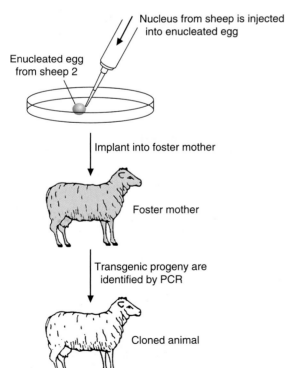

FIGURE 21-10 Organismal cloning of a mammal. PCR, polymerase chain reaction.

CLINICAL CORRELATES **Adverse drug reactions** are the fourth largest killer in the United States, with more than 100,000 deaths and more than 2 million severe reactions per year, and are the largest source of medical malpractice. More than 50% of the population have genetic variants in *CYP* genes affecting drug efficacy.

II. TECHNOLOGY INVOLVING PROTEINS

A. **Strategies for separating proteins**
    1. The **physical characteristics** that define a protein as a sum of all the properties of the **individual amino acids** are used for purifying proteins. This process of separation is done by various methods of **chromatography** (Table 21-1).
    2. Another way of separating proteins with different amino acid composition is by **application of an electric field** termed **electrophoresis** that exploits charge and size of proteins. Different variations are listed in Table 21-2.

B. **Techniques for detecting single proteins (diagnostics)**
    1. **Enzyme-linked immunosorbent assay** (ELISA) is based on antibody–antigen interactions.
        a. Antigens are precoated onto plastic plates. A primary antibody is used to bind to the antigens. If the primary antibody is human, an antihuman immunoglobulin G (IgG) is coupled to an enzyme as a second antibody, binding to human antibodies on the plate.
        b. A substrate (that changes color when cleaved by an enzyme) is added after the second antibody has bound to the plate for detection.

CLINICAL CORRELATES **ELISA** is commonly used as a **test to screen for HIV infection.** HIV antibodies are detected from blood, urine, or buccal washes. ELISA is not sensitive (false-negative) during the initial 3 to 4 weeks of infection or late in the disease when HIV-specific antibody production is low. A positive ELISA occurs 22 to 26 days after acute infection. False-positive results are also possible in multiparous women, people recently vaccinated for hepatitis or influenza, hematologic malignancies, multiple myeloma, alcoholic hepatitis, or primary biliary cirrhosis.

t a b l e **21-1** Chromatographic Techniques for Separating Biomolecules

Name	Separates by	Brief Description
Gel filtration	Size, mass	Apply protein mixture to porous beads. Big molecules are excluded first; small ones are retarded in column.
Ion exchange	Charge	Apply protein mixture to charged beads. Negatively charged proteins stick to positively charged beads. Negatively charged proteins come through. Conversely, positively charged proteins stick to negatively charged beads.
Affinity	Specific ligand	Specific ligands are bound to beads to extract protein from mixture (e.g., antibody to capture antigen, peptide to capture receptor, DNA to "catch" a transcription factor).
Liquid chromatography	Hydrophobicity or charge under pressure	Enhanced column chromatography Separate by size or hydrophobicity under high pressure. Peptides, small proteins, and pieces of DNA (can differentiate 1–base pair difference)

t a b l e 21-2	Electrophoresis Techniques for Separating Biomolecules	
Name	**Separates by**	**Brief Description**
DNA	Mass of DNA on agarose	A porous gel with an electric charge separates DNA by mass because there are uniform negatively charged phosphate groups
Native	Shape (radius)/protein mass; DNA by mass	For DNA, can resolve 1 base pair For proteins dependent on shape of protein and mass so that unfolded proteins can be separated from folded ones
SDS-PAGE	Mass of proteins	Sodium dodecyl sulfate–polyacrylamide gel electrophoresis Denature proteins, add SDS detergent to unfold protein, and place uniform negative charge Electric field separates by mass
Two-dimensional	Isoelectric point (pI) and mass of proteins	First, separate proteins by pI so they stop migrating where there is **no** net charge, and then apply to SDS-PAGE as above Resolves thousands of proteins for proteomics

2. **Western immunoblotting** (Figure 21-2) separates proteins by sodium dodecyl sulfate–polyacrylamide gel electrophoresis (SDS-PAGE) (Table 21-2) and transfers them to a membrane. Often, the membrane is cut into strips for testing patient samples for antibodies directed against the "blotted" protein (antigen).
   a. If antibodies are present directed against one or more of the blotted antigens, those antibodies will bind to the proteins, whereas other antibodies will be washed away.
   b. To detect bound antibodies, anti-IgG is coupled to a reporter, and after excess secondary antibody is washed free, a substrate is added with the conjugate, resulting in a visible band where the primary antibody bound to the protein.

CLINICAL CORRELATES   Western immunoblotting confirms **HIV infection and is more specific than ELISA**. Antibodies are visualized against each viral protein. HIV-infected cells are lysed, electrophoresed, and blotted onto a membrane. Membrane strips are incubated with the serum samples from each patient. If positive, it is confirmed by the presence of HIV viral proteins p24 or p31 *and* gp120 or gp160.

C. Strategies for determining protein structure
   1. **X-ray crystallography** provides a three-dimensional structure by "seeing" how atoms arrange in a protein dictated by their electron density distribution.
   a. Highly purified protein is crystallized and exposed to x-rays.
   b. The diffraction patterns are recorded and analyzed with computers to generate an electron density to fit the amino acid sequence. Energy minimization assures the chemical bonds are correct.

CLINICAL CORRELATES   Determining protein structure by x-ray crystallography aids in drug design. The tyrosine kinase product of bcr-abl is implicated in **chronic myelogenous leukemia** (CML). The **abl kinase inhibitors,** such as imatinib **(Gleevec),** were synthesized.

2. **Nuclear magnetic resonance (NMR)** is complementary to crystallography.
   a. The nuclei of some atoms (^{1}H, ^{13}C, ^{15}N) resonate at specific radiofrequencies, so when atoms are close (<0.5 nm), their distances in relation to secondary structure can be calculated. Although limited to smaller proteins (<45 kD), crystals are not required.
   b. NMR is performed in solution and can measure the dynamic movements of a protein.

3. **Mass spectrometry** measures mass-to-charge ratios of protein accurately and with miniscule amounts of sample to determine the total mass (molecular weight) and the amino acid sequence of a protein.

   a. This has replaced chemical sequencing by Edman degradation, although most protein sequence information comes from translation of gene sequences.

   b. Mass data are used to search sequence databases to identify proteins in a sample.

D. **Proteomics**

1. Proteomics refers to the **PROTE**in complement of the gen**OME,** the gene *products.* Unlike the genome, the proteome changes constantly depending on the physiologic state.

2. First, protein separation occurs by enrichment and two-dimensional gel electrophoresis (Table 21-2). After the proteins are separated, identification of the proteins and their modifications is accomplished by mass spectrometry (see section II.C.3).

3. Diversity and complexity of humans are not due to the genome but instead to the proteome and protein modifications because humans only have about 30,000 genes.

Review Test

Directions: Each of the numbered questions or incomplete statements in this section is followed by answers or by completions of the statement. Select the **one** lettered answer or completion that is **best** in each case.

1. A patient has a disease that leads to hyperexcretion of a protein in the urine. Which methodology is the fastest, easiest, and least expensive to determine the molecular weight of the native protein in the urine?

(A) Ion exchange chromatography
(B) Size exclusion chromatography
(C) X-ray crystallography
(D) NMR
(E) SDS-PAGE

2. An SNP in the coding region of a tumor-suppressor gene was recently discovered. Heterozygous individuals synthesize both the normal and mutant forms of this gene. The normal form codes for a leucine at a particular position within the protein; when the SNP is present, that codon is altered to code for an arginine. Although the SNP was identified at the nucleotide level, you wish to separate and characterize 10 μg of each of the proteins. Assuming you had a mixture of the two forms of the protein, what initial approach would you use to separate these two forms?

(A) Mass spectrometry
(B) X-ray crystallography
(C) NMR
(D) Ion exchange chromatography
(E) Affinity purification on a *KLF-6* polyclonal antibody column

3. A 42-year-old man presents to the emergency room and receives a neurologic consult for a slowly progressing chorea with some rigidity and seizures. These episodes have occurred in the past, and a deceased mother had choreic neurologic episodes and dementia. You suspect the patient might have Huntington disease, and the hospital has a laboratory equipped to perform RFLP analyses. Which of the following techniques is required to carry out RFLP analysis?

(A) Western blot
(B) Northern blot

(C) Southern blot
(D) X-ray crystallography
(E) Mass spectrometry

4. A patient you have been treating for Gaucher disease, a lysosomal storage disease, comes into your office wanting to have her relatives tested to determine whether they are carriers of the disorder. The most predominant β-glucosidase mutation, N370S, is expressed in this family. Wanting to do this in the most expeditious and least costly manner would require the use of which one of the following techniques?

(A) SNP assessment
(B) DNA sequencing
(C) Allele-specific oligonucleotide probe hybridization
(D) RLFP analysis
(E) DNA fingerprinting

5. Which is the best technique to separate oxygenated normal hemoglobin A (HbA) from oxygenated sickle cell hemoglobin (HbS), assuming no protein aggregation?

(A) Native gel electrophoresis
(B) SDS-PAGE
(C) Gel filtration
(D) Affinity chromatography with a C-terminal antibody
(E) Ultracentrifugation

6. A patient coming into an outpatient clinic for metabolic blood work has a portion of his blood subjected to ion exchange chromatography on a carboxymethyl cellulose column. The patient's serum profile indicates less protein is binding than in a normal blood sample. How might this be interpreted?

(A) Some serum proteins of the patient are deficient in sialic acid residues.
(B) Some serum proteins of the patient are deficient in glycosaminoglycan side chains.
(C) The patient's serum contains more negatively charged proteins than normal.

(D) Some serum proteins are deficient in a substituent identical to diethylaminoethyl cellulose.

(E) The patient has a silent mutation in a hemoglobin variant.

7. A PCR assay needs to be developed to determine the HIV status of a newborn in the pediatric intensive care unit whose mother is HIV positive. Which set of primers should be used for the assay?

(A) The primers should consist of antiparallel complements of two parts of a noninfected human genome.

(B) The primers should be designed so that, after annealing with potential infective DNA, the 5′ end of primer 1 would "face" the 3′ end of primer 2.

(C) The primers should be synthesized so that, after annealing with potential infective DNA, the 5′ end of both primers "face" each other.

(D) The primers should be designed to be synthesized with dideoxynucleotides to allow sequencing of the mutation.

(E) The primers should be designed with identical sequences to those in the HIV genome and must bind to DNA in a complementary, antiparallel manner.

8. A patient is referred to you by her obstetrician for genetic counseling for an apparent chromosomal microdeletion. To be able to test the heritability of this disorder by RFLP analyses, what is required?

(A) SDS gel electrophoresis to detect the gene product of normal and diseased individuals

(B) Mutations flanking restriction sites so the entire gene can be sequenced

(C) A unique single-stranded oligonucleotide that can be amplified by successive rounds of heating, cooling, and annealing

(D) Restriction sites closely linked to the mutation causing the disease

(E) Antibodies used with ribonucleotide probes for detection of the altered trait

9. A patient has come in for an HIV test. This test is run in two phases. The first test is an ELISA as a screen, and if two positive test results occur by ELISA, the second test will be run. The second test is a confirmatory Western blot. What do the ELISA and Western blots measure in their respective assays for HIV?

(A) The ELISA is measuring the presence of HIV antigen in the sera, whereas the Western blot is measuring the presence of antibodies to HIV proteins in the sera.

(B) The ELISA is measuring the presence of antibodies to HIV proteins in the sera only, whereas the Western blot is measuring the presence of HIV antigens in the sera.

(C) The ELISA is measuring the presence of HIV antigen in the sera, whereas the Western blot is measuring the presence of HIV antigen in the sera as well.

(D) The ELISA is measuring the presence of antibodies to HIV proteins in the sera only, whereas the Western blot is also measuring the presence of antibodies to HIV proteins in the sera.

(E) The ELISA measures the presence of antibodies directed against human leukocyte antigen (HLA) molecules to HIV, whereas the Western blot measures levels of free, circulating virus in the sera of the patient.

Answers and Explanations

1. **The answer is B.** Size exclusion (gel) chromatography separates proteins by mass. Ion exchange chromatography involves either anion or cation exchange for separating proteins with a net positive or negative charge. No information concerning the mass of a protein results from ion exchange chromatography. NMR spectra and x-ray crystallographic diffraction techniques require laborious effort and are not fast, easy, or inexpensive. SDS-PAGE does not yield the mass of a native protein because the proteins are denatured before being separated by size.

2. **The answer is D.** The key is isolation as well as detection. The change of leucine to arginine alters the charge properties of the protein (leucine has no charge on the side chain, whereas arginine has a +1 charge on the side chain at pH 7). This suggests that ion exchange chromatography, at the appropriate pH, can separate the two forms of the protein. Mass spectrometry can differentiate the masses but cannot obtain separated material for further analyses. Likewise, NMR and X-ray crystallography might detect a difference, but would not provide material for further studies. A polyclonal antibody would not differentiate the two forms, although a monoclonal antibody, if designed properly, might separate the forms. The polyclonal antibody would likely bind to both forms of the protein with equal affinity.

3. **The answer is C.** Because RFLP analyses involve DNA digested with restriction enzymes, and the fragments resolved by gel electrophoresis, a Southern blot needs to be performed to complete the RFLP study. A Western blot is performed on proteins separated by size, and a Northern blot is performed on RNA, also usually separated by size. Mass spectrometry could be used on the isolated protein, as could x-ray crystallography, but it is DNA that is being probed in this question.

4. **The answer is C.** Because the mutation is known and is due to a single nucleotide change, allele-specific oligonucleotides can be synthesized that differentiate between the normal and disease gene. By appropriately labeling the probes, and using stringent hybridization conditions, it can be determined which probe (or probes) will hybridize to sample DNA in a simple experiment. The experiment is to spot sample DNA on nitrocellulose and then probe the sample with the two available probes. If both probes bind to the sample, the patient is a carrier. DNA sequencing, RFLP analysis, and DNA fingerprinting involve electrophoresis on a gel-based material, which will require more time and expense. SNP assessment does not require gel electrophoresis, but the assays are more time-consuming than a simple hybridization experiment.

5. **The answer is A.** Because the difference between HbA and HbS is the sixth amino acid of the Hb β-chain (an E6V mutation), the difference in mass is very small, and separation based on charge will be able to differentiate between the two forms of hemoglobin. Native gel electrophoresis can accomplish this. SDS-PAGE blankets the protein with a uniform negative charge that will mask the inherent difference. Gel filtration and ultracentrifugation are not sensitive enough, and a C-terminal antibody will detect both forms because the difference between the two forms is manifest at the amino-terminal end of the protein.

6. **The answer is C.** A carboxymethyl cellulose column contains a negative charge and binds positively charged proteins. If fewer proteins in the patient's blood are binding to the column, the patient's blood contains either fewer positively charged proteins or an increased amount of negatively charged proteins compared with the normal case. Both sialic acid and glycosaminoglycans are negatively charged. Reducing the levels of both of these agents would increase protein binding to the column. Diethylaminoethyl cellulose is not found on proteins. A silent mutation does not change the charge distribution of a protein.

7. **The answer is E.** For the development of a PCR assay, one requires primers designed to hybridize to the specific HIV target (choice A is incorrect) that are complementary and antiparallel (choices B and C are excluded) and that require deoxyribonucleotides (not dideoxynucleotides,

so choice D is incorrect) because one wants continuous DNA synthesis to occur. If one examines appropriately designed primers, the 3′ ends face each other after hybridization to their respective templates.

8. **The answer is D.** Because a chromosomal microdeletion and subsequent RFLP analysis are based on DNA, the optimal detection is by a Southern blot after digestion with a restriction enzyme that cleaves on sites surrounding the location of the deletion. If a deletion is present, the restriction fragment will be smaller than if the deletion is not present. SDS-PAGE or antibodies will not detect the disorder at the DNA level. Gene sequencing is not required to detect microdeletions. A single-stranded oligonucleotide cannot be amplified by PCR.

9. **The answer is D.** Both an ELISA and Western blot detect host antibodies against HIV antigens. Neither detects the virus or antigens of the virus. Anti-HLA antibodies may be present, but the HIV test is not designed to measure them.

Comprehensive Examination

1. You have a patient who is undergoing workup for a genetic disorder. You receive the results of test that was ordered and the report states, "ΔF508 mutation—absence of the phenylalanine at this position on the protein." What is true about this patient's condition?

(A) The patient will have a positive sweat chloride test.
(B) This patient will develop or has Duchenne muscular dystrophy.
(C) There is a very high likelihood of Alzheimer disease with this mutation.
(D) This patient will develop Marfan syndrome.
(E) This patient has von Willebrand disease.

2. For the management of deep vein thrombi, heparin is a common medication given to patients with myocardial ischemia, derived from either acute coronary syndrome or disseminated intravascular coagulation. Which of the following is true about the structure of this glycosaminoglycan?

(A) It is composed with repeating disaccharide units.
(B) It is composed of a short, branched carbohydrate.
(C) It has NANA residues branching from a linear oligosaccharide chain.
(D) Its base unit is a member of the class of sialic acids.
(E) The structure is seen in ABO blood groups.

3. By what mechanism does digoxin help patients with congestive heart failure?

(A) Stimulates β_1 receptors on myocytes
(B) Decreases intracellular myocyte calcium levels
(C) Activates myocyte Na^+/K^+ ATPase
(D) Increases intracellular myocyte calcium levels
(E) Stimulates α_1 receptors on myocytes

4. In a patient with severe chronic obstructive pulmonary disease (COPD), COPD "flares" are common and result in an inability to ventilate. This leads to the accumulation of carbon dioxide in the body, a primary respiratory acidosis. Of the following mechanisms, which is the most important one for the management of acid-base status?

(A) $CO_2 + H_2O \Longleftrightarrow H_2CO_3 \Longleftrightarrow H^+ + HCO_3^-$
(B) $H^+ + NH_3 \Longleftrightarrow NH_4^+$
(C) $CH_3COOH \Longleftrightarrow CH_3COO^- + H^+$
(D) $H_2O \Longleftrightarrow H^+ + OH^-$
(E) $CH_3CHOHCOOH \Longleftrightarrow CH_3CHOHCOO^- + H^+$

5. A 57-year-old man with a long history of alcohol abuse comes to the emergency room with symptoms of confusion and heptomegaly on examination. The patient also has a flapping tremor at the wrist (asterixis). He is diagnosed with hepatic encephalopathy, which can be partially treated with a diet of branched-chain amino acids. Which of the following sets of amino acids would you suggest?

(A) Tryptophan, phenylalanine, tyrosine
(B) Aspartate, glutamate, asparagine
(C) Valine, leucine, isoleucine
(D) Glycine, alanine, serine
(E) Methionine, proline, cysteine

6. A 28-year-old man complains of a rash on his sun-exposed skin, diarrhea, and loss of balance. His urinalysis results are significant for an increase in neutral amino acids, and he is diagnosed with Hartnup disease. Which one of the following amino acids would have been found in the urine sample?

(A) Lysine
(B) Phenylalanine
(C) Arginine
(D) Histidine
(E) Glutamate

7. A 46-year-old longshoreman is brought to the emergency room with muscle twitching, spasms, and difficulty swallowing. Apparently, the cargo container he was unloading from Indonesia contained the rodenticide strychnine. Strychnine interferes with one of the functions of which of the following nonpolar, aliphatic amino acids?

(A) Tyrosine
(B) Asparagine
(C) Glycine
(D) Glutamate
(E) Lysine

8. A teenager presents to the emergency room (ER) 2 hours after an overdose of salicylic acid (aspirin). In an attempt to alkalinize the urine, the ER physician administers sodium bicarbonate, which results in salicylate anions becoming trapped within the renal tubule and preventing diffusion of the charged salicylate across the renal epithelium into the patient's systemic circulation. What is the ratio of secreted salicylate to trapped salicylate if the renal dialysate has a pH of 6, and the pKa of salicylic acid is about 3?

(A) 10,000:1
(B) 1000:1
(C) 100:1
(D) 1:100
(E) 1:1000

9. A man visits the emergency room with signs of severe dehydration: he is thirsty, has decreased skin turgor, is tachycardic, and is somnolent. According to the patient, he abruptly began to suffer from diarrhea this morning, which he describes as multiple bouts of watery diarrhea. You suspect *Vibrio cholerae* and begin volume resuscitation. By what biochemical mechanism does *Vibrio* lead to these clinical manifestations?

(A) Adenylate cyclase activation
(B) Phospholipase C activation
(C) Phosphodiesterase activation
(D) Tyrosine kinase receptor activation
(E) Serine-threonine kinase activation.

10. A 16-year-old African-American girl comes to the emergency room with complaints of painful muscle cramps. She states that she has sickle cell anemia and that she ran out of her pain medication. A complete blood count and smear rapidly confirm the diagnosis, and she is started on intravenous fluids and pain medications. The molecular defect underlying her disease is which of the following?

(A) A valine rather than a glutamate at position 6 of the β-globin protein
(B) A glutamate rather than a valine at position 6 of the β-globin protein
(C) A valine rather than a glutamine at position 6 of the α-globin protein

(D) A glutamine rather than a valine at position 6 of the α-globin protein
(E) Expansion of a polyglutamine repeat within the β-globin gene

11. A young girl presents to the physician's office for a sports physical before participation in volleyball. She appears to have a perfect habitus for the sport because she is much taller than her peers and has exceptionally long arms and fingers. Auscultation of her heart reveals a midsystolic click. The physician suspects she may have Marfan syndrome, which is a defect in which of the following proteins?

(A) Myosin heavy chain
(B) Spectrin
(C) Ankyrin
(D) Fibrillin
(E) Collagen

12. A 47-year-old woman passes out at work and is brought to the emergency room. Her blood sugar is 24 mg/dL (normal, >70 mg/dL). After her sugar is corrected, she is able to tell you that she has had previous similar episodes and has been dealing with palpitations, one isolated seizure, and bouts of confusion, amnesia, and unconsciousness. Her C-peptide levels are much higher than normal. What is a possible cause of this woman's state?

(A) Anorexia
(B) High-protein diet
(C) Exogenous administration of insulin
(D) Insulin-secreting islet cell tumor
(E) High-glucose diet

13. In 1795, the British navy began to dispense limes during long sea voyages (hence the name "limeys" for British sailors), a measure that was largely successful in preventing scurvy. Scurvy is a condition characterized by general weakness, anemia, gum disease (gingivitis), and skin hemorrhages resulting from a lack of ascorbic acid (vitamin C) in the diet. Ascorbic acid plays a crucial role in which of the following processes in collagen synthesis?

(A) Transcription
(B) Glycosylation
(C) Hydroxylation
(D) Covalent cross-linkage
(E) C-peptide cleavage

14. A social worker refers a 2-year-old child to the physician because of suspected child abuse. On physical examination, the child has blue sclerae and diminished hearing in both ears, and radiographs of the child's extremities show subacute healing long bone fractures. The child is diagnosed with osteogenesis imperfecta. This disorder results from a defect in the synthesis of which of the following proteins?

(A) Transthyretin
(B) Calcitonin
(C) Spectrin
(D) β-Mysosin heavy chain
(E) Collagen

15. An 18-year-old boy works in the circus as a contortionist because of his hypermobile joints that allow for abnormal flexibility. He also has increased elasticity of his skin and bruises easily. This is a typical presentation of Ehlers-Danlos syndrome, resulting from a defect in collagen. Ehlers-Danlos type VI results from a lysyl oxidase deficiency. Which of the following processes will therefore be impaired in this disorder?

(A) Transcription
(B) Glycosylation
(C) Hydroxylation
(D) Covalent cross-linkage
(E) Secretion into the extracellular space

16. A 24-year-old bride prepares for her wedding day. After her manicure and pedicure, her hairdresser uses rollers to create a new style for her hair. To create a "permanent wave," the stylist applies thioglycollate to break apart the –S–S– bonds in the cystine units, reducing them to –SH groups. Which level of protein structure is most greatly affected by this treatment?

(A) Primary structure
(B) Secondary structure
(C) Supersecondary structure
(D) Tertiary structure
(E) α-Helix formation

17. Isoniazid is used in the treatment of tuberculosis but is is metabolized differently by different groups of patients. In comparing two groups of patients, the primary isozyme for metabolizing the drug was found to have a similar K_m, but there is was a threefold difference in V_{max} between the two isozymes. What are the clinical implications of the kinetic properties of these two isozymes?

(A) Patients with the lower V_{max} require lower doses.
(B) Patients with the lower V_{max} require higher doses.

(C) Patients with the higher V_{max} require lower doses.
(D) Patients with the lower V_{max} that are given higher doses have reduced toxicity.
(E) Drug toxicity is not related to V_{max}.

18. Different tissues use different isozymes to phosphorylate glucose. Both glucokinase (K_m = 10 mM) and hexokinase (K_m = 0.10 mM) convert glucose to glucose 6-phosphate. Which of the following is a correct statement based on the kinetic properties of these two enzymes?

(A) Hexokinase will metabolize 100 times more glucose molecules per second than will glucokinase.
(B) Hexokinase will lower the energy of activation of the reaction more than glucokinase.
(C) Hexokinase will have a higher V_{max} than glucokinase.
(D) Hexokinase will reach V_{max} at a lower glucose concentration than glucokinase.
(E) Glucokinase will metabolize 100 times more glucose molecules per second than will hexokinase.

19. An 8-year-old girl presents with precocious puberty, short stature, and large macules the color of coffee with milk. Further history finds the patient to have McCune-Albright syndrome, a result of estrogen production due to the production of excess aromatase from ovarian follicular cysts. As a research project, you synthesize a compound that inhibits aromatase in order to treat the precocious puberty component of her illness. The results of kinetic experiments using aromatase and the inhibitor are presented below.

[Substrate] with Inhibitor	Rate of Reaction (mol/L/s)	[Substrate] without Inhibitor	Rate of Reaction (mol/L/s)
5 mM	5×10^{-7}	5 mM	8×10^{-7}
10 mM	0.5×10^{-6}	10 mM	1.2×10^{-6}
20 mM	1.0×10^{-6}	20 mM	1.8×10^{-6}
40 mM	1.6×10^{-6}	40 mM	1.9×10^{-6}
80 mM	2.0×10^{-6}	80 mM	2.0×10^{-6}

Which answer choice best describes the type of inhibition being observed?

(A) Competitive
(B) Noncompetitive
(C) Uncompetitive
(D) Feedback
(E) There is no inhibition observed.

20. You are in the laboratory and are trying to understand the interaction between lovastatin and HMG-CoA reductase. Analyses reveal that the V_{max} of the reductase is unchanged in the absence or presence of the statin, yet the K_m is increased. Lovastatin is most likely functioning as which of the following?

(A) Competitive inhibitor
(B) Noncompetitive inhibitor
(C) Feedback inhibitor
(D) Allosteric activator
(E) Irreversible inhibitior

21. A 19-year-old woman is running on a treadmill. Exercise increases her respiratory quotient. Which of the following statements is correct concerning the respiratory quotient?

(A) It is higher for fat than carbohydrate.
(B) It is higher for protein than carbohydrate.
(C) It is the ratio of CO_2 produced to O_2 utilized during substrate oxidation.
(D) It is increased in exercise due to enhanced fat metabolism.
(E) It is increased in exercise due to enhanced amino acid metabolism.

22. A 25-year-old man is intubated in the intensive care unit. He is being treated for an overwhelming infection. Through a gastric tube, he is being fed proteins that are broken down to amino acids. When his dietary nitrogen intake exceeds his excreted nitrogen, this is most accurately called which of the following?

(A) Negative nitrogen balance
(B) Positive nitrogen balance
(C) Nitrogen balance
(D) Biosynthesis
(E) An anabolic state

23. A 33-year-old nonalcoholic man is referred to a gastroenterologist for the management of a newly diagnosed α_1-antitrypsin deficiency from a liver biopsy. This enzyme normally inhibits the enzyme elastase but also will inhibit trypsin. Trypsin will cleave proteins at which of the following sites?

(A) The carboxyl side of arginine or lysine
(B) The carboxyl side of aromatic amino acids
(C) The carboxyl side of uncharged amino acids
(D) Aromatic amino acids found at the carboxy terminus
(E) Basic amino acids found at the carboxy terminus

24. A 27-year-old woman with end-stage cystic fibrosis has lost the function of her pancreas. Absorption of which of the following vitamins will not be affected by the loss of pancreatic exocrine function?

(A) Vitamin C
(B) Vitamin A
(C) Vitamin D
(D) Vitamin E
(E) Vitamin K

25. A 23-year-old man develops steatorrhea, weight loss, and a bloody diarrhea. He notes that the diarrhea is worse when he eats breads or cereals. A gastroenterologist performs a biopsy during a colonoscopy, which reveals celiac disease. This disorder is most directly due to which of the following?

(A) Excess lipids in the feces
(B) Deficiency of enterokinase
(C) Defective transport of the amino acid cystine
(D) A defect in the transport of neutral amino acids
(E) Hypersensitivity to the protein gluten

26. A patient comes for an annual check-up with his pediatrician. He has pyruvate kinase deficiency with the typical manifestations, including occasional anemia, a severe episode requiring a blood transfusion, and some symmetric growth delay. Which of the following statements is correct concerning this disorder?

(A) The defect primarily affects erythrocytes and results in cell membrane alterations and splenic sequestration.
(B) Pyruvate kinase deficiency is an autosomal dominant disorder.
(C) Pyruvate kinase deficiency is the most common cause of enzyme deficiency–induced hemolytic anemia.
(D) Clinical manifestations are the result of decreased plasma bilirubin.
(E) In severe forms, erythrocytes must rely on aerobic mechanisms to create adenosine triphosphate (ATP).

27. An 84-year-old woman is in the medical intensive care unit because of septic shock. Her underlying source is pneumonia, and she is doing poorly because of advanced metabolic acidosis. Her laboratory results reveal a lactate of 12.3 (>5 indicates a severe acidosis, normal lactate is ≤ 1 mM), and the values are increasing with each assay. Which of the following statements is true concerning high lactate states?

(A) It reflects a state in which there is a high NADH/NAD$^+$ ratio.

(B) When lactate is high, respiratory compensation is seen with a decrease in the respiratory rate.

(C) High lactate indicates an increased responsiveness to catecholamines.

(D) Lactate cannot be converted to glucose.

(E) Treatment for high lactate includes decreased ventilation.

28. A 58-year-old man is taken to the emergency room after being poisoned with arsenic. Arsenic has several harmful effects, including forming an inactivating complex with α-lipoic acid in pyruvate dehydrogenase. As a result of this poisoning, how many ATP equivalents will the oxidation of glucose yield within the muscle, under aerobic conditions?

(A) 1
(B) 2
(C) 4
(D) 5
(E) 6

29. A child presents with developmental delay of verbal milestones, intermittent ataxia, poor muscle tone, abnormal eye movements, and seizures. The mother notes worsening of these symptoms with exertion. You are concerned that the child has pyruvate dehydrogenase complex deficiency. Which one of the following is true about this disorder?

(A) The patient is unable to form acetyl coenzyme A (CoA) from carbohydrate precursors.

(B) Clinical sequelae are related to an excessive production of citrate.

(C) Underlying neuropathology is usually observed in individuals whose onset is in childhood.

(D) Presentation and progression are predictable and uniform once the diagnosis is confirmed.

(E) An absence of compensatory anaerobic metabolism is seen under low oxygen conditions.

30. A 2-month-old presents to the pediatrician for follow-up care. The child appears abnormal, and the mother states that the baby was small for gestational age and is developing much differently than her other children. The child has difficulty sleeping at night and is frequently short of breath during the day.

In addition, the mother states that the child exhibits abnormal eye movements and does not respond to visual stimuli. On examination, the baby has poor muscle tone, has microcephaly, and is hyperventilating. You suspect a defect in pyruvate carboxylase. Which of the following is true about this disorder?

(A) It is an X-linked disorder.

(B) Clinical sequelae are related to an excessive production of citrate.

(C) Morbidity and mortality can be corrected with early medical intervention.

(D) The patient has an inability to form oxaloacetate from carbohydrates.

(E) Compensatory anaerobic metabolism is absent under low oxygen conditions.

31. An elderly homeless man is brought in by EMS because he was found unresponsive in a cold basement. It's the middle of winter, and according to bystanders, he recently resorted to a wood stove to provide him some relief from the cold. On examination, he exhibits sinus tachycardia (a value of 124, with normal between 60 and 100), displays a pulse oximetry reading of 100% oxygen saturation, is disoriented to person/place/time, and is yelling that his head hurts. You obtain laboratory tests, including an arterial blood gas with co-oximetry, and his carbon monoxide level is 23%. What is the pathophysiology of carbon monoxide toxicity?

(A) Binds to and inhibits ATP synthase activity

(B) Binds to and inhibits the cytochrome oxidase complex

(C) Uncouples oxidative phosphorylation

(D) Binds to and inhibits the ATP-ADP antiportor

(E) Complexes with NADH dehydrogenase and inhibits its activity

32. Which statement is true of glycogen in humans?

(A) Glycogen is a minor form of glucose storage.

(B) Linkages between glucose residues are α-1,4 and α-1,6 at branch points.

(C) Glycogen degradation produces glucose 3-phosphate as its major product.

(D) Glycogen stores in muscle are used to directly form GTP.

(E) Glycogen is formed from fatty acids or glucose.

33. A 3-year-old child presents to the pediatrician for failure to thrive. A workup including an ultrasound of his liver shows cirrhosis. A biopsy of the liver demonstrates a deficiency of glucosyl 4:6 transferase. Which of the following is the most likely glycogen storage disease (GSD) that affects this child?

(A) Type I: von Gierke disease
(B) Type II: Pompe disease
(C) Type III: Cori disease
(D) Type IV: Andersen disease
(E) Type V: McArdle disease

34. An infant was brought into the emergency room after her parents witnessed her having a seizure. The child's blood glucose was 28 mmol/L. After a thorough workup, a glycogen storage disease (GSD) is suspected, and a muscle biopsy is significant for the accumulation of dextrin, a form of glycogen in which the branches only contain a few glucose molecules. Which of the following GSDs is most likely the cause of the hypoglycemia and subsequent seizure?

(A) Type I: von Gierke disease
(B) Type II: Pompe disease
(C) Type III: Cori disease
(D) Type IV: Andersen disease
(E) Type V: McArdle disease

35. A 24-year-old student is training for the track and field events at her college. She presents to her physician with complaints of severe muscle cramps and weakness when training. Muscle biopsy demonstrates glycogen accumulation, liver biopsy is unremarkable, and laboratory tests indicate a deficiency of myophosphorylase (muscle glycogen phosphorylase). Which of the following is the most likely diagnosis?

(A) Andersen disease
(B) Cori disease
(C) McArdle disease
(D) von Gierke disease
(E) Hers disease

36. Which statement regarding glucagon is true?

(A) A high-carbohydrate meal will cause blood glucagon levels to increase.
(B) A high-protein meal will cause blood glucagon levels to decrease.
(C) A high-carbohydrate meal will cause blood glucagon levels to decrease.

(D) Tumors of the β cells of the pancreas are called glucagonomas.
(E) Glucagon secretion is decreased with cholecystokinin.

37. A 56-year-old, newly diagnosed type 2 diabetic patient fails an initial attempt at controlling her diabetes with dietary measures alone. She follows up with her family physician, who starts her on a sulfonylurea. This drug works through which of the following mechanisms?

(A) Stimulating the production of GLUT-2
(B) Stimulating the synthesis of new insulin
(C) Antagonizing the effects of arginine on pancreatic β cells
(D) Inhibiting the release of glucagon
(E) Stimulating the release of preformed insulin

38. A 4-month-old boy presents with frequent episodes of weakness, accompanied by sweating and feelings of dizziness. Physical examination is remarkable for palpably enlarged liver and kidneys. Laboratory tests reveal hypoglycemia and lactic acidemia. The patient is diagnosed with an enzyme deficiency of glucose 6-phosphatase, which is normally only expressed in which of the following?

(A) Liver and muscle
(B) Liver and brain
(C) Liver and kidney
(D) Erythrocytes
(E) Liver and adipose tissue

39. A 14-year-old high school girl who is extremely conscious about her appearance has gone a full day without eating. She hopes by the day of her school dance to fit into a dress she intentionally bought a size too small. Which of the following organs contributes to the glucose that is being synthesized through gluconeogenesis?

(A) Spleen
(B) Red blood cells
(C) Skeletal muscle
(D) Liver
(E) Brain

40. A newborn infant is found to have persistent hypoglycemia despite increased feeding intervals. The child is also irritable with a moderate degree of hepatomegaly. He is found to have normal levels of muscular fructose 1,6-bisphosphatase but decreased levels of the hepatic isoform. Which of the following statements is true of fructose 1,6-bisphosphatase?

(A) Its synthesis is induced by adenosine monophosphate (AMP).
(B) Its synthesis is induced by insulin.
(C) It is inhibited by fructose 2,6-bisphosphate.
(D) Its synthesis is induced in the fed state.
(E) Its synthesis is inhibited during fasting.

41. Which glucose derivative is found in high levels in seminal fluid?

(A) Sorbitol
(B) Fructose
(C) Glycogen
(D) Glucose
(E) Lactose

42. A 23-year-old woman gives birth to a healthy baby and plans on breast-feeding. Prolactin is an important hormone for the synthesis of milk in the breast because it stimulates the synthesis of α-lactalbumin. The function of this protein is to do which of the following?

(A) Convert galactose to galactitol
(B) Lower the K_m of galactosyl transferase for glucose
(C) Add galactose for the glycosylation of proteins
(D) Reduce oxidized glutathione
(E) Form fructose from sorbitol

43. A 5-year-old child presents with Hurler syndrome, which is characterized by dwarfism, hunchback, coarse facies, mental retardation, clouding of the cornea, and sensorineural deafness. The patient also has organomegaly due to the accumulation of which of the following?

(A) Glucocerebroside
(B) Sphingolipids
(C) Heparan sulfate and dermatan sulfate
(D) Glycogen
(E) Galactose 1-phosphate

44. A 75-year-old man presents to his doctor with significant knee pain. He is a former plumber who spent years on his knees and is also an avid tennis player. X-rays demonstrate osteoarthritis, and the patient is considering knee replacement surgery. Which synovial fluid component is important to provide "cushioning" in joints?

(A) Glycosaminoglycans
(B) N-acetylgalactosamine

(C) Dolichol phosphates
(D) Sphingolipids
(E) Collagen

45. A 58-year-old man with a 30-year history of heavy drinking presents with confusion, unstable gait, and nystagmus. On the Mini Mental State Examination, he scores 21/30, and a diagnosis of Wernicke-Korsakoff syndrome is made. Which of the patient's enzymes is working at a reduced activity level due to the patient's condition?

(A) Transaldolase
(B) Phosphopentose isomerase
(C) Transketolase
(D) Phosphopentose epimerase
(E) Glucose 6-phosphate dehydrogenase

46. A 24-year-old man is brought to the emergency room with multiple gunshot wounds. He is rushed immediately to the operating room because of intractable hypotension. His blood type was determined to be B negative, and blood products were ordered. Which of the following carbohydrate units will be found on the reducing end of his red blood cell surface proteins?

(A) N-acetylgalactosamine
(B) N-acetylglucosamine
(C) Galactose
(D) Glucose
(E) Fructose

47. A 2-year-old child is brought for evaluation for developmental delay, mental retardation, and abnormal bleeding. After a thorough workup by a pediatric geneticist, the child is found to have a congenital disorder of N-linked oligosaccharides. Which of the following substances is involved in the synthesis of N-linked glycoproteins?

(A) α-Mannosidase
(B) α-Lactalbumin
(C) Thiamine pyrophosphate
(D) α-Fucosidase
(E) Dolichol phosphate

48. What enzyme deficiency leads to classic galactosemia?

(A) Lactase
(B) Glucose 6-phosphate dehydrogenase
(C) Galactokinase deficiency
(D) Galactose 1-phosphate uridyltransferase
(E) UDP-glucose epimerase

49. Which statement is true regarding pancreatitis?

(A) Grey-Turner and Cullen signs are common findings.
(B) Surgery is a mainstay of treatment.
(C) Gallstones and scorpion bites are not risk factors.
(D) Advanced pancreatitis leads to hypercalcemia.
(E) Hypertriglyceridemia is a cause of pancreatitis, especially with levels higher than 1000 mg/dL.

50. A 53-year-old man presents with xanthomas under his eyes, hepatomegaly, and a triglyceride level almost 8 times the upper limit of normal at 1500 mg/dL. He is diagnosed with type V hyperlipidemia. In which tissue are triacylglycerols primarily synthesized?

(A) Skeletal muscle
(B) Heart muscle
(C) Liver
(D) Spleen
(E) Blood cells

51. A 50-year-old alcoholic man presents with a ruddy face, distended abdomen, and enlarged, fatty liver. Both the liver and adipose tissue can synthesize triglyceride. Which of the following reactions is liver specific for triglyceride synthesis?

(A) Glucose to DHAP
(B) Glycerol to glycerol 3-phosphate
(C) DHAP to glycerol 3-phosphate
(D) Phosphatidic acid to diacylglycerol
(E) Fatty acid to fatty acyl CoA

52. A 40-year-old woman presents with pain in her legs that is elicited upon walking and relieved by rest. Imaging reveals that diffuse atherosclerosis is causing her leg pain. She is found to have no functional apoprotein C-II. Which of the following will be elevated in this patient's blood?

(A) Cholesterol esters
(B) Chylomicrons
(C) LDL
(D) HDL
(E) Cholesterol

53. A 5-year-old boy presents with altered mental status, heart failure, and muscle weakness. His serum levels of ketones and glucose are abnormally low. He is diagnosed with primary carnitine deficiency. What is the primary problem with this disorder?

(A) Activation of fatty acids
(B) Impaired transport of long-chain fatty acids
(C) β-Oxidation
(D) ω-Oxidation
(E) α-Oxidation

54. An infant presents with difficulty moving his limbs, facial abnormalities, and seizures. His blood level of very-long-chain fatty acids is abnormally elevated, and he is diagnosed with Zellweger syndrome. Which of the following is true concerning the oxidation of very-long-chain fatty acids?

(A) Initially occurs in mitochondria
(B) Oxidation occurs at the α-carbon
(C) Produces acetyl CoA
(D) Generates no reduced cofactors
(E) Degraded three carbons at a time

55. A 38-year-old woman is found to have an obstructing gallstone in the common bile duct. What is clinical implication of this obstruction?

(A) Increased formation of chylomicrons
(B) Increased recycling of bile salts
(C) Increased excretion of bile salts
(D) Increased conjugation of bile salts
(E) Increased excretion of fat in the feces

56. A 60-year-old woman had an episode of chest pain radiating to her left arm, which was diagnosed as a myocardial infarction. She was prescribed a statin medication. How does statin treatment lower cholesterol and LDL levels?

(A) It inhibits the rate-limiting step in cholesterol biosynthesis.
(B) It increases synthesis of bile salts to digest cholesterol.
(C) It increases the serum level of HDL.
(D) It inhibits formation of LDL from IDL.
(E) It inhibits synthesis of LDL receptors.

57. A 40-year-old man presents with severe claudication secondary to atherosclerotic plaques in the arteries of his legs. His laboratory tests indicate high levels of cholesterol and LDL. Which of the following is the precursor of LDL?

(A) IDL
(B) Cholesterol
(C) Cholesterol esters
(D) HDL
(E) Chylomicrons

58. Which statement correctly describes a role of HDL?

(A) It is the largest of the lipoproteins, and it eliminates cholesterol esters and triacylglycerol from the serum.

(B) It carries triglyceride from tissue to tissue.

(C) It transports free fatty acids throughout the body.

(D) It serves as a shuttle for cholesterol from the periphery to the liver for metabolism.

(E) It carries amino acids from tissue to tissue.

59. A 15-year-old girl presents with severe menstrual cramping, caused by increased prostaglandin production. Prostaglandins are synthesized most directly from which of the following?

(A) Arachidonic acid
(B) Glucose
(C) Acetyl CoA
(D) Oleic acid
(E) Leukotrienes

60. An 18-year-old girl presents with a lack of secondary sexual characteristics, such as age-appropriate pubic hair growth and breast development. Her history reveals she has never started menses. She is diagnosed with 17-α-hydroxylase deficiency. The levels of various steroid hormones in her serum are found to be abnormal. Steroid hormones are most directly derived from which one of the following?

(A) Acetyl CoA
(B) Cholesterol
(C) Fatty acids
(D) Glucose
(E) Oleic acid

61. A 52-year-old man takes a daily 81-mg aspirin for cardioprotective purposes. Aspirin will inactivate a key enzyme in platelets for which length of time?

(A) 24 hours
(B) Permanently
(C) 12 hours
(D) 48 hours
(E) 72 hours

62. A 1-year-old infant's arms and legs have become spastic and rigid. Analysis shows an abnormally low level of sphingomyelinase activity, causing accumulation of sphingomyelin. Which of the following substrates combine to directly form sphingomyelin?

(A) Serine and palmitoyl CoA
(B) Fatty acyl CoA and sphingosine
(C) Palmitoyl CoA and ceramide
(D) Phosphatidylcholine and ceramide
(E) UDP-galactose and ceramide

63. In the nursery, an infant with blond hair and blue eyes is noted to have a mousy odor to his urine upon diaper changes. As is mandated by the state, all infants are screened for multiple inborn errors of metabolism, and he is found to have phenylketonuria (PKU). The cells of this child are unable to convert phenylalanine to which one of the following?

(A) Tyrosine
(B) Serine
(C) Glycine
(D) Cysteine
(E) Alanine

64. A 45-year-old woman presents with severe dehydration and decreased urine output. Her blood urea nitrogen level is abnormally elevated because her kidneys are not able to properly excrete urea in the urine. Which of the following is an important molecule in urea synthesis?

(A) Serine
(B) Glutamate
(C) Proline
(D) Ornithine
(E) Leucine

65. Which statement is true regarding the excretion of nitrogenous products?

(A) Ninety percent of urea excretion occurs by the liver.

(B) Ninety percent of urea excretion occurs by the kidneys.

(C) Correctly measuring the kidney's functional ability to excrete nitrogenous wastes is difficult.

(D) There is no link between the urea cycle and the TCA cycle.

(E) Liver urea synthesis is not inducible.

66. A 16-year-old girl is found by her parents on the bathroom floor unconscious. There is an empty bottle of acetaminophen in the toilet. She is rushed to the hospital, where she is given several doses of *N*-acetylcysteine. Acetaminophen overdose is potentially life-threatening because it depletes cellular stores of which substance?

(A) Nitric oxide
(B) Histamine
(C) Creatine
(D) Glutathione
(E) Serotonin

67. A 43-year-old man with a long history of poorly controlled hypertension presents to the emergency room with a severe headache. His blood pressure is found to be dramatically elevated at 250/148 mm Hg. Which of the following products, derived from amino acids, can be employed to treat his hypertension?

(A) Melanin
(B) Nitric oxide
(C) GABA
(D) Dopamine
(E) Serotonin

68. A 56-year-old woman develops diarrhea, flushing, wheezing, and a heart murmur. A computed tomography (CT) scan of the abdomen demonstrates a mass in the ileum along with multiple metastatic liver lesions. A biopsy reveals a diagnosis of a carcinoid tumor and displays elevated levels of the serotonin metabolite, 5-hydroxyindole acetic acid (5-HIAA). Serotonin is normally produced from which amino acid?

(A) Tyrosine
(B) Arginine
(C) Histidine
(D) Glycine
(E) Tryptophan

69. A 59-year-old woman develops a shuffling gait and a pill-rolling tremor. She is referred to a neurologist for evaluation. After a thorough workup, a diagnosis of Parkinson disease is made, and the patient is placed on a monoamine oxidase inhibitor (MAOI). The drug is given to Parkinson patients to decrease the degradation of which of the following?

(A) Serotonin
(B) Nicotinamide
(C) 5-HIAA
(D) Endothelium-derived relaxation factor (EDRF)
(E) Dopamine

70. A 12-year-old boy develops convulsions and is referred to a neurologist. After running an electroencephalogram (EEG), it is determined that the child has epilepsy. He is started on a benzodiazepine, which stimulates GABA

activity. GABA is derived from its precursor amino acid via which one of the following types of reactions?

(A) Deamination
(B) Decarboxylation
(C) Hydroxylation
(D) Iodination
(E) Methylation

71. A 63-year-old woman reports a long history of joint pain. Her fingers are severely deformed secondary to rheumatoid arthritis. Upon visiting a rheumatologist, she is started on methotrexate. This drug inhibits which of the following conversions?

(A) Dopamine to norepinephrine
(B) Tyrosine to dopa
(C) Dihydrofolate to tetrahydrofolate
(D) Histamine to formiminoglutamate (FIGLU)
(E) Norepinephrine to vanillylmandelic acid

72. A 5-year-old boy presents with mental retardation and self-mutilation. Blood tests show an elevated uric acid level. He is diagnosed with Lesch-Nyhan syndrome, a disease caused by a defect in hypoxanthine-guanine phosphoribosyl transferase (HGPRT). HGPRT is most significant in which of the following pathways?

(A) Purine synthesis
(B) Purine salvage
(C) Purine degradation
(D) Pyrimidine synthesis
(E) Pyrimidine degradation

73. An infant presents with recurrent infections and a markedly decreased lymphocyte count. Elevated levels of adenosine and deoxyadenosine are found in the serum. X-ray shows the virtual absence of a thymic shadow. The defective reaction in this disease is which one of the following?

(A) AMP to adenosine
(B) Adenosine to inosine
(C) Guanosine to guanine and ribose 1-phosphate
(D) Inosine to hypoxanthine and ribose 1-phosphate
(E) Hypoxanthine to xanthine

74. An infant presents with developmental delay, muscle weakness, and anemia. Urine analysis reveals a high level of excreted orotic acid. Ammonia levels are normal in this patient.

In which of the following pathways is this disease manifest?

(A) Purine synthesis
(B) Purine degradation
(C) Purine salvage
(D) Pyrimidine synthesis
(E) Pyrimidine degradation

75. An infant presents with neonatal jaundice. After several weeks, the jaundice becomes more exaggerated. The patient has an enzyme deficiency that inhibits conjugation of bilirubin. Which of the following reacts with bilirubin in the conjugation reaction?

(A) Vitamin C
(B) Iron
(C) Ceruloplasmin
(D) Porphyrin ring
(E) UDP-glucuronate

76. A 26-year-old woman meets with her family physician to discuss family planning. She is interested in starting a family soon and is looking for advice on what nutritional supplements would be beneficial during pregnancy. The physician suggests which two of the following supplements as being the most important for the health of the fetus?

(A) Selenium and vitamin K
(B) Copper and riboflavin
(C) Iron and folate
(D) Vitamin C and vitamin D
(E) Vitamin A and biotin

77. An intern is scrubbing in to a complicated surgery that is anticipated to last 15 hours. In preparation, the intern has not eaten or drunk anything for the past 15 hours so that he will not have to go to the bathroom in the middle of the surgery. After 30 hours of fasting, which of the following is most important for the maintenance of normal blood glucose levels?

(A) Glycogenolysis
(B) Gluconeogenesis
(C) Triacylglycerol synthesis
(D) Increased insulin release
(E) Decreased muscle protein breakdown

78. Which of the following steroid hormones is secreted in response to angiotensin II?

(A) Cortisol
(B) Aldosterone
(C) Both cortisol and aldosterone

(D) Neither cortisol nor aldosterone
(E) Testosterone

79. Which of the following stimulates the production of progesterone by the corpus luteum?

(A) LH
(B) PRL
(C) TSH
(D) GH
(E) FSH

80. A 30-year-old woman presents to an infertility clinic with her husband stating that she and her husband have been unsuccessfully trying to have a baby for 2 years. Over the next few months, her physician runs some tests, which show that she may not be ovulating. Which of the following is responsible for ovulation?

(A) Increased FSH
(B) Increased estradiol
(C) LH surge
(D) Increased progesterone
(E) Increased progesterone and estradiol

81. One colony of bacteria is split into two Petri plates: one plate with growth medium containing glucose and all 20 amino acids and the other plate with growth medium with one sugar (lactose) and one nitrogen source (NH_4^+). Which one of the following statements is correct concerning cells grown with only lactose and one nitrogen source?

(A) cAMP levels will be lower than cells grown in the presence of glucose and all 20 amino acids.
(B) Catabolite-activator protein (CAP, or cAMP-binding protein) will be bound to the *lac* promoter.
(C) The *lac* repressor will be bound to the *lac* operator.
(D) RNA polymerase will not bind to the *trp* promoter.
(E) Attenuation of transcription of the *trp* operon will increase compared with cells grown in the presence of glucose and all 20 amino acids.

82. A 75-year-old man is brought to the emergency room after being hit by a car. He suffered an open femur fracture that required orthopedic surgery. After several days, a wound infection sets in with a new bacterial organism that is resistant to all antibiotics currently available. The effort toward creating new antibiotics requires targeting of characteristics exclusive to bacteria and not to humans. Which of the following statements is exclusively true of prokaryotes but not eukaryotes?

(A) Transcription and translation are coupled.
(B) Most cells are diploid.
(C) Each gene has its own promoter.
(D) DNA is complexed with histones.
(E) Genes contain introns.

83. Eukaryotic secreted proteins are synthesized on ribosomes attached to the rough endoplasmic reticulum, whereas cytoplasmic proteins are synthesized on cytoplasmic (free) ribosomes. Which one of the following statements does not accurately describe an aspect of secreted protein synthesis?

(A) They are sorted in the endoplasmic reticulum and Golgi apparatus.
(B) A signal sequence is present at the N terminus.
(C) A hydrophilic signal sequence is required.
(D) After entering the endoplasmic reticulum, the signal sequence is removed by signal peptidase.
(E) The protein is secreted via exocytosis.

84. A 47-year-old man, with no known family history of cancer, develops changes in his bowel habits, including pencil-caliber stools with occasional bleeding. A colonoscopy and biopsy confirm the diagnosis of adenocarcinoma of the colon. Furthermore, the tumor is found to express a mutation in the ras protein. Which of the following correctly describes the ras protein?

(A) A nonreceptor tyrosine kinase
(B) A nuclear transcription factor
(C) A polypeptide growth factor
(D) A receptor tyrosine kinase
(E) A guanosine triphosphate (GTP)–binding protein

85. A 53-year-old man presents to the physician because he is fatigued and "not feeling himself." The doctor orders a routine set of tests, which demonstrates a white blood cell count of 85,000/mL (normal, 3000–10,000/mL). Molecular studies suggest that he has chronic myelogenous leukemia (CML). Which of the following translocations is associated with CML?

(A) t(8;14)
(B) t(14;18)
(C) t(11;14)
(D) t(9;22)
(E) t(15;17)

86. A 22-year-old woman, who has had numerous episodes of unprotected intercourse since the age of 12 years, visits a gynecologist for her first Pap smear. The results return positive for atypical cells, indicative of human papilloma virus (HPV) infection. Which of the following correctly describes the effects of HPV on cell growth?

(A) The viral E7 protein degrades cellular *p53*.
(B) The virus causes insertional inactivation of critical genes.
(C) The viral E6 protein perturbs the normal function of cellular *Rb*.
(D) The viral LMP-1 protein prevents the expression of cellular *bcl-2*.
(E) The viral E6 protein degrades cellular *p53*.

87. Which of the following conditions is caused by a trinucleotide repeat?

(A) Hemophilia A
(B) Prader-Willi syndrome
(C) Fragile X syndrome
(D) Angelman syndrome
(E) Leber hereditary optic neuropathy

88. Which of the following statements is correct concerning robertsonian translocations?

(A) Form the basis for genetic imprinting
(B) Failure of the homologous chromosomes to separate during meiosis
(C) Manifest clinically as cri du chat syndrome
(D) When a chromosome experiences two internal breaks with a subsequent rejoining of the internal fragment in the reverse orientation
(E) A variant translocation between two acrocentric chromosomes, whereby two long arms are joined at the centromere with the loss of the two short arms

89. Which statement is true regarding mendelian genetics?

(A) The inheritance pattern of one trait is dependent on the inheritance of another trait.
(B) Independent assortment occurs during anaphase II of meiosis after crossover has occurred.
(C) The offspring inherit one allele at each locus from each of the parents.
(D) The two alleles for each characteristic segregate during fertilization.
(E) In autosomal recessive inheritance, 25% of offspring are carriers.

Answers and Explanations

1. **The answer is A.** This patient has cystic fibrosis (CF), which is a hereditary disease that affects the ability to produce normal mucus in the exocrine glands of the lungs, liver, pancreas, and intestines. CF is most commonly caused by the ΔF508 mutation, which results in the deletion (Δ) of the amino acid phenylalanine (F) at the 508th (508) position on the CFTR protein. This is due to a 3-base deletion within the gene. Diagnosis is possible with newborn screening and confirmed by detecting high levels of salt in a patient's sweat. Duchenne muscular dystrophy is caused by a mutation, most often a large deletion, within the dystrophin gene. Although there is no specific gene yet identified that causes Alzheimer disease (AD), the presence of an abnormally folded protein, called *amyloid precursor protein*, and its proteolysis results in β-amyloid neurofibrillary tangles, which is a pathognomonic finding in AD. Marfan syndrome is caused by mutations in the *FBN-1* gene, which creates an abnormal fibrillin-1 protein, which is normally found in the extracellular matrix. Von Willebrand disease (vWD) is the most common hereditary coagulation abnormality and is caused by a deficiency of von Willebrand factor (vWF), precluding normal platelet adhesion.

2. **The answer is A.** Glyscosaminoglycans are proteoglycans typified by being composed of a large number of repeating disaccharide units with a core protein and long unbranced polysaccharide chain (the lone exception is hyaluronic acid, which does not contain a core protein). Conversely, glycoproteins, for example ABO blood groups, have shorter, more branched carbohydrates and usually contain sialic acid.

3. **The answer is D.** Digoxin increases intracellular myocyte calcium levels, thereby increasing myocyte contractility. This occurs primarily by digoxin's ability to inhibit the extracellular α subunit of the myocyte's Na^+/K^+ ATPase pump. This pump normally transports three sodium ions out of the cell in exchange for two potassium ions entering the cell, at the expense of ATP. By inhibiting the Na^+/K^+ ATPase, intracellular Na^+ levels increase, reducing the rate of calcium extrusion from the cell (the Na^+/Ca^{2+} exchange pump that pumps sodium out of the cell requires a high extracellular Na^+ concentration, which cannot be maintained owing to the inhibition of the Na^+/K^+ ATPase). More intracellular calcium increases the length of phase 4 and 0 action potentials, effectively increasing the contractility of the heart. β- and α-adrenergic receptors belong to a class of G-protein–coupled receptors that are targeted by catecholamines. These include—with varying specificity to the β and α receptors—epinephrine, norepinephrine, phenylephrine, and albuterol, to name a few, and are not used in the standard management of congestive heart failure.

4. **The answer is A.** The primary conversion of carbon dioxide into a soluble form that can be expired (and thereby removed from the body) is through mechanism (A). Mechanism (B) is seen in metabolic acidosis as the kidney tries to excrete hydrogen protons via NH_4^+. An accumulation of acetic acid during metabolic acidosis (e.g., diabetic ketoacidosis, DKA) can result in the reaction seen in mechanism (C). Mechanism (D) is the simple equilibrium reaction of water into its conjugate acid and base. Mechanism (E) is the breakdown reaction of β-hydroxybutyric acid, a "ketone" product seen in DKA.

5. **The answer is C.** The branched-chain amino acids make up the three essential amino acids L-leucine, L-isoleucine, and L-valine. These amino acids are found in proteins of all life forms. Dietary sources of the branched-chain amino acids are principally derived from animal and vegetable proteins. None of the other amino acids suggested as answers falls into the category of branched-chain amino acids.

6. **The answer is B.** Phenylalanine is the only amino acid listed as an answer choice that that does not have an ionizable side chain. The symptoms of dermatitis (rash), diarrhea, and dementia

are the "3 Ds" of pellagra. Pellagra is a congregate of symptoms resulting from vitamin B_3 (niacin) deficiency. In Hartnup disease, the transport of neutral amino acids into intestinal epithelial cells is compromised, and this includes tryptophan. Because tryptophan is a precursor for niacin synthesis, if the patient has a low niacin uptake, the symptoms of pellagra can manifest.

7. **The answer is C.** Strychnine interferes with neurotransmission by the amino acid glycine. Glycine is the only nonpolar amino acid listed as an answer choice. Tyrosine is a polar aromatic amino acid. Asparagine and glutamine are polar, uncharged amino acids. Lysine is an example of a positively charged amino acid.

8. **The answer is B.** Salicylate is excreted when it is uncharged (the AH form) and is trapped in the renal tubule when in charged form (A^-). The Henderson-Hasselbalch equation is pH = pK + log ([AH]/[A$^-$]). Because pH = 6, and pK = 3, the ratio of [AH] to [A$^-$] is 1000:1.

9. **The answer is A.** *Vibrio cholerae* is a comma-shaped gram-negative flagellated rod that is carried in water, food, and, classically, shellfish. This noninvasive organism requires large inoculums and secretes a toxin (AB_5), which ADP-ribosylates a $G_{\alpha s}$ protein, which in turn keeps adenylate cyclase active and increases cAMP levels. The high cAMP causes secretion of chloride ions and decreases sodium absorption, which leads to extensive osmotic losses of water into the intestinal lumen. This leads to "rice-water stools" in which the "rice" is the desquamated intestinal mucosa and the water is the osmotically lost water. Phospholipase C activation occurs in, for example, IgE activation and results in histamine secretion from mast cell degranulation. Phosphodiesterase activation is seen, as an example, when light interacts with rhodopsin, enabling vision. Tyrosine kinase receptor activation is part of the insulin and other growth factor signaling pathways. Serine-threonine kinase activation is also an intracellular signaling pathway that controls several cell functions, including apoptosis. The TGF-β receptor acts through a serine-threonine kinase activity.

10. **The answer is A.** Sickle cell anemia results from a single mutation in the β-globin subunit of hemoglobin, in which a valine rather than a glutamate is present at position 6. There are other abnormalities of hemoglobin that affect the α chain as well as the β chain. Expansion of a polyglutamine repeat occurs in the huntington protein, resulting in Huntington disease, a progressive movement disorder, but is not observed in sickle cell disease.

11. **The answer is D.** Marfan syndrome presents similarly to the case described and results from an autosomal dominant mutation in the structural protein fibrillin. Familial hypertrophic cardiomyopathy is associated with defects in myosin heavy chain. Hereditary spherocytosis is associated with mutations in spectrin or secondary defects in ankyrin. Collagen defects are seen in Ehlers-Danlos syndrome and vitamin C deficiency. Fibrillin is an essential component of microfibrils. The main organ systems affected in Marfan syndrome are the muscuoloskeletal system (arachnodactyly, dolichostenomelia, scoliosis), cardiovascular system (acute aortic dissection, mitral valve prolapse), pulmonary system (spontaneous pneumothorax), and eyes (lens subluxation, decreased nighttime vision).

12. **The answer is D.** The pancreas synthesizes proinsulin, which is cleaved in the Golgi apparatus to form mature insulin and the C-peptide. If the patient is not eating carbohydrates, there will not be a large enough stimulus to result in a high insulin or corresponding C-peptide level. If she were self-administering pharmaceutical insulin, it would not include C-peptide; thus, her serum C-peptide level would not be elevated. Therefore, answer choice D is the most likely answer, and this patient should be evaluated for an insulinoma. Her low blood glucose is due to excessive insulin secretion resulting in the peripheral tissues removing the glucose from circulation. A high glucose diet would not lead to greatly reduced blood glucose levels.

13. **The answer is C.** Vitamin C (ascorbic acid) is an important cofactor for the enzymes prolyl hydroxylase and lysyl hydroxylase. The hydroxylation of proline stabilizes the triple helix stricture of collagen. The hydroxyl group of lysine is often glycosylated with glucose and galactose. Cross-linkage of collagen results from the oxidation of lysine. C-peptide cleavage occurs in insulin processing.

14. **The answer is E.** Osteogenesis imperfecta results from mutations in the gene for type I collagen. As such, the patients have multiple fractures with minimal trauma. The blue sclerae result from defects in the collagen that is found in the eye. Transthyretin forms the amyloid of familial amyloidotic neuropathies, whereas calcitonin forms the amyloid in medullary carcinoma of the thyroid. Spectrin mutations are found in hereditary spherocytosis, and β-myosin heavy-chain mutations are found in familial hypertrophic cardiomyopathy.

15. **The answer is D.** The triple helix of collagen spontaneously associates into collagen fibrils, where the extracellular enzyme, lysyl oxidase, converts lysine to allysine. The newly formed residue then covalently links to the amino group of lysine on a neighboring collagen molecule, giving the fibril increased tensile strength. Lysine oxidase is not involved in the transcription, glycosylation, hydroxylation, or secretion of collagen from the cell. Lysyl hydroxylase is responsible for the hydroxylation of lysine residues in collagen. Glycosylation will occur upon the hydroxylated lysines in collagen.

16. **The answer is D.** The tertiary structure is stabilized by covalent disulfide bonds as well as hydrophobic interactions, electrostatic interactions, and hydrogen bonds. The primary structure is composed of covalent amide bonds. The secondary, supersecondary, and α-helical structures are stabilized by noncovalent interactions. α-Helical structures are a subset of secondary structure.

17. **The answer is A.** Isoniazid is acetylated in the liver in order to detoxify it and prepare it for excretion. The low V_{max} enzyme acetylates the drug at a slower rate than the high V_{max} enzyme (given that the K_m values are the same for each enzyme). Thus, individuals with the low V_{max} enzyme do not excrete the drug as rapidly as those with the high V_{max} enzyme, and a lower dose of drug will be effective in those patients. If given a high dose, those patients would experience potentially toxic levels of the drug because their metabolic clearance of the drug is slow.

18. **The answer is D.** The K_m is the substrate concentration at which 50% maximal velocity is reached. The K_m is related to the V_{max} via the Michaelis-Menton equation and is not a substitute for V_{max}. Thus, because hexokinase has a lower K_m for glucose than glucokinase, hexokinase will reach one-half maximal velocity at a lower substrate concentration than will glucokinase. K_m is not an indicator of the energy of activation of the reaction. Because the V_{max} of the enzymes is not known, one cannot determine whether answer choices A, C, and E are correct.

19. **The answer is A.** The data indicate competitive inhibition because as the substrate concentration is increased, the effects of the inhibitor can be overcome, and the same velocity is obtained as in the absence of inhibitor. This indicates that the substrate and inhibitor are competing for binding to the same site on the enzyme. In noncompetitive and uncompetitive inhibition, the substrate and inhibitor bind at different sites, and once the enzyme is inhibited, adding more substrate cannot reverse the inhibition (thus, the same reaction velocity both in the presence and absence of inhibitor would not be observed). In irreversible inhibition, once the enzyme is inhibited, it cannot be reactivated, indicating that only a reduced velocity (compared with uninhibited) would be observed. Because at low substrate concentrations, in the presence of inhibitor, the velocity of the reaction is reduced, some type of inhibition is occuring in this experiment.

20. **The answer is A.** A competitive inhibitor will compete for binding with the substrate to the enzyme. Thus, in kinetic terms, competitive inhibitors increase the apparent K_m (because it takes increased substrate to displace the inhibitor from the active site), but do not alter the maximal velocity (because at high enough substrate concentrations, the enzyme is saturated with substrate). A noncompetitive, as well as irreversible, inhibitor reduces V_{max} without affecting K_m. Feedback inhibition refers to an end product of a pathway inhibiting a previous step of the pathway; lovastatin is not a product or intermediate of the cholesterol biosynthetic pathway. Because the K_m has been increased in the presence of lovastatin, the drug is not acting as an activator, which usually reduces the K_m, which allows the reaction to proceed at lower substrate concentrations.

21. **The answer is C.** The respiratory quotient (R.Q.) is the ratio of CO_2 produced to O_2 used (CO_2/O_2) by a tissue in oxidation of a foodstuff. The R.Q. for fat is 0.7, 0.8 for protein, and 1 for carbohydrate. R.Q. is increased in exercise owing to enhanced carbohydrate metabolism (glycogen degradation producing glucose for energy needs) compared with fat metabolism (fatty acid oxidation) in the resting state.

22. **The answer is B.** Positive nitrogen balance describes the state when dietary nitrogen exceeds excreted nitrogen. Negative nitrogen balance occurs when dietary nitrogen is less than excreted nitrogen. Nitrogen balance occurs when dietary nitrogen equals excreted nitrogen. Anabolism describes biosynthetic pathways, which require energy. Catabolism describes degradative pathways, some of which yield energy. The patient is most likely in an anabolic, biosynthetic state because of increased antibody synthesis, which requires the use of amino acids. However, the most accurate term used to describe this state is *positive nitrogen balance.*

23. **The answer is A.** Trypsin normally cleaves a peptide on the carboxyl side of arginine or lysine. Chymotrypsin has the ability to cleave a peptide on the carboxyl side of aromatic amino acids. Elastase is actually the major target of α_1-antitrypsin, and elastase cleaves peptides on the carboxyl side of uncharged amino acids. Carboxypeptidase A cleaves aromatic amino acids from the carboxy terminus, whereas carboxypeptidase B cleaves basic amino acids from the carboxy terminus.

24. **The answer is A.** Vitamin C is the only water-soluble vitamin listed and not affected by this patient's pancreatic insufficiency. Vitamins A, D, E, and K are the fat-soluble vitamins that the body needs. Absorption of these is not possible without pancreatic lipase and bile salt secretion, in order to emulsify the lipids and to allow the vitamins to be absorbed by the intestinal epithelial cells.

25. **The answer is E.** Celiac disease, or nontropical sprue, results from hypersensitivity to the grain protein gluten. Biopsy of the intestine demonstrates destruction of the absorptive cells of the gut because gluten stimulates an inflammatory response in the gut. Excess lipids in the feces does result in steatorrhea, which is an effect, not a cause, of celiac disease. Defective transport of cystine in the kidney leads to kidney stones, a condition known as cystinuria. Defects in the transport of neutral amino acids results in Hartnup disease. Enterokinase activates pancreatic zymogens in the intestinal lumen so that digestion can occur. In the absence of enterokinase, protein and fat digestion would be minimal. However, a loss of enterokinase does not lead to destruction of the gut epithelial cells, as occurs in celiac disease.

26. **The answer is A.** Pyruvate kinase deficiency is an autosomal recessive disorder that primarily affects erythrocytes because they rely only on glycolysis to create ATP. With decreased ATP production, the cell is unable to maintain the biconcave cell membrane shape, and the cell is sequestered in the spleen for destruction. Moreover, with an impaired glycolytic pathway, depending on the severity of the enzyme deficiency, patients may have mild to serious manifestations. Hemolysis of defective erythrocytes results in release of bilirubin, so bilirubin levels increase, do not decrease, under these conditions. Pyruvate kinase deficiency is second to glucose 6-phosphate dehydrogenase deficiency for enzyme deficiency–induced hemolytic anemia.

27. **The answer is A.** Lactic acidosis is a common clinical entity and the result of tissue hypoperfusion and oxygenation. On a molecular level, this results in a high $NADH/NAD^+$ ratio and causes shunting to anaerobic metabolism and the accumulation of lactate. In advanced cases as seen in this patient with sepsis, impending cardiopulmonary collapse is a major concern because of decreased responsiveness to catecholamines to maintain adequate blood pressures and respiratory failure from persistent respiratory compensation (tachypnea and increased minute ventilation). Mechanical ventilation, exogenous administration of catecholamines, and correction of the acidosis/volume deficits are the mainstays of treatment.

28. **The answer is D.** With the arrest of the pyruvate dehydrogenase complex, glucose will only provide energy gains from glycolysis. Because the glycerol 3-phosphate shuttle is the major shuttle system in muscle, the two molecules of cytoplasmic NADH produced will yield three ATP equivalents. When added to the two ATP molecules produced at the substrate level, a total of five ATP equivalents will result.

29. **The answer is A.** Pyruvate dehydrogenase complex deficiency (PDCD) is one of the most common neurodegenerative disorders and is caused by abnormal mitochondrial metabolism. Specifically, an inability to convert pyruvate to acetyl CoA leads to decreased downstream synthesis of TCA substrates (e.g., citrate) and cellular conversion from aerobic metabolism to the anaerobic/lactate pathway. Childhood-onset (as opposed to in utero) forms of this disorder result in intermittent periods of decompensation, albeit normal neurologic development. There is significant variability in the severity of the disease based on how defective the enzyme is, resulting in variable phenotypes as extreme as death within 1 year to survival to adulthood. The default pathway without aerobic metabolism (lack of oxygen) is anaerobic metabolism.

30. **The answer is D.** Pyruvate carboxylase deficiency is a rare, difficult to manage disorder that affects neonates and prevents the conversion of pyruvate to oxaloacetate. This forces glucose metabolism down the anaerobic pathway and results in the accumulation of lactic acid. As fatty acid oxidation generates acetyl CoA, pyruvate dehydrogenase activity in the mitochondria will be inhibited. In the presence of a deficient pyruvate carboxylase, pyruvate begins to accumulate and is converted to lactate in order for glycolysis to continue. The inability to generate oxaloacetate results in a slowing of the TCA cycle and inefficient energy production. Decreased ATP production severely affects the developing nervous system, which has high energy needs. The result is progressive motor pathway degeneration (e.g., hypotonia), decreased cerebellar functioning (e.g., ataxia) and respiratory compensation (i.e., respiratory alkalosis via hyperventilation to correct the lactic acid metabolic acidosis).

31. **The answer is B.** Carbon monoxide (and cyanide) combine with cytochrome oxidase and block the transfer of electrons to oxygen in the final step of the electron transport chain (complex III also contains cytochromes, which can bind carbon monoxide). Patients typically present with intentional exposure (e.g., sitting in a running car in an enclosed area) or have accidental exposures to carbon monoxide fumes during cold weather. Patients present with alterations of conciousness, normal oxygen saturations, and the pathognomonic "cherry-red skin." Carbon monoxide does not act as an uncoupler, nor does it inhibit ATP/ADP exchange across the inner mitochondrial membrane.

32. **The answer is B.** Glycogen is a major form of glucose storage and is formed from glucose. The structure of glycogen consists of α-1,4 linkages and α-1,6 linkages at branch points. Glycogen degradation produces glucose 1-phosphate and, at the branch points, free glucose. In the liver, glycogen degradation is used to help maintain proper blood glucose levels during exercise or fasting; in the muscle, glycogen is used to generate ATP to fuel muscle contraction. The degradation of glycogen does not lead directly to the formation of GTP.

33. **The answer is D.** Andersen disease (type IV glycogen storage disease [GSD]) results from a deficiency of glucosyl 4:6 transferase (the branching enzyme, also known as *transglucosidase*). This enzyme is responsible for forming branches in glycogen. The other answer choices are all deficiencies in enzymes responsible for the degradation of glycogen: for example, glucose 6-phosphatase deficiency in von Gierke disease; maltase deficiency in Pompe disease; glycogen debrancher deficiency in Cori disease; and muscle glycogen phosphorylase deficiency in McArdle disease.

34. **The answer is C.** Of the glycogen storage diseases, the presence of dextrin is unique to Cori disease, a deficiency of debranching enzyme activity. Hypoglycemic seizures may occur in the first decade of life. Long-term morbidity arises from hepatic disease and progressive muscle weakness. Von Gierke disease, a deficiency of glucose 6-phosphatase, and Pompe disease, a deficiency of acid α-glucosidase (also known as lysosomal maltase), both result in excessive glycogen with normal structure and cardiomyopathy. McArdle disease also results in excessive glycogen with normal structure, but the deficient muscle phosphorylase results in symptoms of muscle cramps and myoglobinuria. Andersen disease results from the deficiency of the branching enzyme, transglucosidase (glucosyl 4:6 transferase), which is found in all tissue. Because of the abnormal glycogen structure, hepatic deposition (preciptiation) may occur and result in severe cirrhosis, hepatic failure, or neuromuscular failure. It also can present as abnormal liver function tests in its mildest presentation.

35. **The answer is C.** McArdle disease (type V GSD) is due to a defect specific to muscle phosphorylase, with normal expression and activity of liver phosphorylase. A presentation involving muscle failure during demands such as exercise is typical. Many affected individuals also experience myoglobinuria due to rhabdomyolysis. Rhabdomyolysis, with concomitant spillage of myoglobin into the bloodstream, can result in serious renal damage. The diagnosis can be made by observing gross blood in the urine, but lacking red blood cells on microscopic examination. Andersen disease (lack of branching enzyme) primarily affects the liver and skeletal muscle. Cori disease is a deficiency of debranching enzyme. Lastly, von Gierke and Hers diseases primarily target the liver. Von Gierke disease is the lack of glucose 6-phosphatase, whereas Hers disease is a lack of liver glycogen phosphorylase activity (with normal muscle glycogen phosphorylase activity).

36. **The answer is C.** Increased glucose levels in the blood will decrease pancreatic α-cell secretion of glucagon. Other factors that decrease glucagon secretion are insulin and somatostatin. A tumor of the α cells, leading to constant glucagon release, is a glucagonoma. Tumors of the β cells of the pancreas are insulinomas. Factors that increase glucagon secretion include decreased plasma glucose, increased plasma amino acids, catecholamines, and cholecystokinin, a hormone released from the gut when stomach contents enter the small intestine.

37. **The answer is E.** Sulfonylureas stimulate the release of preformed insulin from pancreatic islets (via an alteration in membrane potential) and have been important drugs in the management of diabetes. Sulfonylureas have the same action on β cells as does arginine, in that preformed insulin is released. Neither sulfonylurea nor arginine is capable of stimulating the production of new insulin. No agent listed directly inhibits glucagon secretion. The production of GLUT-2 is insulin independent and would not be altered with sulfonylurea treatment.

38. **The answer is C.** Type 1 glycogen storage disease, von Gierke disease, results from the deficiency of glucose 6-phosphatase. The deficiency blocks the release of glucose from glycogen stores and also obstructs glucose synthesis in the last step of gluconeogenesis. Thus, glucose is only available from the diet, resulting in severe hypoglycemia when fasting. Although muscle is a major storage area for glycogen, the glucose 6-phosphate is converted to glucose *in the liver* before it can be used by muscle as an energy source. Brain and erythrocytes depend on glucose in the serum for their energy source, whereas adipose tissue uses fatty acids entering the Kreb cycle as their main source of energy. The kidney also contains glucose 6-phosphatase activity, and will contribute to gluconeogenesis during starvation conditions.

39. **The answer is D.** The two organs that produce all of the enzymes necessary for gluconeogenesis are the liver and kidneys. Although the kidneys only supply 10% of the newly formed glucose, their participation takes on a major role in starvation. Mature red blood cells lack a nucleus and, therefore, are unable to transcribe the messenger RNA (mRNA) needed to translate and synthesize the needed enzymes for gluconeogenesis. Skeletal muscle and brain tissue also lack the ability to transcribe and translate the gene for glucose 6-phosphatase and must rely on the blood glucose supplied by the diet, gluconeogenesis, and glycogenolysis for their needed energy requirements.

40. **The answer is C.** Fructose 1,6-bisphosphatase is an important regulatory step in gluconeogenesis. Its activity is inhibited by fructose 2,6-bisphosphate. It is also inhibited by AMP. In addition, its synthesis is induced during the fasting state but not in the fed state. Insulin has no direct effect on this critical regulatory enzyme. Because insulin is released in the fed state, it will not lead to increased synthesis of this enzyme.

41. **The answer is B.** Fructose is the major energy source for sperm cells, and low levels contribute to infertility. Sorbitol is a precursor of fructose and is converted into fructose by sorbitol dehydrogenase. Glycogen is formed from glucose in the liver by several enzymes, including glycogen synthase. Glucose is a monosaccharide that functions as a major cellular energy source and metabolic intermediate; lactose is a disaccharide and the source of galactose. Of the sugars listed, fructose is present at the highest concentration in the seminal fluid.

42. **The answer is B.** Prolactin, released from the anterior pituitary, stimulates the synthesis of α-lactalbumin, which reduces the K_m of galactosyl transferase for the substrate glucose. Glucose is then joined to UDP-galactose, thereby forming lactose. The same enzyme, galactosyl

transferase, is also responsible for the glycosylation of proteins. Aldose reductase converts galactose to galactitol. Glutathione reductase is required to reduce glutathione, in a reaction requiring NADPH. Sorbitol is converted to fructose by the action of sorbitol dehydrogenase.

43. The answer is C. Hurler syndrome results from a deficiency of α-L-iduronidase. Children with this illness have progressive mental retardation and have an average life span of 10 years. Death is usually due to accumulation of the glycosaminoglycans, such as heparan sulfate and dermatan sulfate, in the arteries, leading to arterial damage and ischemia. A sphingolipidosis would lead to the accumulation of glucocerebroside (Gaucher disease) or other sphingolipids. A defect in liver phosphorylase (Hers disease) would lead to an accumulation of liver glycogen. A defect in galactose 1-phosphate uridylyl transferase (classic galactosemia) would lead to an accumulation of galactose 1-phosphate.

44. The answer is A. Glycosaminoglycans are found in synovial fluid and the vitreous humor of the eye. Negatively charged uronic acid and sulfate groups contained within the glycosaminoglycans create a very hydrophilic environment, and water strongly associates with these molecules. Compression from outside forces, such as axial loading during walking, lead to water molecules being "squeezed" out, providing a lubricant effect. When the outside force is removed, the negatively charged glycosaminoglycans repair each other, and water reenters the structure, restoring the cushion to the joint. N-acetylgalactosamine, by itself, dolichol phosphates, collagen, or sphingolipids would not behave as the glycosaminoglycans do.

45. The answer is C. Wernicke-Korsakoff syndrome results from a deficiency of thiamine due to any condition resulting in a poor nutritional intake. Heavy, long-term alcohol use is the most common association with Wernicke-Korsakoff syndrome. Thiamine is converted to thiamine pyrophosphate, which serves as a cofactor for several enzymes that function in glucose utilization. These enzymes include transketolase, pyruvate dehydrogenase, and α-ketoglutarate dehydrogenase. None of the other enzymes listed require thiamine pyrophosphate as a cofactor.

46. The answer is C. The human ABO blood types arise from differences in the oligosaccharide content of glycoproteins and glycolipids on the surface of blood cells. Differences in a single sugar on the non-reducing end result in blood types A, B, or O. In all three blood types, a generic oligosaccharide consisting of fucose, galactose, and N-acetylglucosamine is attached to the red blood cell surface proteins. In the absence of an additional sugar, the result is type O. When galactose or N-acetylgalactosamine is covalently bound to the galactose, the types are considered B and A, respectively.

47. The answer is E. Dolichol phosphate is a long-chain alcohol associated with the endoplasmic reticulum that transfers branched polysaccharide chains to proteins during the synthesis of N-linked glycoproteins. Both α-mannosidase and α-fucosidase are enzymes involved in the lysosomal degradation of glycoproteins. α-Lactalbumin is involved in the synthesis of lactose. Thiamine pyrophosphate is a cofactor for transketolase in the pentose phosphate pathway, and also for enzymes that catalyze oxidative decarboxylation reactions (such as pyruvate dehydrogenase).

48. The answer is D. Classic galactosemia is a rare metabolic disorder that results in an inability to metabolize galactose and results in significant long-term effects (e.g., cirrhosis, renal failure, cataracts, and brain damage) if exposed to galactose. There are three forms of galactosemia, with classic galactosemia being the most severe manifestation. Classic galactosemia is caused by a deficiency of galactose 1-phosphate uridyltransferase. Galactokinase deficiency and UDP-galactose epimerase deficiency are two other, less severe forms of galactosemia. Treatment of classic galactosemia includes early detection (typically from mandated newborn screening) and elimination of dietary galactose. Lactase deficiency is seen in lactose-intolerant individuals and is an acquired deficiency of lactase that does not lead to significant long-term sequelae. Glucose 6-phosphate dehydrogenase deficiency is a defect in the hexose monophosphate shunt pathway that leads to hemolytic anemia in the presence of strong oxidizing agents.

49. The answer is E. Pancreatitis is an inflammatory process of the pancreas with significant morbidity and mortality. Gallstones and alcohol consumption are the most common causes, but other causes exist, including trauma, steroids, mumps, autoimmune causes, scorpion and snake venom, endoscopic retrograde cholangiopancreatography (ERCP), and certain drugs (e.g., azathioprine). Prognosis depends on the degree of pancreatitis. Ranson's criteria are helpful to stage the severity with hypocalcemia (not hypercalcemia), an ominous sign of pancreatic paren-chymal saponification. Treatment is largely supportive: nothing by mouth (NPO), intravenous fluids, nasogastric tube, and pain control. Only in advanced cases with evidence of phlegmon on CT are surgical intervention and antibiotics indicated. Grey-Turner (bruising of the flanks) and Cullen signs (bruising around the umbilicus) are not associated with pancreatitis.

50. **The answer is C.** Triacylglycerols are formed primarily in the liver, but they can also be gener-ated in adipose tissue and intestinal cells. In the liver, they are packaged in very-low-density lip-oprotein (VLDL) and are secreted into the blood. Triacylglycerols are stored in adipose tissue. Skeletal muscle does not produce triacylglycerol, nor do the spleen or red blood cells. Type V hy-perlipidemia results from elevated levels of VLDL and chylomicrons.

51. **The answer is B.** The liver can use glycerol to produce glycerol 3-phosphate (G-3-P) by a reaction that requires ATP and is catalyzed by glycerol kinase. The liver can also produce G-3-P by converting glucose through glycolysis to DHAP, which is reduced to G-3-P. Adipose tissue lacks glycerol kinase and thus cannot generate G-3-P from glycerol; therefore, it must convert glucose to DHAP, which is then reduced to G-3-P. Both tissues can convert glucose to DHAP, DHAP to glycerol 3-phosphate, phosphatidic acid to diacylgylcerol, and the activation of free fatty acids to fatty acyl CoA.

52. **The answer is B.** Apoprotein C-II is transferred from HDL to nascent chylomicrons and nascent VLDL. Apoprotein C-II activates lipoprotein lipase, which hydrolyzes the triacylglycerols of chy-lomicrons and VLDL to fatty acids and glycerol. In the absence of C-II activity, chylomicrons and VLDL levels will be increased because the triglyceride cannot be removed from those particles. LDL contains the highest content of cholesterol and its esters, and its levels are not increased in this disorder (LDL is derived from IDL, which is derived from VLDL as the triglyceride content of the particle is reduced). Triglycerides are also elevated because they are the major component of chylomicrons and VLDL.

53. **The answer is B.** Primary carnitine deficiency is caused by a deficiency in the plasma mem-brane carnitine transporter leading to urinary excretion of carnitine. Cells cannot transport car-nitine from the circulation across the plasma membrane and into the cell. This depletion of intracellular carnitine impairs transport of long-chain fatty acids into the mitochondria. Without a route of entry into the mitochondria, fatty acid oxidation is blocked. The lack of energy genera-tion from fatty acid oxidation leads to hypoglycemia and low ketones. Primary carnitine defi-ciency does not directly affect fatty acyl activation, β-oxidation, ω-oxidation, or α-oxidation.

54. **The answer is C.** Oxidation of very-long-chain fatty acids initally occurs in peroxisomes and generates hydrogen peroxide and NADH as reduced cofactors. Oxidation occurs at the α-carbon, and produces acetyl CoA (oxidation occurs two carbons at a time, not three). The last steps of oxidation occur in the mitochondria.

55. **The answer is E.** Obstruction of bile in the biliary tree will prevent the recycling and excretion of bile salts. Reduced excretion of bile salts leads to reduced digestion of fats and decreased for-mation of chylomicrons. As a consequence, ingested fat would not be digested and would remain in the chyme and ultimately in the feces, leading to steatorrhea. The conjugation of bile salts would also decrease because their recycling is also blocked.

56. **The answer is A.** HMG-CoA reductase is the rate-limiting enzyme in cholesterol biosynthesis, and statins block HMG-CoA reductase activity. Inhibition of HMG-CoA reductase results in decreased intracellular cholesterol levels. Decreased intracellular cholesterol levels result in an increased expression of LDL receptors on the surface of hepatocytes. This results in increased intracellular uptake of serum LDL, leading to decreased serum LDL levels. Inhibition of HMG-CoA reductase does not directly affect synthesis of bile salts, HDL, or IDL.

57. **The answer is A.** IDL is degraded to form LDL. Cholesterol is converted to cholesterol esters for storage in cells and HDL particles. HDL does not form LDL (LDL is derived from IDL, which is derived from VLDL). Chylomicrons are synthesized by intestinal epithelial cells.

58. **The answer is D.** HDL is the densest, smallest lipoprotein with a low triglycerol content and high protein content and contains primarily ApoA1. HDL transfers cholesterol ester to other lip-oproteins in exchange for various lipids, which it shuttles back to the liver. Within the liver, the

cholesterol esters are degraded by lysosomal enzymes. HDL does not carry triglyceride to any great extent, fatty acids, or amino acids throughout the body. The triglyceride in HDL arises via the cholesterol ester transfer protein (CETP) reaction, in which HDL exchanges a cholesterol ester for triglyceride with a VLDL particle.

59. The answer is A. Prostaglandins can be synthesized from arachidonic acid (which requires the essential fatty acid, linoleate, for its synthesis). They cannot be directly synthesized from glucose, acetyl CoA, or oleic acid. Leukotrienes are also derived from arachidonic acid. Prostaglandins are not derived from leukotrienes.

60. The answer is B. Steroid hormones, such as progesterone, testosterone, 17-β-estradiol, cortisol, and aldosterone, are most directly formed from cholesterol. Cholesterol forms pregnenolone by cleavage of its side chain. Acetyl CoA is the precursor for cholesterol biosynthesis. Fatty acids (including oleic acid) are not utilized in the de novo synthesis of cholesterol, or steroid hormones.

61. The answer is B. Aspirin inhibits the enzyme cyclooxygenase within platelets and it is a permanent inactivation. Aspirin will form a covalent linkage with the enzyme at the active site, leading to irreversible inhibition. Inhibition of cyclooxygenase blocks the synthesis of prostaglandins and thromboxane A_2.

62. The answer is D. Patients with Niemann-Pick disease have a deficiency of sphingomyelinase activity. Sphingomyelin is formed when phosphatidylcholine reacts with ceramide. Serine and palmitoyl CoA condense to form a precursor of sphingosine. Once sphingosine is formed, a fatty acyl CoA combines with sphingosine and forms ceramide. UDP-galactose and ceramide combine to form galactocerebroside.

63. The answer is A. Phenylalanine hydroxylase converts phenylalanine to tyrosine. A defect in this enzyme results in an accumulation of phenylketones in the urine, which gives urine its characteristic odor. PKU is treated by restriction of phenylalanine in the diet. Phenylalanine is not a precursor for serine, glycine, cysteine, or alanine synthesis.

64. The answer is D. Ornithine serves as a carrier that is regenerated in the urea cycle. Serine, glutamate, proline, and leucine are not involved in the urea cycle or in urea production.

65. The answer is B. Ninety percent of urea excretion occurs by the kidney (about 30 g/day), and the kidney's functional ability to excrete nitrogenous wastes is measured by the blood urea nitrogen (BUN). The liver is responsible for urea synthesis, and its synthesis is variable and dependent on protein intake. A key relationship exists between the urea cycle and the TCA cycle: one of the urea nitrogens supplied to the urea cycle as aspartic acid is formed from the TCA cycle intermediate oxaloacetic acid. The TCA cycle intermediates are formed by cytoplasmic isozymes of the TCA cycle enzymes because these reactions occur in the cytoplasm.

66. The answer is D. Glutathione plays an important role in detoxifying acetaminophen. As cellular stores of glutathione are depleted and hepatocytes are damaged, jaundice, encephalopathy, and accumulation of toxic substances occur. Nitric oxide is an important vasodilator. Histamine mediates HCl release from the stomach as well as bronchoconstriction of the lungs. Creatine is a storage form of high-energy phosphate when phosphorylated. Serotonin is a neurotransmitter involved in mood and depression. *N*-acetylcysteine can be used as a precursor for glutathione (γ-glutamyl-cysteinyl-glycine) biosynthesis.

67. The answer is B. Nitric oxide, also referred to as *endothelium-derived relaxing factor* (EDRF), relaxes the smooth muscle of blood vessels and thus lowers blood pressure. Nitric oxide is derived from arginine. Melanin is the major skin pigment that is derived from tyrosine. GABA is an inhibitory neurotransmitter (derived from glutamic acid), whereas both dopamine and serotonin (dopamine from tyrosine, and serotonin from tryptophan) are normally stimulatory neurotransmitters involved in affecting mood.

68. The answer is E. Serotonin, which is overproduced in carcinoid syndrome, is an indolamine neurotransmitter derived from tryptophan. Tyrosine is the precursor for catecholamine neurotransmitters, including dopamine, norepinephrine, and epinephrine. Nitric oxide, an important vasodilator, is derived from arginine. Histidine forms histamine, which is an important inflammatory mediator. Glycine can function as an inhibitory neurotransmitter.

69. **The answer is E.** Parkinson disease results from a relative deficiency of dopamine. Monoamine oxidase (MAO) and catecholamine *O*-methyltransferase (COMT) are enzymes that degrade catecholamines such as dopamine, epinephrine, and norepinephrine. MAOs can also degrade serotonin, resulting ultimately in the formation of 5-HIAA. MAO inhibitors will allow these neurotransmitters to remain elevated for extended periods of time. Nicotinamide can be synthesized from tryptophan. EDRF is a short-acting substance that rapidly degrades spontaneously.

70. **The answer is B.** Decarboxylation of glutamate results in the formation of the inhibitory neurotransmitter GABA. This is the only reaction type that converts glutamate to GABA. Hydroxylation of tyrosine forms dopa. Thyroid hormone requires iodination of tyrosine molecules. Methylation of norepinephrine forms the adrenal hormone epinephrine. A deaminated metabolite of catecholamines is vanillylmandelic acid, which is excreted in the urine.

71. **The answer is C.** Methotrexate inhibits the enzyme dihydrofolate reductase, which is the enzyme that converts dihydrofolate to tetrahydrofolate. Dopamine β-hydroxylase converts dopamine to norepinephrine. Tyrosine hydroxylase is the enzyme that converts tyrosine to dopa. Histamine is degraded to formiminoglutamate (FIGLU). Norepinephrine is deaminated and methylated by the sequential action of monoamine oxidase (MAO) and catechol *O*-methyl transferase (COMT).

72. **The answer is B.** Hypoxanthine-guanine phosphoribosyl transferase (HGPRT) and adenine phosphoribosyl transferase (APRT) are enzymes associated with the purine-salvage pathway. Purine bases can be salvaged by reacting with PRPP to re-form nucleotides. If purine bases cannot be salvaged because of a defect in one of these enzymes, purines will instead be converted to uric acid, which will rise in the blood, and can lead to gout. The enzyme is not involved in pyrimidine metabolism.

73. **The answer is B.** The child has severe combined immunodeficiency disease (SCID) caused by a deficiency in adenosine deaminase (ADA) activity. ADA converts adenosine to inosine, as well as deoxyadenosine to deoxyinosine. AMP is degraded to adenosine by removal of a phosphate by 5′-nucleotidase. There are two reactions catalyzed by purine nucleoside phosphorylase (PNP): (1) guanosine is converted to guanine and ribose 1-phosphate, and (2) inosine is converted to hypoxanthine and ribose 1-phosphate. Like ADA deficiency, PNP deficiency also results in SCID. However, in PNP deficiency, adenosine and deoxyadenosine do not accumulate. Hypoxanthine is converted to xanthine by xanthine oxidase in the purine degradative pathway. Deoxyadenosine accumulation leads to the inhibition of ribonucleotide reductase and inhibition of immune cell maturation.

74. **The answer is D.** The patient has hereditary orotic aciduria, a defect in the pyrimidine biosynthetic pathway. The defective enzyme is UMP synthase, which converts orotic acid to OMP, and then OMP to UMP. In this disorder, orotic acid accumulates and is released into the blood and then into the urine. A defect in the urea cycle (ornithine transcarbamoylase deficiency) will also lead to orotic aciduria, but is also associated with hyperammonemia. Orotic acid is not formed during purine synthesis or degradation, nor in pyrimidine degradation.

75. **The answer is E.** UDP-glucuronate reacts with bilirubin to form bilirubin monoglucuronide. This reaction is catalyzed by bilirubin uridine diphosphate glucuronyl transferase (UDP-GT). Vitamin C increases uptake of iron in the intestinal tract. Iron is in the center of the porphyrin ring in heme. Ceruloplasmin is involved in the oxidation of iron. None of these other factors interact with bilirubin.

76. **The answer is C.** Pregnancy is a time of increased metabolic demand, and two of the most important supplements are iron, to prevent anemia, and folate, to prevent neurotubule defects in the developing fetus. Copper and selenium are trace elements that are rarely deficient. Riboflavin is often found in grain products. Vitamin C and vitamin D are often obtained appropriately from the diet. Vitamin A derivatives are often teratogenic and, therefore, should be avoided during pregnancy. Vitamin K deficiency is common in newborns, and they are often supplemented at birth.

77. **The answer is B.** About 2 to 3 hours after a meal, the liver maintains normal blood glucose by glycogenolysis. Within 30 hours, liver glycogen stores are depleted, leaving gluconeogenesis as the primary process for maintaining normal blood glucose. Ketone bodies are generated, triacylglycerols are broken down, and muscle protein breakdown increases. In the fed state, insulin increases; in the fasting state, glucagon increases, while insulin decreases.

78. **The answer is B.** Angiotensin II stimulates the synthesis and secretion of aldosterone from the adrenal cortex, but not cortisol or testosterone. Aldosterone is a hormone that instructs the kidneys to retain sodium and excrete potassium.

79. **The answer is A.** Luteinizing hormone (LH) stimulates the corpus luteum to produce progesterone. Prolactin (PRL) stimulates lactogenesis in the breast. Thyroid-stimulating hormone (TSH) is synthesized in the pituitary gland and stimulates the release of T_3 and T_4 from the thyroid gland. Growth hormone is released from the pituitary and does not affect the corpus luteum. Follicle-stimulating hormone (FSH) stimulates the growth of ovarian follicles. It is not involved in progesterone formation.

80. **The answer is C.** A surge of LH at the midpoint of the menstrual cycle stimulates the egg to leave the follicle. Initially, FSH acts on immature follicles to promote maturation. Estradiol causes the endometrium to thicken and vascularize in preparation for implantation. After ovulation, the residual follicle secretes both progesterone and estradiol. Progesterone also causes the endometrium to thicken and vascularize.

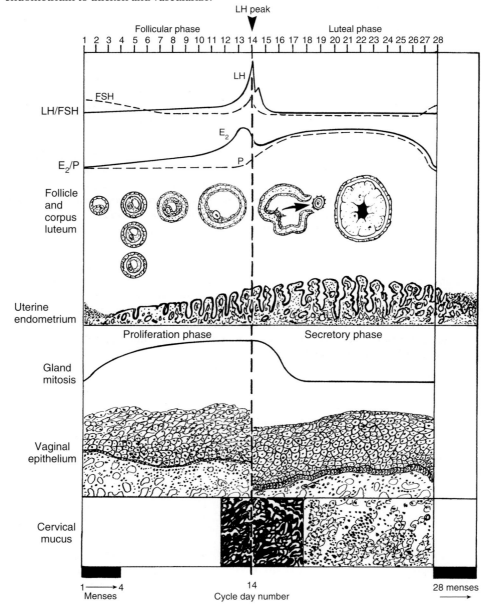

81. **The answer is B.** In the absence of glucose and the presence of lactose, the *lac* repressor will be inactive, cAMP levels will rise, and the CAP protein–cAMP complex will bind to the *lac* promoter, stimulating transcription of the operon. In the absence of amino acids, tryptophan levels in the cell will be low; thus, the repressor for the *trp* operon will be inactive, and the operon will be transcribed by RNA polymerase. Attenuation of transcription of this operon will decrease because of the reduced tryptophan levels.

82. **The answer is A.** In prokaryotes, transcription and translation occur concurrently and are coupled. Eukaryotes contain a membrane bound nuclei, so transcription is separated from translation. In eukaryotes, most cells are diploid, and each gene has its own promoter, DNA is complexed with histones, and genes contain introns. These characteristics are not true of prokaryotes.

83. **The answer is C.** A hydrophobic signal sequence (not hydrophilic) at the N terminus of a secretory protein allows the nascent protein to pass into the lumen of the rough endoplasmic reticulum (RER). The signal sequence is then cleaved, such that the protein may be further processed within the RER and the Golgi apparatus in preparation for exocytosis.

84. **The answer is E.** The ras protein is a guanosine triphosphate (GTP)–binding protein, which is turned on when it is bound to GTP and shut off when it hydrolyzes GTP to guanosine diphosphate (GDP). Mutations that destroy this hydrolytic activity are among the most common in cancer, resulting in continuous growth-promoting signals. The *abl* and *src* genes are two nonreceptor tyrosine kinases, whereas the epidermal growth factor receptor is a receptor tyrosine kinase. The *myc* gene is an example of a nuclear transcription factor. Fibroblast growth factor is a typical example of a polypeptide growth factor implicated in cancer.

85. **The answer is D.** Chronic myelogenous leukemia is associated with t(9;22), a translocation between chromosomes 9 and 22. The resulting chromosome is known as the Philadelphia chromosome, in which the *bcr* gene from chromosome 22 is fused to the *abl* gene on chromosome 9. The aberrant bcr-abl protein is thus created and results in an unregulated tyrosine kinase being activated in the cell. There are several other important chromosomal translocations associated with blood and lymph cancers, including t(8;14) found in Burkitt lymphoma, t(14;18) found in follicular lymphoma, t(11;14) found in mantle cell lymphoma, and finally, t(15;17) found in acute myelogenous leukemia, M3 variant.

86. **The answer is E.** HPV infection causes cervical cancer and is acquired as a sexually transmitted disease. Its oncogenic potential is related to the viral E6 protein, which disrupts cellular growth by degrading cellular *p53*. The viral E7 protein perturbs the normal function of *Rb*. Retroviruses can cause cancer because they can cause insertional inactivation of key growth-controlling genes. The Ebstein-Barr virus (EBV) LMP-1 protein results in cancer through its ability to prevent the expression of *bcl-2*. HPV does not insert into the host genome (it replicates autonomously), nor does it express the LMP-1 protein.

87. **The answer is C.** Fragile X syndrome is the second leading inherited cause of mental retardation and is caused by trinucleotide repeats of CGG (up to 200) within the *FMR-1* gene on the X chromosome. Some other examples of trinucleotide repeat disorders include Huntington disease, spinocerebellar ataxia, Friedreich ataxia, and myotonic dystrophy. Hemophilia A is an X-linked recessive disease that leads to a deficiency of clotting factor VII. Uniparental disomy leads to specific genetic abnormalities: paternal transmission of the del(15)(q11q13) deletion results in Prader-Willi syndrome; maternal transmission of this deletion results in Angelman syndrome. This is the classic example of genetic imprinting. Because all the mitochondria in the developing zygote originate from the ovum, defects in the mitochondrial genome are exclusively maternally transmitted, as seen in Leber hereditary optic neuropathy (LHON). Most often, this disorder results from one of three distinct point mutations in the mitochondrial DNA (mtDNA).

88. **The answer is E.** Robertsonian translocations are variant translocations between two acrocentric chromosomes, whereby two long arms are joined at the centromere with the loss of the two short arms. Parent-specific expression is an example of genetic imprinting and is seen in Prader-Willi syndrome and Angelman syndrome. Both disorders result from a chromosome deletion

(del(15)q11q13). Inheriting the deletion from the father results in Prader-Willi syndrome; inheriting the deletion from the mother results in Angelman syndrome. Failure of the homologous chromosomes to separate during meoisis is an example of a nondisjunction. Cri du chat syndrome is a rare genetic disorder caused by loss of genetic material on the short arm of chromosome 5. Inversions occur when a chromosome experiences two internal breaks with a subsequent rejoining of the internal fragment in the reverse orientation.

89. **The answer is C.** The offspring inherit one allele at each locus from each of the parents. The other answers are incorrect. The inheritance pattern of one trait is *independent* and does not influence the inheritance of another trait (A), independent assortment occurs during *anaphase I* of meiosis after crossover has occurred (B), the two alleles for each characteristic segregate during *gamete production* (D), and in autosomal recessive inheritance, 50% of offspring are carriers (E).

Index

Page numbers followed by t indicate table; those in *italics* indicate figure.

Calcitonin, 27t, 245
Calcitriol, 171, *171*
Calcium, hormones that act through, 233–234, *236*
Calcium metabolism, hormones that regulate, 245
Calmodulin, 104
cAMP
    cascade, 103
    in glycogen degradation, 102, *102*
    G proteins and, 233, *235*
    in protein synthesis, 279
    structure of, *103*
cAMP-CAP complex, 279
Cancer, 305–315
    apoptosis, 308–309, *309*
    DNA repair and carcinogenesis, 313–314, 313t
    molecular carcinogenesis, 311–313
    molecular markers for, 315, 2935t
    molecular progression of, 314–315
        angiogenesis, 314
        invasion, 314
        metastasis, 315
        tumor growth, 314
    oncogenes, 305–307
        cell cycle regulators, 307
        growth factors, 305–306
        nuclear transcription proteins, 307
        proto-oncogenes, 305
        signal transducing proteins, 306, *306*
    oncogenesis mechanisms, 309–311
    tumor-suppressor genes, 307–308
Captopril, 42
Carbamoyl phosphate, in urea cycle, 178, *179*
Carbamoyl phosphate synthase I, 178
    deficiency of, 178
Carbohydrates
    derivatives of, 7, *8*
    dietary requirements for, 215
    digestion of, 50–51, *51*, 60
    glycolysis, 63–71
    glycosides, 6–7
    glycosylation of proteins, 9
    malrotation of, 5, *6*
    monosaccharides, 4–5, *5, 6*
    oxidation of, 7, *8*, 9
    reduction of, 9
    structure of, 4–9, *5–8*
Carbamoyl phosphate, in pyrimidine synthesis, *204*, 207
Carbamoyl phosphate synthetase II, 207
Carbon atoms, 1, *1*
Carbonic anhydrase inhibitors, 3, 21
Carbon monoxide
    electron transport chain and, 89t, 96
    toxicity, 30, 36–37
Carbon-nitrogen groups, *2*
Carbon-oxygen groups, *2*
Carbon-sulfur groups, *2*
Carbon tetrachloride, 91
Carboxylation, of clotting factors, 28t
Carboxypeptidase, 56
Carcinogenesis
    chemical, 311–312, 311t
    DNA repair and, 313–314, 313t
    molecular, 311–313
    radiation, 312
    viral, 312–313
Carcinoid syndrome, 194
Carcinoid tumors, 194

Cardiac creatine kinase, 202
Cardiomyopathy, familial hypertrophic, 31t
Carnitine
    deficiency of, 142
    in fatty acid oxidation, 142, *143*, 150
Carnitine acyltransferase, 140
Carnitine acyl transferase (CAT I), 142–143
    deficiency of, 143
Caspases, 309
Catabolite repression, *278*, 278–279
Catalase, reactive oxygen species and, 92, *92*
Cataracts, 9
Catecholamine *O*-methyltransferase (COMT), 197–198
Catecholamines, *196*, 197–198
Cathode, 23
CDK1, 289
CDK2, 289
CDK4, 288–289, 307
CDK6, 288–289
cDNA, 319
Celiac disease, 54
Cell cycle, 286–288
    anaphase, *287*, 288
    control of, 288–289, *289*
    G_0, 286
    interphase, 287, *287*
    metaphase, *287*, 288
    mitosis, *287*, 287–288
    prophase, *287*, 288
    regulators of, 307
    telophase, *287*, 288
Cell membrane
    functions of, 17–18
    structure of, 16, *16*
Centrioles, 288
Centromere, 286
Ceramide, 166, 194
Cerebrosides, 11
Cervical cancer, 312
cGMP, 193
    degradation of, 205, *206*
    in purine synthesis, 203–204
Chaperone proteins, 25
Charcot-Marie-Tooth disease, 26
Chédiak-Higashi syndrome, 28, 36
Chemical carcinogenesis, 311–312, 311t
Chemokine receptor gene CCR-5, 324
Chenocholic acid, 152, 161
Chief cells, 225
Chimeric protein formation, 310
Chloramphenicol, 7, 275
Cholecalciferol, 171, *171*
Cholecystokinin (CCK), 245
Cholera toxin, 16
Cholesterol, 15
    in steroid hormones synthesis, 169, *170*
    synthesis of, 151, *152*
Cholesterol esters, 158
Cholic acid, 152
Chorionic sampling (CVS), 297
Chromatin, 286
Chromatography, 329, 329t, 334
Chromosomal translocations, 291–292, 302–303
    oncogenesis by, 309–311, *310*
Chromosomes, 286, *287*
    sex, 286, 292

Mismatch pair DNA repair, 260, 313–314
Missense mutations, 271, 284
Mitochondria, 95
    electron transport chain and, 85
    matrix of, 85
Mitochondrial DNA (mtDNA), 85, 253–254, 269–270
    disorders of, 88
Mitochondrial inheritance, 296
Mitosis, *287,* 287–288
Molecular carcinogenesis, 311–313
Monoacylglycerol (monoglyceride), 15, *15*
Monoamine oxidase (MAO), 197–198
Monosaccharides, 4–6, *5, 6*
Morphine, 240, 249
Morquio syndrome, 130t
Mosaic, 292
Mosaicism, 296, 302
Mouth, carbohydrate digestion by, 50, *52*
mRNA (*See* Messenger RNA (mRNA))
Mucopolysaccharides, 130, 130t
Multifactorial inheritance, 296
Multiple endocrine neoplasia (MEN) syndromes, 306
Multiple myeloma, 27, 27t
Muscle
    biochemical functions of, 227
    during fasting, *223,* 223–224
    during fed state, 220, *222*
Muscle-brain isoenzyme, 228
Muscle glycogen, 97, 101, 108
    degradation, *103,* 103–104
    during exercise, *103,* 103–104, 118
    synthesis, 104
Muscle protein, degradation of, 223–224
Muscular dystrophy, 31t
Mutations
    deletions, 259, 272
    in DNA sequencing, 323–325
    in DNA synthesis (replication), 259
    frameshift, 272
    insertions, 259, 272
    missense, 271, 284
    nonsense, 271
    point, 259, 271
        oncogenesis by, 309
    protein synthesis and, 271–272
    silent, 271
    vs. polymorphisms, 323
Mycophenolic acid, 203, 213
myc proto-oncogene, 307, 310
Myelogenous leukemia
    acute, 310t
    chronic, 302–303, 310, 310t, 330
Myeloma, multiple, 27, 27t
Myeloperoxidase, reactive oxygen species and, 90–91, *91*
Myocardial infarction (MI), indicators of, 45
Myoclonus, startle, 25
Myopathy, fatal infantile mitochondrial, 85

N-acetylcysteine, 192, 202
N-acetylgalactosamine, 131
N-acetylglutamate, 180
N-acetylneuraminic acid, 166
N-acetyltransferase, 40
NAD+ (flavin mononucleotide)
    in electron transport chain, 86, *86*
    in lactate formation, 68, *68,* 75–76
    in tricarboxylic acid cycle, 80, 80–81

NADH
    in electron transport chain, *85,* 85–87, 89
    in lactate formation, 68, *68,* 75–76
    in tricarboxylic acid cycle, *80,* 80–81
    in tricarboxylic acid cycle regulation, *80*
NADH dehydrogenase complex, 87
NADH:ubiquinone oxidoreductase, 88
NADP+, in electron transport chain, *86*
NADPH, 217
    in fatty acid synthesis, 137, *138*
    in pentose phosphate pathway, *126,* 128–129
    in triacylglycerol synthesis regulation, 140, *141*
NADPH oxidase
    deficiency of, 90
    reactive oxygen species and, 90, *91*
Na^+-K^+ ATPase, 6
Nerve agent, 42
    antidote for, 48
Neuroblastoma, 280, 311
Neurofibromatosis-1 *(NF-1),* 307, 317
Neutral pH, 3
N-glycosides, 7
Niacin (B₃), 81, 217t, 231
Nicotinamide adenine dinucleotide, reduced (*See* NADH)
Niemann-Pick disease, 168t
Nitrates, 193
Nitric oxide
    functions of, 193
    synthesis of, 193, *193*
Nitric oxide synthase, 193, *193*
Nitrogen
    addition and removal, 176–177, *177*
    transport to liver, 177–178
Nitroglycerine, 193
Nitroprusside, 193, 202
N-*myc,* 311
Noncompetitive inhibitors, 42, *42, 43,* 49
Noncovalent bonds, 25–26
Nonpolyposis colon carcinoma, hereditary, 313t
Nonprogressive hyperglycemia, 66
Nonreceptor tyrosine kinase proteins, 306
Nonsense mutations, 271
Nontropical sprue, 54
Norepinephrine, 197
Northern blots, 319, *320*
Nuclear DNA, 85
Nuclear magnetic resonance (NMR), 330
Nuclear transcription, molecules that regulate, 308
Nuclear transcription proteins, 307
Nucleic acid
    DNA (*See* DNA)
    RNA (*See* RNA)
Nucleosides, *17,* 18
Nucleosomes, 253, *254*
Nucleotide excision DNA repair, 259, *261,* 313
Nucleotides
    functions of, 18
    structure of, *17,* 18

O blood type, 131, *131*
Odd-chain fatty acids, oxidation of, 145
O-glycosides, 6, *7*
Okazaki fragments, 258, *260*
Olestra, 53
Oligomycin, 89t
Oligonucleotides, 319
Oligosaccharides, 6, *7*